Funded by
MISSION COLLEGE
VTEA
Carl D. Perkins Vocational and Technical Education Act Grant

Ethical Practice in Grief Counseling

ABOUT THE AUTHORS

Louis A. Gamino, PhD, ABPP, FT, is a diplomate in clinical psychology with the American Board of Professional Psychology and a fellow in thanatology with the Association for Death Education and Counseling (ADEC). He has been on staff with the Scott & White Clinic and Hospital in Temple, Texas, since obtaining his doctorate from the University of Kansas in 1980. Dr. Gamino is an associate professor of psychiatry and behavioral science, Texas A&M University Health Science Center College of Medicine.

He is program director for the Scott & White Bereavement Conferences held biennially in September (even-numbered years).

Dr. Gamino is former editor of *The Forum,* a journal-style newsletter published by ADEC. Together with Ann Cooney, he is coauthor of *When Your Baby Dies Through Miscarriage or Stillbirth* (2002). Dr. Gamino is principal investigator of the Scott & White Grief Study, and his research program is focused on adaptive grieving after loss. He has published numerous articles and book chapters on bereavement.

In recognition of excellence in clinical care of the dying and the bereaved, Dr. Gamino was the 2008 recipient of ADEC's Clinical Practice Award.

R. Hal Ritter, Jr., PhD, LPC, LMFT, is an ordained Baptist minister who received his PhD from Baylor University with a specialty in the psychology of religion and ethics. He is an associate professor of family medicine in the Texas A&M Health Science Center College of Medicine. Dr. Ritter currently serves as the Family Medicine Residency Behavioral Science Educator at Scott & White Memorial Hospital in Temple, Texas. He also serves on the ethics committee for the Scott & White Memorial Hospital.

Dr. Ritter is a diplomate and training supervisor in the American Association of Pastoral Counselors. Also a licensed marriage and family therapist, Dr. Ritter is a clinical member and approved training supervisor in the American Association for Marriage and Family Therapy.

Academically, Dr. Ritter is adjunct faculty at the George W. Truett Theological Seminary at Baylor University in Waco, Texas. In addition, he has taught graduate classes in marriage and family therapy at Baylor University and at the Tarleton State University of Central Texas in Killeen, Texas. Dr. Ritter serves on the editorial board of *The Journal of Pastoral Care and Counseling.* He has published numerous articles and book reviews related to the topic of psychotherapy.

Ethical Practice in Grief Counseling

LOUIS A. GAMINO, PhD, ABPP, FT
R. HAL RITTER, Jr., PhD, LPC, LMFT

SPRINGER PUBLISHING COMPANY
NEW YORK

Springer Publishing Company, LLC
11 West 42nd Street
New York, NY 10036
www.springerpub.com

Acquisitions Editor: Sheri W. Sussman
Project Manager: Mark Frazier
Cover design: David Levy
Composition: Apex CoVantage, LLC
Ebook ISBN: 978-0-8261-0084-9

09 10 11 12 / 5 4 3 2 1

Library of Congress Cataloging-in-Publication Data

Gamino, Louis A., 1953–
Ethical practice in grief counseling / Louis A. Gamino & R. Hal Ritter.
p. cm.
Includes bibliographical references.
ISBN 978-0-8261-0083-2 (alk. paper)
1. Grief therapy—Moral and ethical aspects. I. Ritter, R. Hal. II. Title.
RC455.4.L67G36 2009
174.2'968914—dc22 2008050934

Printed in the United States of America by Hamilton Printing

In memory of my father, Joseph Gilbert Gamino (1917–2007)
In honor of my mother, Mabel Rose (Long) Gamino
&
Dedicated to my loving wife, Marla Ann (Yarnell) Gamino
L.A.G.

In memory of my father, Robert Harrold Ritter (1918–1996)
In honor of my mother, Nina (Mathews) Ritter,
who was at Dad's side when he died peacefully at home
&
Dedicated to my faithful wife, Michaela Jane (Lorfing) Ritter,
who prayerfully stood by my side when I almost died in 1983
R.H.R., Jr.

Contents

Foreword

When I began my practice in clinical psychology in 1968, my annual professional liability insurance was $70. Forty years later, it has escalated to 30 times that amount, *with annual increases.* Some of this increase is the result of inflation and the rising cost of health care. Some of the increase is the result of society's litigious bent. Some reflects the increasing technology used in the field of mental health. Counseling over the Internet was nonexistent 40 years ago because there was no Internet. In this book, Louis Gamino and Hal Ritter present the whole gamut of areas where thanatologists and grief counselors may face ethical dilemmas and concerns, many of which they may not have thought of before now.

One complex area where ethics intersects thanatological practice is the "right to die." Giving dying persons a choice in their final months of life has been an important discussion over the past 4 decades. Some years ago, I worked with the Concern for Dying group in New York where we crafted a living will. This document and other advanced directives have given dying patients much more autonomy over end-of-life choices. However, as medical technology develops, some of these choices are not as clear-cut as some would want us to believe. The emergence of hospice during this same time period, with its focus on palliative care, makes some of these choices clearer and easier to manage.

Another area of ethical controversy in thanatology is physician-assisted suicide. I served as a consultant to the American Psychological Association when it tried to come up with a formal position on this issue. Discussions in this area can obviously generate a lot of heat. Because depression and pain management can be factors in the choice to die, patients may change their minds, making this a very murky area. I remember consulting with the staff at Massachusetts General Hospital when an elderly man repeatedly shouted that he did not want his gangrenous leg removed. He wanted to die. During my suicide evaluation of him, he told me the same thing. Ultimately, his leg was removed. When

I spoke with him later, he denied saying that he wanted to die and was very happy to be alive.

Gamino and Ritter make the case that grief counselors and those working with patients and families in end-of-life care need to explore their own mortality before letting this affect their ethical decisions. I couldn't agree more. Back in the early 1970s, many physicians were not doing a stellar job with end-of-life care because they saw the death of a patient as a failure. Unfortunately, many physicians still operate with that mindset. Dr. Ned Cassem and I created an elective course for second-year medical students at Harvard where students could meet with dying patients and their families and hone their skills for working with this population. An important objective of this course was to help these students explore their own mortality—how it might influence their motivation for entering medicine and how it might affect their work with dying patients. The class was well attended and I later published the exercises in a book, *Personal Death Awareness* (1976). A related area of ethical concern is grief counselors who have not worked through a loss in their own life, which can cloud their judgment when working with bereaved clients. Thanatologists, death educators, and grief counselors are well advised to consider whether they have the requisite "death competence" described by Gamino and Ritter that is so crucial when working with the dying and the bereaved.

With the increase in disasters, both man-made and natural, there is a tendency for grief counselors to want to rush in and help. However well-intended their motivation, without adequate training all kinds of ethical problems can emerge. I had just moved from Boston to California when a commercial jet collided with a smaller plane, killing all on board and raining debris on one particular community. I decided that I needed to help with this disaster and just showed up on the scene. I was an experienced grief counselor trained in stress debriefing, but I was not part of a formal response team. This limited my helpfulness and opened me to possible ethical violations. I recognized this and soon exited. I took home one important lesson about disasters—know the community where you are trying to work. This was a largely Latino community and many of the behaviors around grief and loss were clearly different from those I knew so well from practicing in Boston. People working disasters need to understand the community in terms of class, religion, and ethnicity if they are to be effective with their interventions. Gamino and Ritter outline carefully how grief counselors can and should respond to community disasters, including being part of a response team such as the Red

Cross. Critical incident stress debriefing should be the approach of first responders; grief counseling may not be needed early in a disaster and may not be appropriate for everyone. Good intentions are not enough. Incidentally, the media often confuses stress debriefing with grief counseling and calls *any* intervention after a disaster "grief counseling." We need to help educate them.

An alluring area of work for some grief counselors is the arena of forensic and legal testimony, often because the fees for service are high. I am frequently asked by lawyers to be an expert witness for cases on which they are working involving death and loss. I try to steer away from the forensic area because the research data is often soft and can be refuted by crafty lawyers who get chuckles from making the counselor look inept. However, there are times when grief counselors must become involved in legal action to which their own clients are party. This is quite a different situation from testifying as an expert consultant. Gamino and Ritter provide excellent guidelines for how to handle this necessary type of legal involvement and how to navigate through the ethical dilemmas presented by giving testimony in a court of law.

The ethical areas that thanatologists and grief counselors need to consider are many and varied, including legal responsibility for patient records, conflicting dual relationships, informed consent, patient confidentiality, Internet counseling, moving or closing a practice, and infraction reporting. Gamino and Ritter do an excellent job of providing timely advice and helpful suggestions for how professionals can manage ethical dilemmas that arise from the practice of grief counseling. The authors present a model for ethical decision making—the Five P Model—that will lead grief counselors through five distinct areas that need to be addressed when faced with *any* ethical decision.

Like the old Baptist hymn says, "What more can be said to you than has been given?" This book is comprehensive and the case studies flesh out the concepts, making the book interesting and readable. Even the most experienced grief counselors need to read this book as it will shine a light on some of our practices that we may never have considered. For me it was conversations with clients between the counseling room and the outside door. Does a discussion about my Boston Celtics in that space constitute the dual relationship of patient and friend? Interesting.

Finally, it is heartening to me to realize how our profession of thanatology has matured over the last 4 decades. We have well-known volumes on the technique and practice of grief counseling. We have our own code of ethics through the Association for Death Education and

Counseling. Now, Gamino and Ritter have provided an invaluable resource on ethics for professionals who certainly will struggle with ethical dilemmas while practicing grief counseling in a contemporary environment. I think it shows the maturity of our field when we ask ourselves not only how to do effective clinical work but also how to practice with the highest ethical standards.

J. William Worden, PhD, ABPP
Clinical Psychologist
Laguna Niguel, California

Preface

During graduate school at the University of Kansas in the 1970s, the clinical psychology program's intramural basketball team was named "Ethics." This moniker derived from the introductory course on assessment in which the professor continually emphasized the importance of ethics in clinical practice, long before ethics courses were required in graduate curricula. Prior to one game, a player from the opposing team questioned the meaning of that nickname, "What is 'ethics'?" Psychology teammates shared a good laugh at the rival's expense, musing over how someone could be ethical without even knowing what the word meant.

Grief counselors and those working with the dying and the bereaved know that ethics in practice is no laughing matter. Concern with what is the right and proper course of action in death-related dilemmas cannot simply be relegated to philosophers, medical ethicists, licensing boards, or ethics committees. Grief counselors must know the principles and standards that govern their work domain and, ideally, operate from a proven system of values and morals.

Unfortunately, even conscientious mental health providers, beleaguered by the prospect of satisfying their annual ethics requirement for licensure, may perceive a disconnect between what constitutes good ethical practice and the enterprise of therapeutically effective counseling. In reality, no such disconnect exists. It is our contention and a major theme of this book that *sound ethical practice is good counseling practice, and good counseling practice requires sound ethical practice.*

Busy grief counselors focused on client care may be tempted to reduce the notion of sound ethical practice to a solely defensive posture, that is, practice that is free of ethical error or missteps that lead to professional liability, risk management concerns, ethics committee investigations, or a malpractice insurance nightmare. However, such a mindset dangerously overlooks the nexus between ethics and practice that is crucial to provision of efficacious counseling. Instead, we propose that sound ethical practice is integral to intervening effectively.

What is unique to ethics in grief counseling? A specialized domain of ethical challenges can arise when counselors grapple with issues pertaining to dying, death, and bereavement. It is the authors' aim to provide, in a comprehensive text, a compilation of these major areas of ethical concern and to address them with a level of specificity beyond that typically found in generic texts on ethics in medicine or mental health. In addition, the Code of Ethics adopted by the Association for Death Education and Counseling (ADEC, 2006; Appendix A), an interdisciplinary thanatology organization, will be invoked as a *domain-specific* standard of care for dilemmas related to dying, death, and bereavement that can be used adjunctively with *discipline-specific* ethics codes that govern various professional groups. (Please note, in this book we cite repeatedly the current ADEC Code of Ethics. Therefore, we have omitted referencing the date of publication in all but this initial citation because to do so would be tedious and unnecessarily redundant.)

For whom is this book written? This volume is designed for grief counselors, mental health clinicians, death educators, health care providers, hospice workers, clergy, those in the funeral and aftercare industry, and anyone concerned with how to better educate and care for the dying and the bereaved. We anticipate that our readers share as their common denominator a dedication to working with death-related problems and issues, rather than sharing the same professional affiliation or training. It is our contention that ethical challenges inevitably arise in everyday practice and that the information in this volume can facilitate a seamless blending of sound ethical decision making with effective practice of grief counseling.

In the interest of disclosing personal biases, it is important for readers to know that both authors of this book hold life values grounded in our respective religious belief systems. Louis Gamino is a lifelong practicing Roman Catholic, and Hal Ritter is an ordained minister of the Southern Baptist Convention. Each of us considers our spiritual values inseparable from the conduct of our lives, both personal and professional. We find the "spirit of the law" embodied in our faith traditions to harmonize quite well with the secular professional codes upon which the reasoning in this text is based. Our Five P Model for ethical decision making maintains fidelity to those secular codes of ethics that inform our professional judgment. It is not based on religious beliefs. Instead, we conceptualize faith beliefs to be a dimension of the grief counselor *as human agent* when determining a specific course of action in response to an ethical dilemma. All codes of ethics call for integrity in deportment and decision making, and for us, integrity is grounded in a Christian value system.

Acknowledgments

No project of this magnitude is possible without encouragement from many sources and support from many helping hands. Both authors express heartfelt appreciation to Sheri Sussman and the editorial staff at Springer Publishing for their encouragement, support, and diligent assistance throughout the preparation of this book.

Louis Gamino

I am deeply appreciative of administrative encouragement from Kathryn Kotrla, Bill Meek, Judy Hyer, Bob Pryor, Bill Hamilton, and Bob Probe as well as support from all my colleagues at Scott & White. Invaluable assistance came from Penny Worley, Stephanie Fondy, June Lubowinski, Julie Bolin, Jeff Swindoll, and Christina Labra. I thank my sister, Denise Gamino, who painstakingly copyedited early drafts of several chapters. I have relied shamelessly on readers of preliminary drafts or sections of the manuscript, including Beryl Lawn, Jane Bissler, Ida Gonzales, Randy Moore, Bill Rae, Connie Fournier, and Illene Noppe. Special help came from Glen Cryer, Paul Ogden, Steve Raines, Steve Garrigan, and Dorothy Winkler. I am so grateful for the support of Nancy Hogan, Bill Worden, Harold Ivan Smith, Bob Neimeyer, Jon Reid, and all the members of my ADEC family too numerous to mention here. Many personal friends lent support as well. Even my in-laws, Frank and Marilyn Yarnell, assisted in the final push by watching over the household while my wife Marla, convalesced and I worked on the manuscript.

This book could not have been finished in a timely manner without the benefit of my "mini-sabbatical" supported by a private gift from my father's estate. I am indebted to both of my parents for making this possible. In the end, I offer humble thanks for the magnanimous love of my wife, Marla Ann, and my children, Gabriel, Claire, and Dominic, who generously shared the kitchen table, the family computer, and their Saturday mornings to make it possible for me to write this book.

Hal Ritter

Any writing project takes time and understanding by those who are not involved in the project. I really express appreciation to my wife, Michaela Ritter, who was a constant encouragement, but who also expressed unlimited understanding and patience. I appreciate her patience for all the times she had to attend various functions by herself, because of my writing schedule.

I also express my appreciation to the various teachers and professors of ethics who taught me academically and also mentored me in the decision-making process. In addition, I appreciate the many clients and patients with whom I have worked as a counselor and therapist. They have taught me many aspects of the decision-making process, for a client's work is primarily that of making decisions that have the possibility of significant life changes. After all, therapy really is a decision-making process, sometimes more ethically significant than others. Some decisions are morally neutral and are based more on circumstances and preferences. However, some decisions are highly significant morally, particularly regarding issues that must be resolved for the forward movement of life. My clients and patients who have engaged in these significant moral decisions have trusted me to share that journey into wholeness with them.

LAG & RHR, Jr.
October 13, 2008
Temple, Texas

1 Introduction

Most health care practitioners, mental health providers, and human services workers have a connotative understanding of what is meant by ethical practice. Strictly defined, ethics is the discipline dealing with what is good and bad and with moral duty and obligation, particularly the principles of conduct governing an individual or group. Ethical practice of grief counseling means helping clients and their families while operating from an internalized code of conduct and adhering to the highest level of professional standards and mores. To do so, grief counselors must start from a position of personal integrity and responsibility and then be aware of and follow ethics codes, statutory regulations, and case law that pertain to their realm of practice.

DEFINITIONS

In the popular press, *grief counseling* is an umbrella term typically employed to describe activities such as providing comfort or consolation to those suffering losses from illness, accidents, violence, natural disasters, terrorism, or war. Grief counselors may be credited with possessing special knowledge or ability to help mourners that goes beyond customary social responses of extending sympathy, offering support, providing companionship, or participating in religious rituals. However, exactly what constitutes this expertise or how grief counselors apply their special skills often remains unclear to the general public.

Depictions of grief counselors in the popular press are not always favorable. For example, one pundit drew an editorial cartoon depicting grief counselors as carrion birds ready to descend and feed from the misery of aggrieved survivors following a fatal school shooting. Thus in popular literature, not only is there ambiguity associated with the concept of grief counseling, but also there may be polarized opinions about its necessity or usefulness. All of this contributes to fuzziness about what is meant by grief counseling.

One of the landmark texts for professionals in the field, William Worden's (2009) *Grief Counseling and Grief Therapy,* distinguishes between *grief counseling* (e.g., psycho-education, supportive listening, normalizing bereavement-related symptoms) for those with uncomplicated bereavement and *grief therapy* for individuals whose grieving is complicated, such as prolonged, delayed, exaggerated, or masked. The latter is thought to require more sophisticated clinical acumen and advanced therapeutic techniques on the part of the provider. However, Worden's distinction may be lost on lay persons or even blurred by professionals who use the terms grief counseling and grief therapy interchangeably.

Because the purpose of this text is to provide professionals working with issues of dying, death, and bereavement a comprehensive handbook for navigating ethical dilemmas that may arise in the course of their work, we embrace a broad definition of grief counseling and eschew fine-grained distinctions based on the level of clinical expertise applied. In this text, the term grief counseling refers to any professional endeavor aimed at relieving personal suffering (e.g., emotional, psychological, physical, spiritual) brought about by the experiences of dying, death, and bereavement. Thus, grief counseling may include a wide spectrum of grief-related services including education, counseling, therapy, consultation, support, and advocacy provided in a variety of locations such as clinics, offices, hospitals, nursing homes, private homes, pastoral settings, funeral homes, schools, or work settings.

Because this book is devoted to domain-specific ethical problems, we use the term *grief counselor* in an umbrella fashion to refer to practitioners licensed in any of several professional disciplines. Thus, grief counselors may be psychologists, social workers, counselors, marriage and family therapists, nurses, physicians, clergy, or funeral directors. Even unlicensed volunteers or paraprofessionals who have received focal training in bereavement support may face some of the ethical dilemmas addressed in this text and therefore can benefit from its content.

Finally, for the sake of clarity and readability, we use the terms *client* and *clients* to refer to those individuals who are the recipients of grief counseling services. The designation of client is intended to be inclusive of those seen in traditional counseling practices as well as others: patients of physicians, nurses, or clinical psychologists; congregants in pastoral settings; customers in funeral home settings; and, when applicable, students and trainees in educational environments. The only exceptions made to this general rule are in discussions specific to hospitals or hospices, where the term *patient* is used by convention.

CASE EXAMPLES

Throughout the text, we include numerous case examples to underscore the commonplace nature of ethical dilemmas in the everyday practice of grief counseling and to illustrate the complexity that many of these situations entail. Some of the cases are purely fictional. Others were inspired by case material conveyed to us by colleagues around the country or from our own case files. In each instance, the circumstances and details of the case have been deliberately altered and reworked so as to remove any potentially identifying information. Our goal is to preserve the authenticity of the case examples for teaching purposes while at the same time to protect the privacy of the original parties involved. In no instances have cases been described verbatim without such modifications. With these precautions in place, any perceived similarity between case examples in this text and instances known to readers are most likely a function of the ubiquity of ethical dilemmas in counseling.

BLIND SPOTS

All grief counselors are subject to blind spots. Even the most ethically conscientious grief counselor can get in a hurry, skip an important step, make an erroneous assumption, overlook a conflict of interest, neglect to consider a consequence, or rationalize an action as good for the client when it is really the counselor's own interests that are being served. The best defense against blind spots is to keep constantly in mind that everyone, *even you*, can fall prey to a blind spot.

Novices in the field are most vulnerable to blind spots because of inexperience. In their eagerness to do a good job, please clients, and cultivate a practice, beginners may act in well-intended ways that have unintended ethical consequences. What starts out as a good-faith attempt to help becomes an ethical misstep when complications arise. For example, there was the beginning counselor who saw a client individually for bereavement-related issues and then agreed to include the client's spouse in some of the sessions in order to facilitate how the spouse could better support the grieving client. When serious marital conflict erupted in the process, the original client became disillusioned and no longer wanted conjoint meetings. However, the counselor was unclear about who was the client at that point—the original client or the couple? Even though the spouse withdrew, the bereaved client felt alienated and distrustful about continuing with the counselor, who was perceived to have mixed allegiances. Because those boundaries were not clear, the original client ended up dropping out of treatment. This is a good illustration of why working with a mentor early in one's career can provide an invaluable form of check and balance against potential blind spots. As risk managers are quick to point out, avoiding a problem in the first place is one of the best strategies for minimizing liability.

Experienced grief counselors are more vulnerable to the blind spot of thinking of themselves as ethically infallible. With good training, considerable practice experience, a favorable reputation, admiration from peers, and a waiting list of clients wanting to be scheduled, one can be lulled into a false sense of ethical security. Believing that nothing untoward will occur in such a successful professional practice is dangerous thinking. Even at the top of one's game or at the height of one's profession, grief counselors can still fall prey to a blind spot.

Consider the situation of the highly esteemed grief counselor who helped a young couple after the devastating loss of their first child following an unanticipated birth complication. So appreciative and grateful was the couple for the grief counselor's deft assistance during their travail that, when they had a healthy second baby, they asked the grief counselor to be one of the godparents at their infant's christening. The honor conveyed by the couple's request temporarily blinded the grief counselor to the untenable role conflicts inherent in their proposal, and the invitation was initially accepted. After reflection and discussion with a colleague, the grief counselor realized that the contradictions posed by a simultaneous professional and personal relationship were ethically inadvisable, and the invitation was subsequently declined.

This shows why not only novices but also experienced grief counselors need to make arrangements for regular consultation with a trusted colleague who can function as an extra pair of eyes and ears to help detect when something might go awry or when an ethical problem is brewing. Many practicing grief counselors meet their ongoing consultation needs using the professional buddy system. That is, they meet periodically for lunch or coffee with a colleague who is not afraid to respond candidly to their questions and doubts. Often, it is a reciprocal relationship wherein they do the same for their colleague. Such an arrangement can keep even the most prestigious grief counselor humble and help ensure that one's therapeutic relationships with clients are not jeopardized by unanticipated or unrecognized ethical violations.

HOW TO USE THIS BOOK

Whether readers are psychologists, social workers, counselors, marriage and family therapists, nurses, physicians, clergy, or funeral directors, all must first faithfully follow their *discipline-specific* codes of ethics and professional standards. In this book, we build on those guidelines by implementing the *domain-specific* ethical standards of the Association for Death Education and Counseling (ADEC), which are designed to inform and guide professionals encountering ethical dilemmas when death and bereavement are the therapeutic focus. This recommendation is consistent with current trends in the field of ethics wherein scholarly literature addressing specific problems in ethics constitutes one of many resources to be consulted when faced with a particular dilemma (Welfel, 2006).

In Chapter 2, we outline our customized process for ethical decision making in care of the dying and the bereaved, the Five P Model, and follow that with an exposition of the concept of death competence for grief counselors in Chapter 3. Chapters 4 and 5 cover consent and confidentiality, respectively, topics important to all mental health providers but which present some special challenges to grief counselors. Then, in subsequent chapters, we address major content areas specific to the enterprise of grief counseling: end-of-life dilemmas (Chapter 6); multiple relationships in thanatology (Chapter 7); ethnic, cultural, and spiritual considerations (Chapter 8); Internet counseling (Chapter 9); ethical controversies in grief counseling (Chapter 10); potential pitfalls of public service (Chapter 11); grief counselor as expert witness (Chapter 12); and moving or closing a professional practice (Chapter 13). The text concludes with Chapter 14 on reporting a colleague or facing a complaint. Having identified the areas of ethics most salient for those working with the dying and the bereaved, we seek to model how discipline-specific and domain-specific ethics codes, used together, contribute to a stance of professional accountability and a timely resolution of ethical problems.

Of course, no book can provide an answer for every occasion. We strive to offer clear guidelines for how to resolve ethical dilemmas in grief counseling given the enormously complex contextual variables that often surround these cases. Readers of preliminary drafts of our book have responded uniformly that the text was thought-provoking and informative, leading them to consider carefully how they would apply its concepts in their own work settings with their unique circumstances. This is precisely our goal—to inform an active, vital, creative, and thoughtful response on the part of grief counselors to the ethical challenges they face everyday. For us, the end result should be a response characterized by uncompromising professional integrity that incorporates thorough knowledge of ethical principles, standards, and precedents together with sensitivity to and compassion for the suffering person.

2 Ethical Decision Making: The Five P Model

Various traditions and models exist for ethical decision making in health care. Although no single model can claim status as the ultimate key to solving every dilemma, every ethically conscious health care professional needs to be familiar with at least one working model to apply when confronted with an ethical dilemma. The ethics code of the American Counseling Association (ACA, 2005a) states succinctly this obligation.

> When counselors are faced with ethical dilemmas that are difficult to resolve, they are expected to engage in a carefully considered ethical decision-making process. . . . While there is no specific ethical decision-making model that is most effective, counselors are expected to be familiar with a credible model of decision-making that can bear public scrutiny and its application. (ACA Code of Ethics, Purpose)

In this chapter, we first review some of the major streams of thought in the field of health care ethics in order to provide a conceptual context for introducing our customized model of ethical decision making. The Five P Model, which adapts and extends the pioneering work of Helen Perlman (1957), is specifically crafted to provide a practical approach for the thoughtful consideration and resolution of the everyday ethical challenges faced by mental health practitioners. We employ the Five P

Model throughout this text and encourage grief counselors to consider it as the credible model they adopt personally.

THEORIES FOR ETHICAL DECISION MAKING

A good theory offers several advantages to the decision maker. First, it provides a methodology for organizing diverse data into a coherent whole. Second, a good theory will provide a user-friendly process for actually making a decision, without resorting to some vague abstraction. In this regard, most ethical theories define the ultimate goal as decision making. Finally, a good theory provides the decision maker with a clear understanding of why the decision is being made, that is, a rationale for the decision. Thus, a good theory can help prevent the cart-before-the-horse phenomenon in ethical reasoning—reaching a conclusion about an ethical matter according to some tacit process and then searching for an ethical principle or law to justify the conclusion (cf. Haidt, 2001). Kitchener (1984) proposed that ethical theory helps the decision maker move beyond immediate, intuitive judgments and actions to a critical-evaluative level of reasoning that incorporates professional codes of ethics and moral principles in a reflective process suitable for addressing novel or complex dilemmas.

Now we review five basic theories for ethical decision making: virtue ethics, rule deontological ethics, principle ethics, utilitarian ethics, and feminist ethics.

Virtue Ethics

Virtue ethics, sometimes called character ethics, is a process of decision making based not only on information but also on one's personal integrity. Virtue ethics is focused on the individual making the decision, as well as the primary group to which one belongs. Tracing its origins back to the Greek philosopher Aristotle, virtue ethics has also enjoyed a contemporary revival (Pellegrino & Thomasma, 1993). The virtue ethics approach asks the question, "Who is a virtuous person?" In other words, how is the person's identity and integrity evident in the decision being made?

What if a grief counselor is asked by a family to falsify information conveyed to the client? In one case, for example, the client's spouse cautioned the counselor before test results were delivered, "We only want *hopeful* information." Unfortunately, the test results clearly indicated a worsening of the client's condition. The counselor's response was, "You need *accurate* information in order to know exactly what you're dealing with so you can prepare adequately." In effect, the counselor was saying, "I cannot lie to the client. My personal integrity does not allow me to lie. What kind of person will people think I am if they know I will lie to another person? And what kind of grief counselor will people think I am if they know I will lie to a client?" In this case, withholding bad news is the equivalent of lying, and the counselor believes that lying compromises personal integrity.

Because virtue ethics asks, "What is a virtuous person?" it is concerned with evaluating good traits of character. In ethics courses, the question may be asked, "Which traits of character or virtue are important for a grief counselor?" (Pence, 2004). Many believe traits such as wisdom and compassion are important. Although knowledge and skill can be learned, wisdom is seen as necessary for the beneficial application of knowledge, and compassion refers to the character of the provider when applying specialized skills.

Hauerwas (1981) espouses a version of virtue ethics that he calls *character ethics,* based on Aristotle's theory. For Hauerwas, the ethical question is, "What kind of people will we be for the decisions that we make?" In other words, the ethical decision not only reflects the personal integrity of the decision maker but also shapes the kind of person that decision maker will be in the future. Decision making molds personhood. In addition, Hauerwas views the ethical question in the context of the community to which one belongs. For Hauerwas, it is the Christian community. However, the context can be any applicable community, such as the broader community of thanatologists: death educators, bereavement researchers, and grief counselors. When Hauerwas asks what kind of people "we" will be, he means that the decision shapes both the personhood of the individual and the identity of the community of which one is a member. In other words, individual grief counselors represent not only themselves but also the community of thanatologists of which they are part.

If the question of virtue ethics is applied to a social issue, such as physician-assisted suicide, the answer becomes one that reflects both the character of the person making the decision and the character of the reference group of which one is a member. For example, if a health care organization supports physician-assisted suicide, what does that decision say about the organization if it also claims to support hospice and progressive palliative care? Is it assisting the dying to live each day until they die, or is it facilitating dying when the terminally ill no longer have quality of life? And who judges the quality of that life?

Families sometimes reflect virtue ethics when they are asked to make end-of-life decisions for a loved one. Various family members may ask, "What does this say about us, as a family, if we terminate care for Mom? Will others say we killed or murdered our mother? I do not like how that feels. That is not what I want to think about this decision." Others may say, "What does this say about us, as a family, if we unnecessarily prolong Mom's life, knowing she is in terrible pain?" In either case, the ethical question is about the identity of the family group, as well as those individual, decision-making family members.

Rule Deontological Ethics

Rule ethics is a form of decision making that seeks to know the "correct" rule for the decision being made. Deontological is from the Latin word *deontos,* which means "duty" (Pence, 2004). The ethical issue is one's "duty" to do "right." The notion of rule ethics was developed by the 18th century German writer Immanuel Kant (1959/1789). For Kant, why an act is done is more important than its consequences. In this regard, personal motive is an important part of determining the rightness of an ethical decision, so the value of an action is determined by the quality of the intention behind the action.

For example, one may give money to the Hospice Foundation of America (HFA) for purposes of getting a tax deduction. Tax-wise, it may be a smart decision. However, it is not a morally virtuous decision. On the other hand, one may give money to the HFA believing in a duty to help those who are dying and their families. In this case, the decision is morally virtuous. In both examples, giving to the HFA has the same consequences: helping dying people and getting a tax deduction. However, the higher motivation of helping dying patients, rather than just getting a tax deduction, makes one decision more virtuous than the other. An additional principle from Kant is that people have value, and they should never be treated as disposable or as merely the means to some other end or consequence. In other words, the higher ethical principle is that which says that people have worth and dignity.

Kant's (1959/1789) approach to rules for decision making included his application of a universalizing principle known as the *categorical imperative.* The categorical imperative insists that any act can be ethical only if it is based on a rational reason or principle that can be recommended as universal law. In other words, it can be proposed for everyone. For example, should people contribute money to the HFA for altruistic reasons? Yes, because helping provide information and resources regarding palliative care and end-of-life decision making is a universal principle for good. What about blackmail as a reason for getting money for the HFA? No, I cannot recommend blackmail as a universal principle because it violates the law as well as human dignity. In other words, supporting the HFA is a sound moral decision. However, to use blackmail or extortion to raise money for the HFA is not morally virtuous because individuals will be devalued and harmed in the process of blackmailing them. In this case, Kant's use of the categorical imperative is a constructive way of helping people think about ethical decisions.

One variation of rule deontological ethics is knowing what one's religious tradition considers to be the right rule to follow. Some will seek out help from sacred texts, from respected fellow faith members, or from clergy to inform their notions of what is right and wrong. Regardless of religious affiliation, a decision maker using rule ethics often seeks out the *right* thing to do in a given situation. Even when the result is a poor outcome, rule ethicists may comment, "Well, it may not have worked out the way we wanted, but at least we know we did the *right* thing." In other words, even though the outcome of the decision was not preferred, there is no second guessing or residual guilt about the decision because the decision makers know they "did the right thing"; that is, they followed the correct rule.

Other variations of rule deontological ethics are company rules or agency policies, state laws, and the regulations of one's profession. Regardless of the origin of the rules that one follows, *most important is the intent to do the right thing.* The assumption is that rules are made to protect individuals and communities. Rules prescribe desirable decisions and proscribe undesirable ones. If the rule says that clients have the right to all aspects of health care information about their individual care, then withholding information about an exam or test result is a violation of the rule. If giving the client the troubling information results in an uncomfortable or distressing emotional response, the person giving the information can still be assured that "at least we know we did the right thing" by giving the information. The person giving the information may say, "I am sorry for the discomfort this has caused, but at least we know you have been told the truth."

Principle or Value Ethics

Many people state they have certain principles that are formative for their lives and foundational for decision making. For some, there is one central principle, such as love, or peace, or life. They will use this organizing principle to consider all the various aspects of any decision, such as "I believe in peace, so I want this to be the most peaceful, or the least violent, decision." In the case of elective medical procedures, violence may be understood as the infliction of pain from the recommended procedure. Although it is realized that some pain is part of life, the intent of decisions is always for the least amount of pain (i.e., violence) and for the pursuit of peace and tranquility (i.e., pain reduction).

If someone values life, he or she may say that he or she wants everything possible done in order to preserve life. Any discussion of premature termination of life by withholding various mechanical or nutritional supports is seen as devaluing life and leading toward a view of human life as expendable when it is inconvenient. Valuing life often divides families in end-of-life dilemmas. There may be one person or group who says, "Do everything possible to keep Dad alive. That's what he would want. He always fought for us when we were growing up, and he taught us to believe in life. He'd never agree to giving up. You never know when a new drug will be discovered." Another person or group may say, "You're right, Dad always fought hard for us. But the fight is over. Dad is in terrible pain, and there is no hope for him getting any better. Living for him, like this, is not life. We need to let him go and let nature take its course."

In this example, some of the family believe that any limits to care are the same as "giving up" and may also be a violation of the principle of the value of life, as it has been taught to them by their father. Conversely, others view the merciful end of a painful, medically debilitated life as a better option for one who always affirmed life. They believe that because there is no hope of recovery, their father should be allowed to die by letting nature take its course. Their decision to "let go" is an affirmation of a life well lived. What the previous group views as "prolonging living" is something they view as "prolonging dying."

Biomedical ethics has embraced the principle or value ethics approach, in large part because of the influential work of Beauchamp and Childress (2008). To guide decision making, they champion four basic ethical principles: *nonmaleficence, beneficence, autonomy,* and *justice.* Their approach is the subject of a later section of this chapter.

Utilitarian Ethics

Utilitarian ethics, or consequentialism, has a long history, particularly in the United States with its philosophy of pragmatism. Pragmatism says that if a particular procedure or activity works out positively, then it must be the best decision. Utilitarianism is a variation on pragmatism—it says that the best ethical decision is one that brings the greatest good to the greatest number. Philosopher John Stuart Mill (1972/1859) is the one who most clearly developed a theory of utilitarianism, "the greater good for all."

Some have argued that the notion of utilitarianism developed historically within the United States because of its traditions in Christianity, with its attendant views of charity, love, and caring for others. In other words, utilitarian ethics pull for the majority to receive the greatest benefit or greatest good, with charity toward all, including one's enemies. Certainly, this is consonant with the democratic system in the United States. Yet one of the limitations of utilitarianism is that the majority may not consider the needs of the minority. With multiple cultures and ethnicities in one society, how does one consider the greatest good for the greatest number?

The greater good for one person or group may be very different from the greater good for another person or group. For some, there is no consideration of the benefit for the larger group. For them, the only consideration is how the decision will benefit some smaller group, such as the elite, or the wealthiest, or the most educated. Alternately, a cultural minority or a religious sect may reject utilitarianism because it excludes or marginalizes its interests (see Chapter 8, "Ethnic, Cultural, and Spiritual Considerations," for a more detailed discussion of how to honor such individual differences in ethical decision making).

In end-of-life issues, the utilitarian approach first views the needs of the patient. What is good and beneficial for this person? What does the patient view as good? How does the patient view quality of life? If capable of medical decision making, what does the patient want? If there is a medical decision being made for the patient by another person, a surrogate or proxy decision maker, the question remains, "What is best for this patient?" It is not what the surrogate decision maker wants for the patient but what the surrogate understands to be the patient's wishes. Although some individual family members may want to keep a loved one on life support, that may not be what is best for the patient or what the patient would want. In such end-of-life examples, utilitarian ethics also ask what is good for the greatest number and how the patient's wants may affect other stakeholders in the decision.

For example, utilitarian ethics often come into play when considering how to allocate scarce medical resources. If the patient with limited life expectancy cannot breathe without a respirator, how long is the patient's choice to continue living supported if there are other critically ill patients with a better chance of recovery who may need that respirator? In the arena of organ transplant, the question arises of who most deserves to receive a preciously limited commodity, such as a cadaver's kidney. The ethic of "the greatest good for the greatest number" may favor giving the kidney to a young adult mother of three minor children whose kidney disease resulted from a congenital birth defect versus an older, single male whose former alcoholism ruined his kidneys.

Feminist Ethics

Feminist philosophy offers a sharp counterpoint to the more traditional ethical theories presented thus far. The feminist perspective prizes relationships as an ethical value (Farley, 1985; Lebacqz, 1985) and seeks to equalize power among people by dismantling social norms and institutions that establish and maintain gendered hierarchies (Donchin, 2004). Feminists posit that most ethical theories have been developed by men, who tend to put a premium on autonomy and individualism. Alternately, Gilligan (1982) put forward caring—managing and maintaining relationships through love, care, and responsibility—as a core ethical value.

Feminists also argue that men have a privileged position in society, which means that men have more power than women, just because of male gender. Especially in Western society, White men tend to have more authority than men of color. The result is that the voices and opinions of others, such as minorities, immigrants, or refugees, are often silenced or marginalized. For this reason, feminists focus on understanding power differentials and their interconnections with gender, race, culture, class, physical ability, sexual orientation, age, religion, and ethnic heritage (Ballou, Hill, & West, 2008; Feminist Therapy Institute, 2000). Eradicating oppression in all its forms, respecting diversity, and advocating for social change when societal or communal attitudes and practices harm an individual's growth potential are core values in feminist ethics.

A good example of how feminist ethics can be applied to ethical decision making in a health care environment is the method proposed by Verkerk et al. (2004). Drawing heavily on Walker's (1998) feminist ethics, they reject a notion of morality as discrete, codified knowledge. Instead, Verkerk et al. view morality as a fluid, interpersonal, socially constructed reality: "It is a way of expressing who we are, of understanding others, and holding others and ourselves to moral account" (p. 32).

In confronting any ethical dilemma, Verkerk et al. (2004) first ask professionals to reflect on their own individual sensibilities and reactions in a given situation, similar to starting with Kitchener's (1984) immediate, intuitive response. Then they guide professionals toward understanding that they are part of a clinical practice that involves multiple perspectives and positions, that is, beginning the critical-evaluative process described by Kitchener. Verkerk et al. use a "reflection square" in which one key perspective is considered in each quadrant: the agent's (i.e., the health care professional's) core values and beliefs, the agent's actions, social norms, and consequences of social norms. Their goal is to enhance consensus-building among professionals working together as a team to attain "moral competence: the ability to see what is morally relevant in a situation, knowing the point of view from which one sees it, understanding that others may see it differently, and then, with others, responding well to what one sees" (p. 37). To some, this may sound like the essence of moral relativism. Yet it is based on core feminist values—mutual respect among health care professionals, sensitivity to the perspectives of others, collaborative rather than hierarchical decision making—and provides a working example of how feminist ethics can be applied to ethical decision making.

ETHICS IN MEDICINE

Ethics in the professional fields of counseling and mental health evolved from the larger rubric of medical ethics. The original impetus for ethics in biomedical and behavioral research emerged after World War II and the Nuremberg War Trials. In Nazi Germany, some medical doctors conducted cruel biomedical experiments on concentration camp prisoners, without their permission. The Nuremberg Code of 1947 resulted from the trials and established standards for biomedical ethics (Grodin, 1992). It was followed by other international efforts to guide physicians in ethical conduct of biomedical research involving human subjects, such as the 1964 Declaration of Helsinki, now in its fifth revision (World Medical Association, 2000).

In the United States, the infamous Tuskegee Syphilis Study, initiated in 1932, exploited poor, rural Southern black males to investigate the long-term effects of the disease and deprived its experimental subjects of the benefits of a cure that was discovered partway through the study, namely, penicillin (Jones, 1981). Public awareness of the study in 1972 brought an outcry for reform (Centers for Disease Control and Prevention, 2008; Tuskegee University, 2008).

In 1974 the U.S. Congress passed the National Research Law (Pub. L. 93–348), which codified into the Federal Register guidelines for protecting human subjects involved in biomedical and behavioral research. These regulations were recently revised (U.S. Department of Health and Human Services, 2005). The original law created the National Commission for the Protection of Human Subjects of Biomedical and Behavioral Research. One of the charges to the commission was to establish guidelines for research at all levels in the United States: What are the boundaries between the routine practice of medicine and biomedical or behavioral research? How is risk–benefit to be assessed when using human subjects? How are human subjects to be selected for research? What is informed consent for the purposes of research on human subjects? (Miser, 2005).

In 1976 the Smithsonian Institution's Belmont Conference convened for an intensive 4-day study of the new guidelines, followed by monthly meetings over the next few years. In 1979 the commission issued its directives as the *Belmont Report* (National Commission for the Protection of Human Subjects of Biomedical and Behavioral Research, 1979). Three ethical principles, or general prescriptive judgments, relevant to research involving human subjects were identified in the *Belmont Report*: respect for persons, beneficence, and justice. In the original Belmont report, *beneficence* encompassed the tandem concern of "first, do no harm," or *nonmaleficence* (Miser, 2005).

One result of the establishment of these four ethical principles is that they apply to all health care situations, including physical medicine and mental health care. Whether in biomedical or behavioral research or in clinical care, the concept of informed consent is given great prominence (see Chapter 4, "Consent"). Consent for nontherapeutic research, which generally seeks healthy volunteers for the purpose of gaining knowledge to further medical options and does not directly benefit the participant, has more stringent requirements to be sure the person is fully free to give consent. Children, prisoners, military recruits, and even medical students are morally excluded from all but the most risk-free research on the grounds that their freedom to refuse is limited or compromised (Wheeler, 1996). On the other hand, therapeutic research, which is often experimental in nature, has a less stringent level of consent because people with end-stage diseases are often willing to accept the potential risks of untried medical interventions when no other treatment options are available.

Biomedical Ethics

Beauchamp and Childress (2008) reformulated the three ethical principles from the *Belmont Report* in slightly different terminology that is in general use today. Respect for persons is now considered under the principle of autonomy. Nonmaleficence and beneficence are now parsed as separate principles. Thus, the four principles they advocate are nonmaleficence, beneficence, autonomy, and justice. Some ethicists will add an additional principle, such as fidelity or professional relationship, but these four are the traditional standard for biomedical ethics. Some professional disciplines have adopted versions of these four, or five, principles as aspirational goals for their members (cf. American Psychological Association, 2002).

Nonmaleficence is based in the oft-repeated principle "first, do no harm" (in Latin, *primum non nocere*). In other words, if nothing can be done to benefit a patient, at least do nothing that will harm the patient. If cure and return to a quality life are not possible, then do not do anything to make the situation worse. The other side of avoiding any harm is the principle of *beneficence*—doing something that will improve the patient's life, even if it means providing only comfort or palliative care. Beneficence is nicely summarized in the doctor's adage "Cure sometimes, alleviate [suffering] often, comfort always" (Roberts, 1997, p. 360).

Autonomy is based in the occidental philosophy of valuing the individual, which comes to the West particularly through the writings of Immanuel Kant (1959/1789). Autonomy is based in the notion of respect for the person, where the individual is the determining agent for decision making. The individual has the right to full disclosure of all information regarding treatment options, as well as information regarding the potential consequences of no treatment. Autonomy is not a democratic process, where the majority of the interested parties make the decision. In other words, the family cannot overrule or outvote the desires of the individual patient who is capable of making an independent decision.

The fourth principle in medical ethics is *justice.* Justice means fairness, that is, all patients will be treated fairly and holistically within the bounds of the resources that are available. It does not mean that all patients will be treated the same because the same resources are not available to every person. However, within the context of what resources are available, treatment should not be limited or withheld based on income, social standing, education, race, gender, ethnicity, disability, or religion. In the field of medicine, the international humanitarian group Doctors Without Borders is a good example of justice in action. These physicians will travel anyplace in the world to provide care, within their ability, regardless of the politics of the geographical area or the politics of the individuals they treat.

Those who include the fifth principle, *fidelity,* believe that being truthful with a patient and maintaining confidentiality are important obligations in any professional relationship. Health care professionals enter into a fiduciary relationship with patients—one with a deep sense of trust embedded in it—that carries with it a qualitatively different level of obligation than would a nonprofessional association. Fidelity means counselors honor the caregiver–client relationship by behaving in a manner worthy of the faith and trust placed in them. Loyalty is another aspect of fidelity—professionals are expected to advocate for clients when appropriate, and they never abandon their clients. Honesty, integrity, trustworthiness, responsibility, and loyalty are all dimensions implied by the principle of fidelity.

Clinical Ethics

Jonsen, Siegler, and Winslade (2004) developed a model specifically for making ethical decisions in clinical medicine. This model, sometimes referred to as the "four box" method, begins by organizing the facts of the case into four discrete categories: medical indications, patient preferences, quality of life, and contextual features. Medical indications include all relevant medical information pertaining to the illness: diagnosis, prognosis, treatment options, and consequences of no treatment. The ethical principles related to medical indications are nonmaleficence and beneficence. Patient preferences consider how the patient with the illness wants to be treated. The ethical principle of autonomy, or respect for the individual as a decision-making agent, is most pertinent. Quality of life can be difficult to determine. After all, who decides what is perceived as quality—the patient, the family, or the staff? The ethical principles most applicable to quality of life determinations include autonomy, nonmaleficence, and beneficence. Contextual features include mediating factors such as religion, economics, family, race, ethnicity, and gender. The prevailing ethical principle here is justice, ensuring that patients are treated well and treated fairly. Because the Jonsen et al. approach is most applicable for clinical cases in medicine, it is less applicable in counseling and therapy (G. McGee, personal communication, December 2006).

ETHICS OF GRIEF

The ethics of grief allow people to mourn individually. Although many risk factors (Gamino, Sewell, & Easterling, 1998, 2000; Parkes & Weiss, 1983; Rando, 1993; Raphael, 1983) and mediating variables (Worden, 2009) influence mourning, the value and quality of the attachment to the deceased person is a principal determinant of the character and depth of grieving. Although much has been written about stages of grief and tasks of grieving (cf. Neimeyer & Gamino, 2003), evolving conceptual models reify the notion that grieving is very much a personal, subjective process (Neimeyer, 1998). Some have attempted to define normative styles of grieving, such as intuitive versus instrumental grievers (Martin & Doka, 1999; Martin & Wang, 2006), whereas others target pathological variations of grief as absent, delayed, or prolonged (Boelen & Prigerson, 2007; Goldsmith, Morrison, Vanderwerker, & Prigerson, 2008; Rando, 1993; Worden, 2009). From one cultural perspective, Muslim physician Muhammed Ayub observed, "If people do not weep now (for their loss), their organs will weep and produce disease later" (Ritter, Smith, Santibanez, Ayub, & Tayi, 2005, p. 260).

Ethically conscious grief counselors adhere to a position of pluralism wherein the sensibilities, preferences, and traditions of each individual mourner are respected. The ADEC Code of Ethics states this quite clearly in its "Basic Tenets."

> The member takes care to know the student or client. Good education and counseling are based upon an understanding of, and a respect for, the student's or client's cultural background, developmental status, perceptions, and other individual differences and needs. (ADEC Code of Ethics, Basic Tenets, 3)
>
> The member strives to present various views of a death-related question, indicating the member's own values if appropriate, and respecting the student's or client's choice among alternatives. (ADEC Code of Ethics, Basic Tenets, 6)

This respect for people's individuality in grieving and in their decision making reflects the fundamental ethical principle of autonomy. Rigidly applying a unitary formula or an external standard of how grieving should progress may constitute a violation of the principle of nonmaleficence, "do no harm."

This is not to say that innovative theory and research have no place in grief counseling. Quite the opposite, they figure prominently for practitioners who stay current in their field. Theory and research can be applied flexibly while still respecting individual differences. For example, we often use Stroebe and Schut's (1999) dual process model of grieving to illustrate for bereaved clients that oscillating between grief work and going on with life is considered normal and to give permission for that oscillation dynamic to express itself in very individual ways. Similarly, in counseling bereaved parents who wonder why their time trajectory of grief seems so different from those mourning other kinds of losses, we use Klass's (2001) qualitative study of bereaved parents in support groups to exemplify categorizations that the parentally bereaved *assign themselves* to describe their grief journeys. However, we portray Klass's findings as a sample, not an invariant template. In each instance, the ultimate goal is to help the struggling griever, which is the ethical principle of beneficence in action.

Sometimes loss brings up old conflicts and animosities within groups, for example, schisms among family members. Grieving may also elicit untapped resources and mobilize latent strengths of which persons were unaware. These crosscurrents are inherent in the nature of grief and thus are to be anticipated in the practice of grief counseling when ethical decisions must be made. Evenhandedly mediating conflicts, promoting fairness in the treatment of the dying or the bereaved, and advocating for open access to resources enacts the ethical principle of justice. The ADEC Code of Ethics endorses this important aspect of ethical practice.

> The member serves in an advocacy role to assist the individual or society to cope with death-related issues. The member intervenes to prevent exploitation of the student or client and is obligated: (a) to be available to the student or client; and (b) to educate or counsel regarding rights, responsibilities and options with their possible consequences. (ADEC Code of Ethics, Basic Tenets, 5)

THE FIVE P MODEL

The preceding discussion of ethical theories and time-honored principles of health care ethics is foundational for how grief counselors think about ethical decision making. In any ethical dilemma, there is the who, what, where, and how of the decision. The *who* includes the client and others involved in the decision. The *what* is defining the problem as well as the contextual variables that surround the problem. The *where* entails venue-specific or location-driven aspects to take into account. The *how* refers to the relevant ethical principles employed as well as the actual process that will be followed for making the decision. Unfortunately, some ethical theories seem to address one dimension of decision making more than another, and some theories seem abstract rather than practical. For these reasons, we propose a five-step model for ethical decision making that addresses the who, what, where, and how of the decision and that is designed to be especially applicable for ethical dilemmas in grieving and end-of-life situations.

A seminal work for us is a social work text by Helen Perlman (1957). In addressing the task of social casework, Perlman defined a four-part problem-solving process, taking into consideration the person, the problem, the place or social context, and the helping process. It is important to note that Perlman was not addressing the idea of ethics or ethical decision making. Nonetheless, her ideas form the nidus of our model. Adapting and extending Perlman's work, we include a fifth element—ethical principles—that transforms her problem-solving process into a decision-making model for ethical reasoning. Thus, our Five P Model can be stated succinctly as follows: "A *person* with a challenging ethical *problem* in a particular contextual *place* applies appropriate ethical *principles* in a deliberate decision-making *process.*" A schematic representation of the Five P Model is presented in Figure 2.1.

The essential elements of the Five P Model for ethical decision making are summarized in Table 2.1.

Person

The first consideration is the person or persons affected by the decision to be made. *Who* is this person? What is the individual's age, educational background, occupational history, and socioeconomic standing? Are there cultural, ethnic, or religious considerations? What kind of interpersonal relationships does the person have in terms of family, friends, and social connections? What experience with loss or losses has the person had? Oates (1982) comments that people's grief, meaning, and recovery are cumulative so that each loss, successively, is a reminder of previous losses. Further, does the person have capacity for decision making? Is

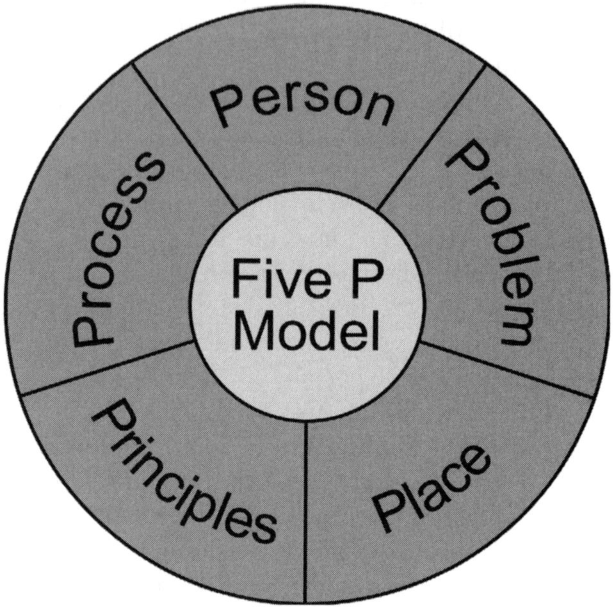

Figure 2.1 Schematic representation of the Five P Model for ethical decision-making

the person's capacity adequate for understanding the subtle nuances and complexities of the ethical issue as it is being formulated?

What decision-making style does the person bring to the process? Some people are more intuitive, believing they just know or feel what the right answer is, and do not question their inner convictions. Deductive decision makers want to first collect data and gather information before deciding. They do not want to overlook a potentially crucial piece of information and prefer to have all the facts to weigh. Then, there are non-deciders who, because of denial or dependency, do not want to take responsibility for decisions that need to be made. In all these things, it is important to have a clear understanding of who is the person in the dilemma.

Problem

The second consideration is the problem. This is the *what* of the decision-making process. What is the specific ethical issue that needs to be resolved? How is the problem understood, and is it properly stated? Is the problem formulated differently by various stakeholders? For example, one person may want to spend the family savings on an elaborate funeral to honor

Table 2.1

FIVE P MODEL FOR ETHICAL DECISION MAKING

"A *person* with a challenging ethical *problem* in a particular contextual *place* applies appropriate ethical *principles* in a deliberate decision-making *process*."

1. *Person:* Who is this person?
Age. Sex. Education. Work history. Economic background.
Single, married, partnered. Home/family. Friends. Social support.
Ethnicity, culture, religion. Community/civic activities.
Strengths/resources. Personal resilience.
Other personal history (e.g., previous losses, decision-making style).

2. *Problem:* What is the specific ethical challenge to be resolved?
Statement of the problem. What is the ethical dilemma?
Who is formulating the problem? Who else has an interest in the problem?
Is the problem properly stated? Other variables?

3. *Place:* Where is the ethical dilemma manifested?
Physical location. Medical setting: clinic, hospital, hospice, nursing home?
Other: private home, funeral home, place of worship, educational setting?
Public or private place? Are there agency/institutional considerations?

4. *Principles:* What ethical principles are the focus of the problem?
Ethical principles: autonomy, beneficence, nonmaleficence, justice, fidelity.
Ethics of the profession. ADEC Code of Ethics.
State/federal laws. Personal narrative. Religious, ethnic, cultural "rules."

5. *Process:* How will the decision be made?
How will information be gathered? How will all voices be heard?
Time limitations. Ethical theory. Resolution of the dilemma.

the deceased. However, other family members may want a simple funeral without incurring significant cost. The important factor is to clearly focus the problem and determine what information must be gathered in order to fully understand the decision. Who will provide the information? What resources are available for gathering the information?

It is always important to distinguish the person from the problem. Counseling theories universally encourage a nonjudgmental acceptance of the person apart from the problem (cf. Rogers, 1957). In particular, narrative approaches to counseling emphasize that the person is not the problem, but the problem is the problem (White & Epston, 1990). In other words, the griever may be very upset and distressed, but the ethical dilemma to be faced and the decisions that need to be made must be evaluated with some objectivity and without being overwhelmed by the emotions of the moment.

Place

The third aspect of ethical decision making is consideration for the context of place wherein the ethical dilemma is manifested. This is the *where* of the decision-making process. Where does the ethical issue occur? Is it a private or public place? Often, the determination of place provides some information regarding who is involved in the decision. Is it a public policy matter? Are there agency, institutional, or venue-specific regulations or contingencies involved, or is it an individual or family decision? Does the dilemma locate itself in a medical environment of some kind, such as a hospital or nursing home? In each of these settings, place determines important contextual cues for the decision-making process.

Principles

Which ethical principles operate is the fourth aspect of ethical decision making. This is part of *how* the decision is made. Is the focus one or more of the major ethical principles for decision making—nonmaleficence, beneficence, autonomy, justice, and fidelity? Are there other considerations, such as religious regulations or ethnic sensibilities, customs, or laws? For example, in respecting the rights of the individual according to the principle of autonomy, some people are very careful to be sure that the decision is made by that individual or agent. Those of Anglo-European descent may be more attuned to individual decision making. On the other hand, for some, no decision is made without the input and consideration of those in close relationship to the agent, particularly family members. For many from Hispanic lineage, no decision is truly individual because all live in a relational matrix with other people who are an important part of one's identity and decisions.

For grief counselors, ethical decisions will be based on allegiance to a discipline-specific code of ethics from their respective professional organization as well as on working familiarity with the domain-specific ADEC Code of Ethics.

Process

The final element of decision making is determining the process that will be followed for resolving the issue. This is another aspect of *how* the decision is made. How will the information that has been gathered be prioritized? What ethical theory and which principles are applicable to the process? If there are several, how will they be prioritized as to which one will carry more decisional weight? Is it to be a democratic decision where the greatest good for the greatest number, such as family members, prevails? How will the minority voices be respected rather than marginalized? Does a rule need to be applied? If two or more provisions of the grief counselor's professional code of ethics appear to give conflicting guidance, how will the discrepancy be resolved? Are there particular legal issues to consider? In other words, a significant part of making the ethical decision is determining what the process will be. Another factor is the temporal aspect of the process. Is it a decision that needs to be made quickly because of some urgency to the problem? Or, is there more time for reflection and contemplation of how the information will be gathered and used? All of these considerations affect the process to be used in ethical decision making.

CASE EXAMPLE

Maria is a 16-year-old Hispanic female who lives at home with her parents and a younger brother. They are a strong Christian family and members of a charismatic church that believes in faith healing. Maria is in the final stages of cancer, currently hospitalized, and in much pain. The medical staff's recommendation is for her to be transferred to hospice care. Maria has been clear about her feelings. Even though she is young, she has been through a lot with radiation and chemotherapy. She now says, "I'm okay. Just let me go."

Maria's maternal uncle, her mother's brother, is the minister of their church. He actively proclaims evangelism and faith healing. He believes that Jesus is going to perform a miracle of healing for Maria, his niece, who is named for Mary, the mother of Jesus. He admonishes the family not to give up. He tells them they must have faith and believe that God is a healer who advocates for life.

The medical staff is in agreement that comfort care is the only viable option for Maria at this stage of her disease. Maria has indicated her personal preference not to continue suffering, but to *allow natural death* (AND) to take its course. However, Maria's parents have always been swayed by the teachings of their church, as presented to them by Maria's uncle. Therefore, her parents are praying for a miracle and want to do whatever is necessary for Maria to live until such a miracle can occur "in God's time." Curiously, Maria's younger brother seems to empathize more directly with his sister's suffering and wants to let her go.

The medical staff wants to help Maria by suspending further medical interventions and by providing palliative pain control and psychosocial support through hospice care. They respect Maria's position and view her as an incredibly courageous young woman whose wish to die should be honored. However, they also know that Maria, at age 16, is still a minor child, and that her parents have the final say in medical decisions for her. They seek the assistance of a grief counselor with experience in end-of-life decision making to help bring the medical staff, Maria, and her family to consensus, if at all possible.

Person

In the Five P Model, consideration of person is first. In the case example, the protagonist is Maria, a 16-year-old Hispanic female with end-stage cancer. She is a minor child who is unmarried and lives at home with her mother, father, and brother. She is fully cognizant of her condition and the futility of additional treatment. Yet, because she is a dependent minor, her parents still have legal authority for her medical decisions. Culturally, Maria and her family endorse an ethic of solidarity where they do not abandon or leave behind one of their own. Also, they are members of a charismatic Christian church that believes in faith healing. In short, for legal, cultural, and religious reasons, Maria's wishes cannot be considered independently from those of her family and faith community.

Besides the extensive support of Maria's family and the expertise of the health care team, the involvement of the grief counselor constitutes an outside resource brought to bear on the ethical dilemma posed by Maria's situation. In addition, the hospital bioethics committee is available to advise, consult, or mediate.

Problem

The second dimension of the Five P Model is the problem. Here, the ethical problem lies in the fact that the patient, Maria, and the health care team favor hospice care for her terminal cancer, whereas her parents and church family want more aggressive medical treatment to prolong her life while praying for the miracle they seek. Thus, the two sides are deadlocked on how to proceed with Maria's care. The medical staff does not want to inflict further suffering on Maria—that is, by "prolonging dying" with use of a respirator and Intensive Care Unit (ICU) technology. Maria's parents insist on "prolonging living" because they fervently believe that their prayers for a miracle will be rewarded with a dramatic turnaround in her condition; therefore, they cannot "give up."

A complicating aspect of the ethical problem is the issue of Maria's capacity for medical decision making. As a mature minor, her preferences generally are given serious consideration, but the final decision still rests with her parents (for a detailed discussion of minors' capacity for their health care decisions, see Chapter 6 on end-of-life issues).

Place

The place where an ethical problem occurs is the third part of the Five P Model. Maria is currently hospitalized. Transferring to hospice probably means hospice home care. However, prolonging her life probably means the ICU. Location in a hospital setting has significant implications for the outcome of the medical decision. The health care team is in its home court and cannot be compelled to deliver treatments they deem unwise, unduly burdensome, or futile. Although charged to be an advisory body only, the bioethics committee may well have an eye toward preventing the hospital's liability and could be perceived as "in the pocket" of the medical staff. Their neutrality would have to be clarified.

Likewise, the grief counselor has a staff affiliation at the hospital that allows the counselor to assume a professional role with Maria and her family. Does this affiliation influence the grief counselor's objectivity? Because the hospital staff requested the counselor's participation, will the counselor's efforts be focused on the staff or on Maria and her family, or both, as the recipients of the grief counselor's expertise? Is it possible for the grief counselor to function as a true ombudsman for conflict resolution with these location-driven parameters? (See Chapter 7, "Multiple Relationships in Thanatology," for an extended discussion of how to handle such mixed allegiances.)

Principle(s)

Several ethical principles, the fourth aspect of the Five P Model, apply to this case example. Autonomy appears to be the most prominent principle in play. To what extent will Maria's clearly expressed wishes about her treatment affect the final medical decision? In other words, will her parents afford her some degree of self-determination in choosing comfort care over continuing treatment? Maria's level of autonomy is incomplete, legally speaking, because of her status as a minor; the autonomous decision really belongs to her parents, and not to her. Pragmatically, her autonomy is also limited by cultural and religious factors that promote inclusion of her natural family and her faith family in decisions about Maria's health care.

The concerns of the medical staff show that the ethical principles of beneficence and nonmaleficence are also in the picture. Their understanding of how to help a dying teenager (i.e., beneficence) is to make her as comfortable as possible by controlling her pain and providing social and emotional support. Nonmaleficence demands that non-curative medical treatments, which induce patient discomfort to administer and create unpleasant side effects afterward, are not pressed upon a vulnerable person with a terminal prognosis. Additionally, Maria should be protected as much as possible from the emotional distress accompanying the disagreement about her treatment.

The ethical principle of justice also figures in this case scenario. The grief counselor may point out that justice demands all voices in the debate be heard and respected. Further, justice includes deliberation about allocating resources. Should an ICU bed be made available for Maria, who is expected to die despite treatment efforts, rather than reserved for someone with an acute illness who has a chance of recovery?

Process

Amid the crosscurrents of these many considerations, determining the process for reaching a decision is the last step of the Five P Model. Although Maria is the patient, several people are involved in the medical decision making for her. The process may have to include all of them. The grief counselor, in concert with the health care team, can provide an invaluable service by meeting with the family members in various stages. For example, an initial meeting may include the minister-uncle along with Maria's parents, brother, and others. However, a subsequent meeting without the uncle may be important for clarifying the parents' position. The brother may figure prominently in the discussion given that he understands closely what Maria wants for herself. His input may counterbalance the uncle's influence. Finally, the counselor may talk with Maria herself about her personal preference and how she understands her parents' thinking in the matter. Such "shuttle diplomacy" can sometimes prepare conflicting parties for a mediated compromise.

In this example, there is a real sense of urgency that the decision must be made without delay. Given that Maria is dying, a course of action needs to be determined for how to handle her physical deterioration. The grief counselor, together with a representative of the medical team (e.g., oncologist, primary care physician, or hospice nurse), may participate in a bedside conversation with Maria to verify her wishes. Also, a similar meeting could include the grief counselor, the doctor, the parents, and Maria in order to finalize a plan. Perhaps some reframing could help the parents accept hospice care for Maria without feeling that they are compromising their religious faith—for example, limiting what medical treatments are pursued does *not* limit what their deity may deign to accomplish for Maria in the way of healing or cure (cf. Jacobs, Burns, & Jacobs, 2008).

SUMMARY

Overall, ethics is about decision making. In making decisions, there are always underlying values represented. Our review of the ethical theories in this chapter is intended to help readers recognize underlying values that they embrace when making ethical decisions. It should be obvious that there is no single perspective or ethical theory that is all-encompassing or always right. Certainly, the tradition of ethics in medicine has much to contribute to our understanding of the foundational principles involved in making well-reasoned, sensitive, and ethically sound decisions in the everyday practice of grief counseling.

Adopting a credible model for ethical decision making is imperative if grief counselors expect to resolve their own ethical dilemmas as well as help facilitate client and family decisions that often have to be made within a very short period of time. The Five P Model is proposed as one such model for ethical decision making that is particularly applicable to dilemmas that arise in grief counseling. It takes into account five elements fundamental to every ethical decision: person, problem, place, principles, and process. Appendix B contains a worksheet modification of Table 2.1 that the authors make available as a tool for ethical decision making with the Five P Model: "A *person* with a challenging ethical *problem* in a particular contextual *place* applies appropriate ethical *principles* in a deliberate decision-making *process*."

3 Death Competence

Because of the special requirements posed by working with the dying and the bereaved, we submit that well-rounded *death competence* on the part of the grief counselor is a crucial component for ethical practice of grief counseling. What is death competence? We define the term to mean the counselor's *specialized skill in tolerating and managing clients' problems related to dying, death, and bereavement.* A vital part of death competence is how grief counselors use their personal loss experience, along with all other life experience, in performing their professional work. Ideally, the counselor's own losses should inform and even enrich a counseling practice rather than impede or detract from it.

In introducing this concept, we propose that death competence is best understood as part of a multifaceted, hierarchical model of professional competence illustrated in Figure 3.1. Much like a three-layer cake, death competence rests on a bedrock of cognitive competence and is supported by a solid stratum of emotional competence. All three layers functioning together constitute the death competence needed for counseling the dying and the bereaved. The substance of this chapter is an exposition of what death competence entails and its implications for self-care, specialty certification, and deployment of a Professional Will.

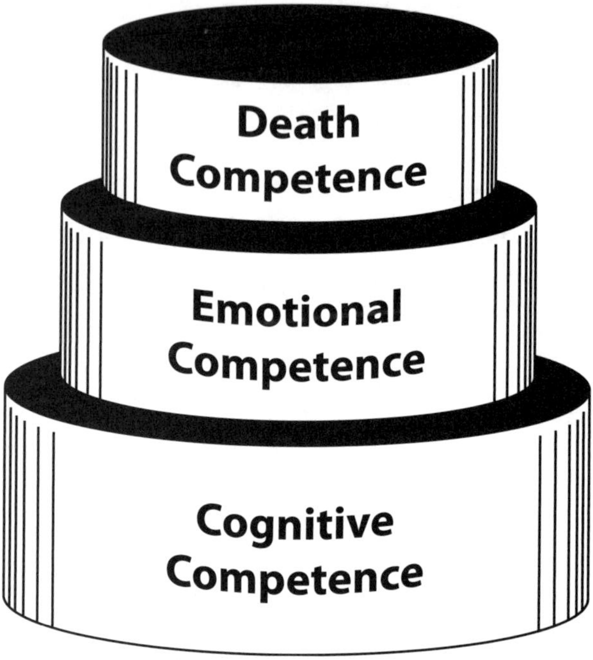

Figure 3.1 Hierarchical model of death competence.

COMPETENCE AS A COGNITIVE VARIABLE

Generally, discussions of a counselor's competence begin with consideration of academic training, supervised learning experiences, and proven proficiencies, in short, what the counselor knows. The explicit assumption that a counselor possesses expert knowledge and skill is the basis for professional licensing and for societal authority to receive payment for rendering services that require such knowledge and skill. Every professional discipline in health care has a code of ethics calling for members to base their practice on the body of knowledge that defines that discipline (American Association for Marriage and Family Therapy, 2001; ACA, 2005a; American Medical Association, 2002; American Nurses Association, 2001; American Psychological Association, 2002; Association of Professional Chaplains, 2000; National Association of Social Workers, 1999). To do otherwise is fraudulent self-representation and inherently unethical.

Grief counseling constitutes a subspecialty domain and, as such, requires scholarly knowledge in thanatology—the study of dying, death, and bereavement. The ADEC Code of Ethics defines this subspecialty.

> Death education and grief counseling are based upon a thorough knowledge of valid death-related data, methodology, and theory rather than stereotypes or untested hypotheses. Thus the practice of death education and/or grief counseling requires knowledge of current thanatological literature. (ADEC Code of Ethics, Basic Tenets, 1)

Furthermore, the notion of competent practice embodies the standard that grief counselors will confine their professional work to activities within their realm of expertise. No practitioner is a master of every therapy method or equally adept at treating different age groups or diverse populations. Most counselors have practice areas they know best and are most comfortable addressing, together with other areas in which their competence is adequate, albeit not so deeply developed. Also, most counselors recognize areas for which they have not received training or have had little formal preparation or supervision. Accurate self-knowledge and judicious discrimination of where one's realm of competence lies serve as important guideposts when counselors determine which cases to accept or decline.

The ADEC Code of Ethics contains several provisions regarding competence on the part of grief counselors and death educators. Its main points include the following:

> Members continually strive to attain higher levels of competence. Each member is obliged to pursue continuing educational and professional growth in all possible and appropriate ways . . . pursuing learning activities that lead to professional certification and licensure when available. (ADEC Code of Ethics, II. Competence, A)
>
> When called upon to deliver professional services, members accept only those positions and assignments for which they are professionally qualified. (ADEC Code of Ethics, II. Competence, B)
>
> Members are aware of the limits and boundaries of their professional competence and in no way represent themselves as having qualifications beyond those which they possess. Each member is responsible for correcting any misrepresentation other persons may make regarding that member's professional qualifications. (ADEC Code of Ethics, II. Competence, C)

> Members provide only those services and use only those techniques for which their training and experience qualifies them. (ADEC Code of Ethics, II. Competence, D)
>
> Members do not engage in professional activities when it is likely that personal problems or impairment may prevent them from performing such activities in a competent manner. (ADEC Code of Ethics, II. Competence, E)
>
> Members accept only those assignments that are within their competency. (ADEC Code of Ethics, V. Responsibility to Employers, D)

Additionally, there are specific provisions in the ADEC Code of Ethics regarding competence among professionals in a position to act as death educators and trainers:

> Members assuming educative functions do so within their professional competence. (ADEC Code of Ethics, DE-II. Standards of Professional Competence, A)
>
> Members teach only in areas in which they have received professional preparation. (ADEC Code of Ethics, DE-II. Standards of Professional Competence, B)
>
> Members engage in continuous study and professional development in order to insure that they provide instruction based on the most current information available in the profession. (ADEC Code of Ethics, DE-II. Standards of Professional Competence, C)

However, in the practice of grief counseling, these considerations about cognitive knowledge as a basis of competence are only the starting point for establishing more comprehensive death competence.

COMPETENCE AS AN EMOTIONAL VARIABLE

"If you can't stand the heat, get out of the kitchen!" This familiar saying conveys an essential truth—mere possession of intellectual knowledge does not guarantee that a person will be able to apply it in a given situation, particularly when the physical environment is taxing, expectations are high, multiple things are occurring at once, coordination with others is critical, and timing is everything. Often this is equated with having the "intestinal fortitude" for a certain task or endeavor. The emotional intensity of grief counseling can be like that hot, bustling kitchen where complex therapeutic demands tax even the most adept counselor.

Pope and Vasquez (2007) make the case rather eloquently that the endeavors of psychotherapy and counseling require emotional competence on the part of the professional provider. Besides cognitive competence, counselors and therapists need to be able to endure the emotional rigors of the therapy process, with its attendant graphic discussions of conflict, trauma, loss, anguish, and suffering. Such interchanges incite emotional responses in any counselor possessing an adequate degree of empathy. How well a grief counselor can tolerate the "heat" generated by such therapeutic material, including monitoring and managing one's own affect, is the real question. Pope and Vasquez argue that personal history of abuse or the effects of inadequate self-care on the part of professional providers can lead to deleterious outcomes such as disrespecting clients, disrespecting work, making more mistakes, lacking energy, working too much (or too little), and losing interest in professional work.

Charles Figley (1995) wrote convincingly about how compassion fatigue can afflict psychotherapists working with trauma-related problems. He warned that therapists and counselors are subject to a secondary form of traumatic stress disorder that he tallied as the "cost to caring" (p. 1). Most vulnerable are those counselors who have the greatest capacity for empathy and who are exposed vicariously to clients' traumas during retelling and reliving in psychotherapy sessions.

To minimize the risk of compassion fatigue as a form of burnout, Figley (1995) calls for therapists to practice strategic self-care: realistic appraisal of one's abilities and competencies; adequate consultation with colleagues; establishment of balance between work and play; and responsible stewardship of one's physical health. Becvar (2003) echoed many of these ideas in calling for therapists who focus their practices on dying, death, and bereavement to attend even more diligently to self-care because of risks associated with compassion fatigue and vicarious traumatization (cf. Gamble, 2002).

There are three key factors involved in maintaining emotional competence for grief counseling. First, good mental health and emotional resilience on the part of the provider are required. Second, adequate strategies for ongoing self-care are needed, together with a reasonable plan for balancing work demands with life's other priorities such as love relationships, recreational needs, community participation, and spiritual development. Third, for many counselors, support from other colleagues "in the trenches" provides strategic reinforcement for maintaining their emotional equilibrium during the stresses of professional practice (Pope & Vasquez, 2007).

Norcross and Barnett (2008) deem self-care for mental health professionals to be an ethical imperative. They ask pointedly how therapists can effectively care for the psychological and emotional needs of their clients unless they themselves adequately care for their own physical and mental health. Indeed, the ACA Code of Ethics (ACA, 2005a) admonishes counselors to maintain self-care as part of their professional responsibility: "Counselors engage in self-care activities to maintain and promote their emotional, physical, mental, and spiritual well-being to best meet their professional responsibilities" (p. 9). Norcross and Barnett enumerate 12 self-care strategies for use both at the office and away from the office, starting with valuing self. Others include minding one's body, nurturing relationships, setting boundaries, checking unrealistic expectations, "escaping" in healthy ways, cultivating spirituality, and fostering creativity. Readers needing more direction in this area can peruse a detailed compilation by Norcross and Guy (2007).

Having established that the counselor possesses cognitive competence for the task and emotional competence for the process, we can turn to a robust notion of death competence required for ethical practice of grief counseling.

DEATH COMPETENCE

As the maxim goes, "Into every life some pain shall come." Everyone sustains losses—rejections, betrayals, disappointments, missed opportunities, terminations, or disasters of some form—during his or her lifetime. Sometimes these ubiquitous loss experiences are referred to as "little deaths" in contrast to the actual physical death of a cherished loved one or one's own death. All of these experiences, small and large, constitute the loss history of an individual (Viorst, 1986). Worden and Proctor (1976) discussed the importance of personal loss history in determining one's level of death awareness, including the attributions and connotations one assigns to the phenomenon of death. Grief counselors are no exception.

What is required for death competence in grief counseling is that practitioners understand and accept their own loss history and manage the emotions associated with these losses. Additionally, death-competent grief counselors continuously self-monitor for personal reactions elicited during counseling and creatively utilize their internal responses to enhance therapeutic effectiveness, all the while maintaining appropriate objectivity and perspective.

Talking to grief counselors about why they have chosen this particular field of professional endeavor will often lead to an admission that the death of a cherished loved one played a part in that decision. In and of itself, this may be admirable. After all, Vaillant (1993) identified service as a form of altruism, a characteristic of psychologically mature and mentally healthy individuals. However, certainly not every grief counselor is prompted to enter the field because of personal loss. Yet where one's own losses *are* an aspect of motivation, there are additional obligations incurred to demonstrate death competence.

Sustaining the loss of a cherished loved one demands that grief counselors emotionally integrate that experience within their personal history and, in the process, acquire deeper self-understanding and a more acute grasp of the realities of the human condition. Doing so promotes development of a richer matrix of life experience, leading to heightened sensitivity and deeper understanding from which to generate cogent treatment recommendations. Living through loss can sensitize the astute counselor to the rigors and nuances of what it is like to lose a loved one, thus resulting in more attuned listening, greater emotional empathy for the pain and suffering of a fellow griever, more perceptive questioning, and more thoughtful suggestion giving.

The ADEC Code of Ethics speaks to the responsibility of grief counselors in regard to their own loss history.

> The member strives to understand his or her death-related feelings and experiences and the ways in which these may impact his or her thinking and work in the field. (ADEC Code of Ethics, Basic Tenets, 2)

Unfortunately, sometimes well-intended individuals enter the field of grief counseling with impediments to death competence. Some potential impediments include unfinished business regarding the death of a loved one, inordinate death anxiety, overgeneralizing from one's own loss experience, or lacking a personal loss history.

Unfinished Business Regarding Death of a Loved One

Some grief counselors may be attempting to come to terms with their own losses by virtue of helping others who are dying or bereaved. They are attracted to this work because they sense an opportunity for themselves to grapple further with their own confounding experiences with loss. They hope that in the process of trying to help others, they will heal themselves. Although it is widely acknowledged that helping professionals gain something themselves in the process of aiding others, *individuals who deliberately try to solve their own problems in grieving through the professional role of grief counselor are really clients masquerading as counselors.* Those individuals lack the objectivity and perspective needed to address clients' problems without personalizing them or adopting clients' problems as their own cause. Instead, addressing the client's pain becomes a collective emotional experience. Like a novice swimmer trying to save someone who is drowning in choppy seas, the effort is doomed to fail.

A litmus test of whether unfinished business with one's own losses is hampering efforts to provide grief counseling occurs when counselors cry with clients. As a rule, crying with clients is neither prohibited nor required. Yet when grief counselors with unfinished business find themselves crying with their clients, often they are crying *for themselves* rather than crying in empathy with their clients' stories. Death-competent grief counselors know well their own loss history and use it creatively to inform their practice, but they do not impose their own raw grieving on the therapy encounter.

Because death and loss happen throughout the life cycle, no grief counselor is immune from sustaining fresh losses over the course of a professional career. So what is the conscientious counselor to do? The sensible answer employs two previously cited concepts: accurate self-awareness and adequate self-care. Processing and understanding how a given death or loss has impacted one is primary. Taking time to grieve and adjust, finding healthy ways to recharge, and taking time off work may be important steps for exercising adequate self-care. Sanders (1984) warned that "therapists too, need to grieve" and highlighted the importance of self-care for the caregiver to avoid jeopardizing one's professional functioning.

Consider the case of a respected grief counselor whose treasured father died. Initially intent on keeping a busy counseling practice going (in part out of concern over time taken off during the father's illness), the counselor mentioned to a trusted colleague the plan to return to work the day after the father's funeral. The colleague cautioned the counselor about returning too soon rather than taking sufficient time off for emotional recuperation. With the colleague's input, the grief counselor was able to see the wisdom in arranging a longer break before resuming practice and modeling for clients appropriate self-care following bereavement. This is another instance verifying that good counseling practice is sound ethical practice and demonstrating how support from a colleague can help sustain a counselor's resilience (cf. Pope & Vasquez, 2007).

It is also true that some deaths impact us less than might be expected (Bonanno, 2004; Gamino, Sewell, Hogan, & Mason, 2008; Wortman & Silver, 1989). Or the death of a difficult person in one's life can yield more a sense of relief than grief, a tacit acknowledgment that life may be appreciably less problematic with that person gone. In these instances, the apparently diminished emotional impact does not necessarily represent unfinished business such as delayed or inhibited mourning (Rando, 1993), or grief "gone underground" as in traditional psychodynamic thinking. Instead, it can be an appropriate response to the loss in light of the predeath relationship, or an indication of high resilience. All of these examples illustrate how grief counselors need to understand and integrate the various losses in their own lives in order to counsel other grievers effectively.

Inordinate Death Anxiety

Paradoxical as it may seem, sometimes individuals with higher levels of death anxiety matriculate into the field of grief counseling. Certainly, grief counselors are not immune to death anxiety or death denial (Becker, 1973). From an existential position, fear of death is universal, and some consider it the basis of all other fears such as abandonment or annihilation (Yalom, 1980). There has been a tremendous amount of empirical research conducted on the topic of death anxiety and its correlates (Fortner & Neimeyer, 1999; Neimeyer, Wittkowski, & Moser, 2004; Templer et al., 2006). Germane to our purposes are the findings that death anxiety is lower among individuals with good psychological adjustment (i.e., higher levels of ego integrity and lower levels of psychological problems) and that, as a cohort, older adults evidence lower death anxiety than middle-age adults. Viorst (1986) posits that elders have had numerous experiences of loss over time—not only deaths of close relatives and friends but also losses of youth, health, or opportunity—and therefore their life perspective affords them reduced death anxiety.

In the neighboring field of medicine, physicians with higher levels of death anxiety demonstrate more negative attitudes toward dying patients (Kvale, Berg, Groff, & Lange, 1999) as well as more difficulty disclosing a terminal prognosis to patients and interacting with families of dying patients (Cochrane, Levy, Fryer, & Oglesby, 1990–1991). In the field of counseling, Kirchberg and Neimeyer (1991) found that beginning counselors ranked client situations involving death and loss significantly more uncomfortable to confront than other crises such as sexual assault or substance abuse. On the other hand, those with many years of experience counseling the dying and bereaved rated such situations as quite comfortable and responded very empathically (Terry, Bivens, & Neimeyer, 1995). Thus, empirical evidence suggests that death anxiety on the part of the professional provider can impede care delivery, whereas experience dealing with problems related to dying and death can promote a counselor's facility in handling such issues. As stated by Worden and Proctor (1976), "The more we examine a potentially ominous subject, the less threatening it often seems" (p. 35).

What do these findings mean for the grief counselor? When one's death anxiety is inordinately high, it can interfere with good practice of grief counseling, thus creating a potential ethical problem. Counselors lacking an adequate comfort level with matters related to dying, death, bereavement, and loss will inevitably shy away from the topic, shift the discussion elsewhere, overlook important historical material, or fail to ask difficult questions about living and dying—precisely the questions that a client may need expert help to formulate and answer.

Ordinarily, the therapeutic inquiry of grief counseling includes questions such as the following: What frightens you most about the prospect of dying? How do you think your family is handling your approaching death? Are you having trouble dealing with your loved one's death? What has been most difficult for you after losing your loved one? What has it been like without [name] here? What does the future without [name] look like to you? When the would-be-counselor's death anxiety is so intense that the counselor cannot risk asking such questions because of resulting discomfort, the counseling will falter. The death-anxious counselor cannot possibly assuage clients' fears and concerns about dying, death, and bereavement. In these instances, the breach of ethical duty comes from what the counselor *fails to do* rather than from an overt misstep or misconduct. Though more difficult to detect, these omissions are no less real ethical lapses.

Another indication that a grief counselor is not unduly burdened by either death anxiety or death denial is the ability to use direct language such as "dying," "death," "died," or "killed," rather than poetic euphemisms such as "passed on," "slipped away," or "gone home." Likewise, death competence means eschewing medical jargon (e.g., cardiac arrest, massive hemorrhage, deep laceration) that camouflages the reality of death behind a barricade of technical terminology. Such jargon does not help clients, nor does it soften the blow. Its clinical precision serves only to protect professional caregivers from their own death anxiety. Looking death squarely in the face and naming it with plain language, albeit using a gentle and compassionate delivery, conveys a healthy acceptance of fatal outcomes and demonstrates one's comfort level addressing the associated counseling issues.

Perhaps the point about death anxiety is best illustrated by the experience of one of our students a few years ago. This trainee had a special interest in bereavement issues and, after doing introductory reading in the field, made some home visits with a seasoned hospice chaplain. Afterward, the student reported astonishment at the conversations witnessed between the dying patients and the chaplain. It seems no stone was left unturned, especially during affect-filled moments in the interviews when the patients' own fears of death surfaced, or the patients expressed thoughts and feelings they had not yet ventured to share with their families or friends. Our student was enterprising enough to ask how the chaplain was able to craft such probing yet sensitive inquiries. The chaplain explained that, from training and experience, "I am just very, very comfortable with the whole idea of death, including my own, and with talking to folks about it." Clearly, the chaplain's low level of death anxiety greatly facilitated grief counseling with the dying. Not every counselor may match this chaplain's exemplary standard, but the take-home lesson is that the grief counselor's death anxiety should not preclude or interfere with effective practice.

Overgeneralizing From One's Own Loss Experience

Another obstacle to death competence among grief counselors is when the counselor's experience of losing a loved one becomes the primary thanatological data on which to base interventions. Such a counselor operates as if everyone's grief trajectory will invariably be some derivative of what the counselor experienced and, therefore, can be understood accurately through the counselor's frame of reference. This inherently egocentric or "counselor-centric" approach leads to formulaic, one-size-fits-all thinking as well as to prescriptive suggestions consistent with the counselor's personal value system rather than tailored interventions based on an empathic understanding of the griever's worldview. Trying to counsel others based primarily on one's own experience of bereavement and loss is shortsighted and unethical because it restricts and limits the many possible ways that people experience and express their grief.

How does this tendency to overgeneralize from one's own loss experience come about? We have been aware of two distinct situations in which this counselor-centric style emerges. The first is when the counselor's own loss experience has been so profoundly and personally life-changing that the counselor becomes an unquestioning devotee eager to lead others through a similar transformative experience. In these cases, the life lessons learned are so prized that they are not critically examined; therefore, these counselors have a hard time thinking outside the box of their own hard-won wisdom. In other words, the counselor operates as if there is only a single common pathway in grieving. Even though the counselor's path to postbereavement personal growth indeed may be laudable, it does not necessarily generalize to all grievers.

The second instance of overgeneralizing from one's own loss experience occurs when the nascent grief counselor possesses too shallow a knowledge base in thanatology and tries to compensate by relying too heavily on idiosyncratic experiences to make up the difference. This can happen with well-meaning volunteers who come into the field as a result of living through loss. Or bereaved individuals who have had good experiences as clients in grief counseling may decide they want to perform that same service for others. It happens also with professionals who migrate into grief counseling from some other sector of medicine or mental health after losing a loved one. In each of these scenarios, the would-be grief counselors simply have not acquired sufficient conceptual or methodological tools to do the work, so they fall prey to overgeneralizing for reasons of expediency. In other words, their death competence fails because their cognitive competence is faulty. These unfortunate situations bring to mind the old adage, "When one's only tool is a hammer, all the world is a nail." Obviously, this is not ethical practice of grief counseling.

By contrast, notable American psychologist Gordon Allport admonished his graduate students to remember that "each man is like all other men; each man is like some other men; each man is like no other man" (J. W. Worden, personal communication, July 9, 2007). The death-competent grief counselor keeps in mind that every client has some unique characteristics and seeks to discover those in the course of the therapeutic dialogue. This means honoring the client's sensibilities, even if they diverge from the counselor's personal views. The ADEC Code of Ethics clearly delineates the grief counselor's responsibility to recognize and respect individual differences:

> The member strives to present various views of a death-related question, indicating the member's own values if appropriate, and respecting the student's or client's choice among alternatives. (ADEC Code of Ethics, Basic Tenets, 6)

Lack of a Personal Loss History

Not every grief counselor has sustained a major loss such as the death of a dear loved one. In particular, graduate-level trainees, entry-level professionals who are young adults, or anyone with a trouble-free personal history may fall into this category. (Sometimes cynical veterans in the field pejoratively refer to those uninitiated into the pain of loss as "death virgins.") The lack of a personal loss history does not necessarily preclude a grief counselor from working effectively with the dying and bereaved. However, it does stand as a reminder that the counselor's expertise must come from sources other than personal loss experience.

Remember, skilled surgeons can perform operations that they themselves have never required. Similarly, a well-trained grief counselor can intervene therapeutically with individuals who have sustained losses the counselor has never endured. Traditionally, counselor training has depended on a fundamental triad: an appropriate course of scholarly study, sufficient supervised practicum experience, and, for many, personal participation as a client in counseling. Dedicated pursuit of such formal training can enable a grief counselor to develop a satisfactory level of death competence even when there has been no substantive personal history of loss.

We recall the trial-by-fire experience of one of our trainees confronted by an angry bereaved client whose son had completed suicide. The client questioned the trainee's capacity to counsel effectively with the argument, "How can you understand if you've never lost a child?" The trainee accurately read the feelings of powerlessness behind the bereaved parent's protest and responded nondefensively and without reprisal. Instead, the trainee patiently acknowledged that, indeed, it was impossible to understand firsthand the pain that the client was experiencing. The trainee pledged to be open to learning what the client had endured, to work earnestly to merit trust, and, with the guidance of a supervisor, to do everything possible to aid and assist the grieving parent. The client was reassured sufficiently to complete the initial interview and chose to continue with counseling because the trainee was honest and "cared."

To summarize, nothing mentioned thus far should be construed by the reader as a mandate that only those healers wounded by loss or trauma (cf. Nouwen, 1979) can be grief counselors. When grief counselors have sustained a major loss, it is incumbent on them to cope with their experience and use it to inform their work but not to use their work for healing themselves. Grief counselors who lack a personal loss history need to follow formal training curricula in order to acquire the death competence needed for working with the dying and the bereaved. Accurate self-awareness and candid observations from supervisors and colleagues can help confirm when the novice has attained the death competence needed for ethical practice of grief counseling.

CERTIFICATION

Clients suffering from grief and loss, as either the primary or the secondary focus of counseling, find their way to practitioners in a variety of treatment venues. As mentioned in the introduction to this book, grief counseling may be provided by professionals from any of several academic disciplines: psychology, counseling, medicine, nursing, social work, ministry, marriage and family therapy, or funeral direction. Because training curricula vary depending on one's academic institution and faculty, not every mental health professional or health care provider comes to the endeavor of grief counseling with the same preparation. So how do earnest professionals from diverse backgrounds ensure that their knowledge of thanatology constitutes sufficient cognitive competence for developing the death competence needed to practice grief counseling?

One avenue is the certification programs offered by the ADEC (Balk, Wogrin, Thornton, & Meagher, 2007), which are designed to recognize practitioners and educators who meet specified knowledge requirements in the domain-specific realm of dying, death, and bereavement. The foundation credential, Certification in Thanatology (CT), is for practitioners with at least a bachelor's degree and 2 years of verified experience in the field. They must demonstrate their competence through a standardized test on a core body of knowledge: dying; end-of-life decision making; loss, grief, and mourning; assessment and intervention; traumatic death; and death education.

The advanced credential, Fellow in Thanatology (FT), is for professionals who hold a master's or doctorate degree, who have at least 5 years of experience in the field of thanatology, who have met specified knowledge requirements measured through a standardized test, and who demonstrate advanced levels of competency via a professional portfolio of achievements including licensure, clinical service, publications, teaching, supervision, professional leadership, and other awards or distinctions.

Newcomers to the field of grief counseling, graduating students, and those who work or volunteer in the field without formal credentials are urged to consider ADEC's certification programs as a vehicle for developing the death competence necessary for the ethical practice of grief counseling. Detailed information can be found at http://www.adec.org.

PROFESSIONAL WILL

Working in the field of dying, death, and bereavement forces grief counselors to confront their own mortality on a regular basis. Whether death results from natural causes such as illness or unnatural causes such as accidents, homicide, or suicide, the reality of death is always present. Death-competent grief counselors are able to acknowledge their own mortality and plan for the possibility that sudden death or disability may preempt retirement and preclude an orderly end to their professional practice. The ADEC Code of Ethics addresses the contingency of untimely termination of one's professional practice.

> Members take reasonable precautions to protect the confidentiality of clients/students in the event of the member's termination of practice, incapacitation or death. (1) Members insure confidentiality of client/student records; (2) Members either transfer client/student records to another professional, or assure secure storage of the records; (3) Clients/students or their legal guardians are informed about the termination of practice and about the transfer/storage of records. (ADEC Code of Ethics, III. Responsibilities to Those Served, F)

A Professional Will is a plan for what happens if the grief counselor dies suddenly or becomes incapacitated (Pope & Vasquez, 2007). Much like a last will and testament that clarifies and mandates what is to be done with one's estate at death, a Professional Will instructs a designated colleague on how to notify clients, handle confidential records, and manage outstanding business matters related to the grief counselor's practice. Having a Professional Will is most urgent for grief counselors in private or solo practices, whereas those working in agencies or group practices often have informal agreements to provide such services for each other (Barnett, 2007). In short, grief counselors are ethically obligated to make provisions for their professional affairs in the event of death or disability, just as they make arrangements for their personal affairs.

Personal Account—Hal Ritter's Story

The following account of the second author's (RHR) personal story is based on a version that first appeared in the *Journal of Pastoral Care* (Ritter, 1990).

In 1983 I was severely injured when a man ran a stop sign and crashed into my car. He walked away unhurt, and he had no insurance. My back was broken and my spinal cord injured. I had a left hemisphere concussion, a crushed left shoulder, and a dislocated left hip. Today, I am a paraplegic. My lower body is paralyzed, although I do have some movement in my right leg. For several years I was able to walk with a cane. However, as of more recently, I have to use a walker. I also live with chronic pain from the injury.

On the afternoon of my injury, I had just left my counseling office. I had a small, part-time practice of counseling while I was completing my doctoral work. At the time of my accident, I still had one course to complete, my comprehensive doctoral exams to take, and a dissertation to write. I went to work that day and came home five months later.

The first few days in the hospital were horrific, as I struggled to live while believing I would die. In intensive care, I told my wife that, because we had no will, we needed to act quickly in case I did not survive. Our Sunday school teacher at that time was an attorney. My wife contacted him, and he came to the intensive care unit of the hospital. There, he visited with us about what we needed and wanted in the will. In addition to our property, we had two small children. Our attorney friend left to prepare the will and returned to the hospital with it. We signed it and had it witnessed by a nurse's aide in the intensive care unit.

After 20 days in an acute care hospital, I was finally stabilized. I was then moved by ambulance to a rehabilitation hospital 100 miles away. My wife was suddenly a single parent to two small children whose father went to work one day and did not come home for five months. I was in a wheelchair for much of that time. When I came out of the rehabilitation hospital, I still had to complete my doctoral studies and write my dissertation. It was a long journey.

But there was another problem. What about my clients? Because I was working only part-time as a counselor, the few clients I had were transferred to my colleagues at our agency. They were gracious enough to send my wife the income from the counseling until the clients completed their work. It was a big help, given that the financial burden of the family suddenly fell entirely on her. When I finally came home, we reviewed the will we had written in the hospital and rewrote it. We also wrote living wills and durable powers of attorney for health care and mental health care.

What if I had been full-time, with a case load of 30–40 clients? What if I had been in private practice, or in practice with only one other person? What would have happened to my clients then? Another situation arose for me 3 years later when I was diagnosed with malignant melanoma. Fortunately, I was out only a short time for surgery, and there was no need for long-term cancer treatment. But what if it had come to that, with chemotherapy and radiation? What would have happened to my practice then?

Through interviewing various therapists, I have found that very few have given much thought to their own mortality or to the consequences it may have for their work with clients. Some do have a will, and some do have life insurance. But often there are no specific plans for what to do with their professional practice. My story illustrates the necessity for a Professional Will to ensure that clients are cared for and that treatment records are preserved in the event of untimely death or disability.

Elements of a Professional Will

So many questions arise when a professional grief counselor is suddenly incapacitated or dies. Where is the list of contact information for present and former clients? What are the procedures for informing clients of the counselor's fate? Who oversees the process of contacting clients, offering them the opportunity for referral, and transferring or storing their records? How is client confidentiality protected? What happens to the business aspects of the practice, such as clients who still owe fees and bills that are due? A host of pragmatic questions apply also. Where are the keys to the office and the secure files? What are the passwords to access computer records? Where is the appointment book or calendar showing which clients are scheduled to be seen? A sound Professional Will provides the answers to all these pressing questions. Appendix C contains a sample template for a Professional Will, together with detailed instructions for the grief counselor and the designated executor. The following discussion explains what elements are needed in a Professional Will, and why.

The grief counselor's Professional Will should first designate a trusted colleague to act as executor, someone who is familiar with the counselor's work and who is authorized by the will to carry out its provisions (Pope & Vasquez, 2007). One of the most important aspects of a Professional Will is the process to be followed immediately upon a crisis. Clients need to be notified, preferably by telephone or by letter, starting with those whose appointments are most imminent. The caller needs to be prepared to deal with the reactions of clients receiving bad news (cf. Buckman, 1992), keeping in mind that these clients, who are already bereaved, are thrust into the role of griever yet again by virtue of losing their counselor. That is why calls are best made by a trusted colleague who would know how to handle such situations or by a staff member who knows the clients personally and can break the news gently. Similarly, the grief counselor may have supervised trainees, and they too need to be contacted and informed. Both active clients and supervisees need to be offered alternative arrangements for continuing counseling or supervision with another professional.

Less immediate but no less important is contacting other collateral parties. Inactive clients, such as those who have terminated their counseling, are most appropriately notified by mail. Licensing and certification boards, professional associations, malpractice insurance carriers, and referring professionals should also be notified by mail regarding the grief counselor's death or disability.

The terms of the Professional Will must include clear instructions about how to access clients' appointment records, treatment records, and billing records. Appointment records are needed to determine who should be called by telephone and who can be notified by letter, as well as how to contact them. Billing records may contain client contact information and also indicate any outstanding payments. Treatment records need to be maintained confidentially and either transferred to a different provider or stored securely. Treatment records that are older than the retention period required by state law (see Chapter 5, "Confidentiality") can be destroyed if that is the best judgment of the designated colleague.

Because assets, or debts, connected to a counseling practice are part of one's estate at death, the executor of one's personal will has fiduciary responsibility for managing financial affairs pertaining to the practice. Thus, the colleague designated by the Professional Will should be ready to work closely with the executor of the estate in handling accounts receivable, creditors, and other billing-related matters.

When drawing up a Professional Will, it is a good idea for the grief counselor to review its provisions with the designated colleague and conduct a walk-through simulation to make sure all questions and contingencies have been adequately considered. Making mention in one's informed consent document of the designated colleague who would function like an executor in the event of the grief counselor's death or disability is recommended (see Chapter 4, "Consent"). Also, it is advisable to have one's attorney for professional practice issues review the will for completeness and conformity to state or jurisdictional law. Additionally, it is helpful to review one's Professional Will and personal will side by side to ensure that they are consistent (Pope & Vasquez, 2007). Copies of the Professional Will should be given to the designated colleague, office staff of the grief counselor, the grief counselor's attorney, and the executor named in the grief counselor's personal will.

From this discussion of the numerous complications incurred when a grief counselor becomes incapacitated or dies unexpectedly, it should be apparent that *honestly facing one's own vulnerability and mortality demands a Professional Will.* Having a Professional Will is the ethically responsible thing to do and is one indication of genuine death competence on the part of the grief counselor.

CHECKLIST FOR DEATH COMPETENCE

Because of the importance we place on grief counselors practicing with an adequate level of death competence, we provide the following checklist for readers to take inventory of their skill set. It is our position that the death-competent grief counselor will answer affirmatively to each of the following 10 questions:

1. Are you comfortable contemplating the prospect of your own death?

2. Can you recall and visualize the death of an important loved one in your life without undue sadness or overwhelming emotion?
3. When clients present problems of loss and bereavement, can you steer into an appropriate discussion of their experience and their affect?
4. Do you have the temperament and emotional capacity to empathize with the dying and the bereaved?
5. Can you tolerate clients' descriptions of deaths that are traumatic, gruesome, horrific, or violent without having to guard your own sensibilities?
6. In working with clients who are dying or bereaved, are you able to monitor and moderate your own feelings elicited by descriptions of their loss experiences?
7. Are you able to discuss nonjudgmentally with clients their suicidal thoughts, feelings, and behaviors?
8. Can you accept that clients have diverse ways of grieving, respect their individuality, and refrain from insisting on a single common pathway in grief?
9. After intense work with the dying and bereaved, can you unwind in healthy ways (e.g., exercising, enjoying nature, socializing with family or friends, meeting with colleagues, engaging in distracting activities such as crafts, hobbies, music, or reading) *without* resorting to drinking too much, using illicit substances, gambling excessively, binge eating, viewing pornography, spending unwisely, or engaging in reckless behavior?
10. Recognizing your own mortality, have you drawn up a Professional Will stipulating how to care for your clients and your practice in the event of your untimely death or disability?

4 Consent

Most ethicists in mental health and medicine agree that informed consent for treatment is not merely a perfunctory ritual of signing forms but a dynamic process. We propose that genuine *informed consent is a continuous consensual process between grief counselor and client that imposes obligations on both parties.* Clients need to understand and agree with the methods to be used based on clear explanations by providers. Although consent can be secured in a variety of ways, all approaches depend on clear communication with the client about the provider's intent, not only when services commence, but also throughout the duration of care. Additionally, for clients to give informed consent, they must know the parameters of confidentiality, including when and why exceptions to this ethical duty are made. Thus, these two integral features of grief counseling—consent and confidentiality—are intertwined. The responsibilities of the grief counselor for obtaining informed consent are the substance of this chapter. Confidentiality is the subject of the following chapter.

DEFINING CONSENT

In their study of biomedical ethics, Beauchamp and Childress (2008) list five components of informed consent. First is *competence* to give consent, meaning the person has the psychological capacity and the legal standing for autonomous decision making, both prerequisites for valid consent. Second is *disclosure* by the provider in a manner that meets a "subjective standard" of addressing the informational needs of the specific person involved, in other words, at a level the person can access. Third is *understanding* by the person who comprehends the information and grasps its implications. Fourth is *voluntariness,* that is, free consent without control or coercion by anyone else, including the provider. Fifth is the act of *consent.*

When Beauchamp and Childress (2008) endorse a "subjective standard" for disclosure by the health care provider, they depart from more traditional interpretations of disclosure obligations. One is the *reasonable person standard,* that is, what information a hypothetical reasonable person would need to make an informed decision, also known as the *client-based standard.* Another is the *professional practice standard,* that is, what is customary for professionals in this specialty to disclose about their services, also known as the *provider-based standard.* States and jurisdictions vary on which of these two standards apply during adjudication of cases disputing informed consent. Yet both of these traditional interpretations place the burden of the informing on the provider.

Newer models in the health care field propose cooperative participation in the informed consent process, termed *shared decision making* by some (Kaplan, 2004; King & Moulton, 2006; Resnik, 2001). Shared decision making is a process in which the provider discloses all the relevant information about the proposed treatment, including potential benefits as well as risks, and the client discloses all the relevant personal information that might determine which of several treatment alternatives might be more advantageous or preferred. Thus, both parties use the information to come to a mutual decision.

Writing from a mental health counselor's perspective, Welfel (2006) proposed two aspects central to the informed consent process: disclosure of relevant information the client needs to make a reasoned decision about whether to engage in counseling and the client's free consent to do so, without coercion or undue pressure. Welfel's concept of disclosure subsumes both disclosure and understanding from the Beauchamp and Childress (2008) scheme, just as her concept of free consent subsumes their notions of voluntariness and consent while at the same time implying client competence for decision making.

Our definition of genuine informed consent as a continuous consensual process between grief counselor and client that imposes obligations on both parties rests on these two essential elements: full disclosure by the counselor and free choice by the client that is established at the beginning of counseling and reestablished periodically throughout the cycle of care. Our definition moves toward the shared decision-making concept.

Grief counselors are obliged to set forth in understandable language and concepts what counseling entails, including reciprocal role behaviors. Counselors ask questions, listen attentively, formulate the problem, field questions and concerns, pose alternatives, and give advice. Clients express their concerns, ask questions, provide information, state their preferences and sensibilities, and consider recommendations. The *consensual* aspect of informed consent is satisfied once these respective role behaviors are understood and, after weighing the potential benefits as well as the limitations of counseling, the client freely chooses to proceed.

The *continuous* aspect of informed consent means that these consensual functions are ongoing and part of a dynamic, evolving interchange throughout the counseling. Some call this a process model of consent (Handelsman, 2001). In other words, obtaining informed consent is not a single, onetime event ratified by signing forms or verbalizing agreement as a precursor to counseling. In a process model, consent is revisited in numerous iterations as grief counseling progresses over time, becoming part of the counseling itself rather than an administrative add-on.

CONSENT AND THE FIVE P MODEL

Using the Five P Model can elucidate for grief counselors some of the common ethical dilemmas that may arise in this all-important aspect of informed consent for counseling.

Person

The person giving consent for counseling must have both the capacity to understand fully the information provided about the proposed service and the legal standing to act as a free agent in making decisions based on that information (cf. Beauchamp & Childress, 2008). The legal term for this is *competence*. However, when disputes arise, such as a contested will, a final determination of competence can be made only by a judge or a court of law. That determination is often based on an opinion provided by a medical or mental health professional who has examined the person for purposes of assessing competence. Elsewhere in this volume, we tackle the issues of capacity and competence for making decisions about health care treatments (see Chapter 6, "Ethical Dilemmas at End of Life").

Ordinarily, an adult client of reasonable intelligence who seeks grief counseling on an elective basis is considered able to give informed consent, although it remains the obligation of the grief counselor to explain the process in language suitable for that client (i.e., the subjective standard). However, if the client is a minor or a disabled person, the grief counselor must obtain consent for treatment from the parent, guardian, or custodian who is empowered to make such determinations for that individual. Common examples of this would be children attending bereavement summer camps or support groups for grievers with special needs (e.g., grievers with Down syndrome).

Problem

Typically, when problems occur with informed consent for grief counseling, they involve faulty procedures that omit, truncate, or otherwise short-circuit full disclosure by the provider or subversive procedures that undermine the client's free choice to make a decision. These two types of problems are illustrated in the case examples provided in the next section of this chapter.

Place

Just as no two grief counselors practice identically, no two practice settings are exactly the same. Place can factor into problems with informed consent in several ways. Mental health agencies or institutions may have evolved customary ways of handling informed consent that vary from current standards of practice in the field, leaving the ethically conscientious grief counselor with procedures that are inadequate. Independent counseling practices that operate informally may take a lax, or even arrogant, approach to informed consent, resulting in misunderstandings later when clients did not realize all that was involved. In some settings—for example, funeral homes, places of worship, or educational settings—the concept of informed consent for services may be somewhat alien or unfamiliar and thus ignored altogether.

Principle

Informed consent is based on the ethical principle of autonomy—respect for an individual's right to self-determination. Regarding informed consent for grief counseling, autonomy demands that clients exercise free choice to accept or decline participation according to what they deem in their best interest. For the practitioner, ensuring client autonomy means adhering to what the client wants and decides rather than trying to mold the client's decisions to fit the practitioner's wishes and preferences.

Process

The ethical challenge with informed consent is ensuring that the principle of autonomy (fourth P) operates in the process (fifth P) of obtaining consent that is free and informed. So what does that process look like? Does the client read and sign a form attesting that he or she wants grief counseling? Does a simple verbal discussion of how grief counseling works suffice? How much information about what counseling entails is enough, and how much is too much? In answer, we suggest a pragmatic approach to the process of obtaining informed consent that augments verbal explanations with appropriately designed written materials.

OBTAINING INFORMED CONSENT

There are many variations in how practitioners handle informed consent in the real world of grief counseling. Using the Five P Model can help resolve dilemmas about obtaining informed consent and about whether the necessary conditions of full disclosure and free choice have been met. To begin, we consider the following case examples, which illustrate various shortcomings in the process of obtaining informed consent for grief counseling.

Case Examples

- A client is referred by a local minister to a grief counselor in an independent office practice. Prior to the intake session, the client receives by mail a packet of information sheets to fill out, including an informed-consent document requiring a signature. In signing, the client attests to reading and understanding the forms and gives consent for counseling. When the packet is brought to the intake session, the counselor asks the client if there are any questions. Hearing none, the counselor proceeds with an intake interview that focuses on the client's loss and subsequent adjustment without any further mention of consent or the limits of confidentiality.

- A family physician refers the client to a grief counselor on faculty in the psychiatry department of a medical school. In this medically oriented environment, presence at an appointment is taken as implicit consent for evaluation and treatment. Signed informed consent documents are not used unless a procedure is biologically invasive, such as electroconvulsive therapy (i.e., shock treatments), or the session is to be recorded by audio or videotape. Thus, grief counseling is seen in the same context as other routine medical appointments, and there is no explicit discussion of informed consent.
- A patient in a hospital's palliative care unit is visited by a grief counselor who is part of a multidisciplinary treatment team. During introductions at bedside, the reason for the counselor's visit is explained, and the patient's cooperation is elicited through conversation: "Hello, I'm Jane Smith, a clinical social worker, and I'm here to see how you're doing with your illness. I'd like to ask you a few questions. . . ." Unless the patient specifically objects or declines, implied consent is assumed, and the encounter continues.
- A hospice chaplain makes a home visit as part of the comprehensive program of care. Even though the hospice model was explained to both the patient and the family at intake, the patient seems surprised to see the chaplain and registers uncertainty about the visit. In trying earnestly to focus on the emotional, social, and spiritual aspects of living with a terminal illness, the chaplain moves from exchanging pleasantries to more probing inquiries in a fairly seamless manner. Rather than directly discussing the patient's prerogative to participate in the interview, the chaplain attempts to gauge the patient's receptivity to the discussion as it goes along.

Each of these examples illustrates weaknesses, loopholes, and omissions in the process of obtaining true informed consent. Having the client sign a consent form without discussion, as in the example of the grief counselor in independent practice, is insufficient. One cannot rely exclusively on forms to achieve the ethical aims of informed consent (Welfel, 2006). Thus, whenever informed consent documents are used, sound ethical practice requires that the conceptual content of the documents be discussed verbally with the client, regardless of whether the client is asked to sign the form. Without knowing exactly what is involved because of inadequate disclosure by the practitioner, the client lacks the basis to make an informed choice. Readability of the form and personalizing the explanation are both important considerations in facilitating a client's understanding (Wagner, Davis, & Handelsman, 1998).

In the example of the medical school clinic, inferring consent from the client's presence without really explaining what grief counseling involves cuts corners in the area of full disclosure by the provider and is presumptive, at best, about free choice. This violates the ethical principle of autonomy. Certainly, sophisticated clients or those experienced with mental health treatment may quickly grasp the structure and purpose of grief counseling and readily elect to press forward. However, many other clients will require a more thorough explanation of what grief counseling is, together with an opportunity to ask questions or clarify their understanding, before their consent is truly informed. This may be the case with less sophisticated consumers, those with no previous experience with mental health services, individuals with a concrete thinking style, or those whose distress is predominantly somatic, such as insomnia, crying spells, diffuse pain, or fatigue. Nagy (2000) suggests a "plain English" explanation of what psychotherapy entails: "Consider telling them what you might want a good friend to know about the nature, structure and anticipated course of treatment" (p. 89).

The examples from the hospital palliative care unit and the hospice home visit, where client consent was merely implied, show that attempting to initiate a grief counseling session without opportunity for the client to clearly and freely consent to the process subverts the autonomy principle on which informed consent is based. Iserson (2001) has encouraged thinking of informed consent as an educational process that ensures the client's autonomy is preserved. Educating the client about the proposed (counseling) procedure facilitates a full and adequate understanding of what is involved, a process that could be labeled "educated consent" or "informed autonomy."

Formalizing Consent

So how does the ethically conscientious grief counselor ensure that clients both understand what is involved in the counseling endeavor and have a reasonable opportunity to accept or decline without undue pressure? There are several legitimate ways to formalize a client's consent for counseling. In some venues, informed consent documents are signed after the provisions of counseling have been explained thoroughly and agreed to by the client. In other settings, brochures or information sheets outline the grief counseling process, and then the counselor discusses and clarifies the information prior to actual interviewing. Sometimes, informed consent rests solely on a verbal understanding between counselor and client as to the nature of grief counseling, its objectives, and its limitations. If so, at a minimum, it must be documented in the counselor's notes that such a discussion took place. What is crucial is that clients understand fully what they are embarking on and give consent without coercion and with the provision that they may withdraw at any time if they do not wish to proceed any further.

As a general rule, oral explanations as the vehicle for obtaining informed consent in grief counseling have the advantage of allowing the counselor to tailor the information to the individual client. The main disadvantages are twofold. First, counselors run the risk of omitting something significant in an oral explanation, possibly because of hasty streamlining or unfounded assumptions about what a client knows or understands, or because they overlook the vast difference in information they possess about what is involved in grief counseling compared to most clients. Second, counselors may depend too heavily on the client's cognitive processing and recall, which can be compromised all too easily by the client's level of distress (Welfel, 2006).

Despite these potential disadvantages, empirical evidence shows that many psychotherapists have relied primarily on verbal discussion to secure informed consent (Somberg, Stone, & Clairborn, 1993). Yet, recall based on auditory memory alone—that is, remembering what was *heard*—is inferior to recall for material presented both visually and vocally (i.e., remembering what was *seen and heard*). That is why many established grief counselors use brochures with new client information (cf. Koocher & Keith-Spiegel, 2008; Zuckerman, 2003) or pamphlets of frequently asked questions (Pomerantz & Handelsman, 2004) to ease the informed consent process. Printed materials can prompt discussions, improve efficiency, and help counselors avoid omissions during the informed-consent process.

Schuck (1994) argued persuasively that there is an "informed consent gap" or discrepancy between how informed consent is described in theory (i.e., the law "in books") and how it is actually practiced in the field (i.e., the law "in action"). Schuck attributes the gap to a disparity in how "idealists" and "realists" view informed consent. Idealists, often judges and medical ethicists, endorse a rather expansive conception of a provider's obligation to talk with consumers. In their scholarly view, informed consent discussions are individually tailored to each client's specific cognitive capacities and emotional needs and cover an extensive scope and sequence. This is intended to ensure full client comprehension and genuine autonomy. Realists, who are primarily practitioners, agree that informed consent is needed but question whether most clients really want the kind of exhaustive dialogue that idealists propose. Realists believe that such cerebral exercises exploring all the ways a planned procedure could go wrong induce needless anxiety and confusion. In their workaday view, the additional time required is simply not justified. So just how much discussion of informed consent between counselor and client is really needed?

We prefer a pragmatic approach to formalizing informed consent that represents a balance between the positions of idealists and realists. Experience tells us that many clients who come electively to grief counseling do not want a long explanation of the subtleties of informed consent because it reduces precious consultation time for which a pricey professional fee has been paid. Of course, ambivalent clients require more extended discussion, and any time devoted to talking about the provisions of informed consent, how grief counseling works, or whether to proceed at all is time well spent. At the other end of the spectrum, we abhor any semblance of the "cowboy mentality" toward informed consent, where the counselor gallops ahead with the interview without paying proper attention to the client's understanding of how grief counseling works and securing the client's consent.

In our opinion, a pragmatic method combining oral explanations that meet the subjective standard together with printed materials, or their equivalents in easy-to-access formats such as videotape or DVD, should constitute the current standard of practice when obtaining consent for grief counseling. We recommend clients arrive at least 20–30 minutes early to their initial appointment to complete office records and financial transactions and then to read a brochure on informed consent, confidentiality, and office policies. This is also the time to provide clients with a notice of privacy practices required by the federal government's Health Insurance Portability and Accountability Act (HIPAA, 1996). Briefly, this outlines what the client can expect regarding confidentiality of protected health information conveyed to the counselor. HIPAA and its requirements are addressed in greater detail in Chapter 5, "Confidentiality."

Thus, when the appointment begins, the grief counselor can more efficiently discuss informed consent with those clients essentially ready to proceed. For clients who are ambivalent or who have questions or concerns about consent, the counselor can more strategically focus extended discussion on the aspects or issues that need clarification. Typically, this combined approach encompasses the initial discussion of informed consent within the first 5–15 minutes of the counseling session, leaving ample time to explore the client's loss experience and take initial history. Before the session ends, counselor and client can revisit the topic of consent for any further counseling, if needed.

Welcomed Versus Tolerated

In seeking informed consent for grief counseling, it is helpful to discriminate between a procedure that is welcomed and one that is tolerated. For example, when an individual consults the family physician because of an acute infection, oral medicines may be prescribed or an injection given to combat the infection. The pills may be a welcome treatment because they are easy to swallow and will resolve the infection. An injection may not be welcomed because of the pain inflicted or a fear of needles but may still be tolerated in the interest of clearing the infection more rapidly or more definitively.

The same distinction between welcomed and tolerated applies to grief counseling. Some clients eagerly seek services because of a strong drive to unburden themselves of distress, a deep longing to receive compassion from someone who will really listen, or a pressing need to obtain advice or have questions answered. Clients like these give consent readily and welcome the counseling, consistent with their high motivation. Other clients may be more hesitant or skeptical, perhaps because the referral was someone else's idea rather than their own. Or they may be intimidated by the intensely personal nature of counseling or the prospect of accessing emotions or memories they know will be upsetting. They agree to undertake grief counseling, knowing it will be uncomfortable or painful, in order to achieve relief from their distress. In these cases, clients tolerate counseling. Ideally, all our clients would enthusiastically welcome grief counseling, but even agreeing to tolerate it is a sufficient basis for informed consent if it is a free decision.

Portability

Portability is also an important aspect of how informed consent is continuously elicited from the client. Portability does not mean possessing a ready copy of written consent forms wherever the counselor goes. Rather, it means grief counselors carry with them all that is needed to establish, and reestablish, informed consent in whatever venue counseling occurs. In today's stratified health care system, it is possible to encounter the same client or family in multiple settings: an office, a hospital, a hospice, the client's residence, a funeral home, or a place of worship. Any change of venue requires reestablishing the counselor–client relationship and reviewing informed consent. (See Chapter 7, "Multiple Relationships in Thanatology," for a comprehensive discussion of how the third P, place, influences the counselor–client relationship.)

The importance of contextualizing informed consent (cf. Schuck, 1994) to the specific demands of a given counseling setting cannot be overemphasized. Grief counselors must acknowledge that certain locations, especially hospitals, can impose constraints on confidentiality, record keeping, fees, and a host of other structural aspects of grief counseling. The necessity for portability in maintaining informed consent across different counseling venues is perhaps best expressed by paraphrasing a popular advertising slogan, "Don't leave your office without it."

SAMPLE TEMPLATE

For those just entering the field of grief counseling, students who have recently graduated, or practitioners who have not yet implemented use of written materials in their informed consent process, we offer a sample template of a client information brochure for informed consent for grief counseling in appendix D. This form is intended to educate prospective clients about grief counseling and prompt verbal discussion as a basis for consent that is both fully informed and freely given. It could be used with or without signature blocks for the client and counselor to sign and date. In either case, documenting in the client's record that the informed consent process was followed, together with notation of any particular concerns or questions voiced by the client, is important.

In drafting this sample template, we have incorporated the major content areas mandated by the ADEC Code of Ethics, specifically, the subsection for grief counselors and therapists that enumerates responsibilities regarding informed consent.

> Before members enter into professional relationships with potential clients, members inform clients/legal guardians about their expertise, techniques

> and other practices that may be used and that may affect the client's well being. Members clarify client/legal guardian goals and the purpose and expectations of the services they provide. (ADEC Code of Ethics, GC-I. Responsibility to Those Served, C)
>
> Clients/legal guardians are informed verbally and in writing at the time of the first interview about the limits of confidentiality as stipulated by law, regulation, or organizational process. (ADEC Code of Ethics, GC-I. Responsibility to Those Served, D)
>
> Prior to initiation of services, members notify clients/legal guardians of all financial responsibilities assumed by client/guardian or counselor. Fees for services, and any changes, must be identified and agreed to prior to services rendered. (ADEC Code of Ethics, GC-I. Responsibility to Those Served, E)
>
> When members agree to provide services to clients at the requests of third parties, the nature of each of the relationships of the involved parties is clarified, accepted by all, and documented as such. Any limitations to confidentiality will be noted as well. (ADEC Code of Ethics, GC-I. Responsibility to Those Served, G)

Additionally, the ACA Code of Ethics (ACA, 2005a) is helpful in spelling out clearly the spirit of shared decision making involved in obtaining informed consent.

> Clients have the freedom to choose whether to enter into or remain in a counseling relationship and need adequate information about the counseling process and the counselor. Counselors have an obligation to review in writing and verbally with clients the rights and responsibilities of both the counselor and the client. Informed consent is an ongoing part of the counseling process and counselors appropriately document discussions of informed consent throughout the counseling relationship. (ACA Code of Ethics, A.2. Informed Consent in the Counseling Relationship, A.2.a. Informed Consent)

The ACA Code of Ethics also identifies several necessary components of informed consent: the purposes, goals, and techniques of counseling; potential benefits and risks; the counselor's credentials; fees and billing arrangements; the extent and limits of confidentiality; record keeping; and clients' rights of refusal.

Along similar lines, Pomerantz and Handelsman (2004) identified seven general areas to be addressed by informed consent information given to clients. These areas include the following: the nature of the therapy together with risks and benefits; alternative treatments, including psychoactive medicines; appointments and emergencies; confidentiality and its limits, including those mandated by HIPAA (1996); fees; insurance and managed care issues; and the counselor's credentials as well as where to go with unresolved complaints about the counseling.

We intend our sample template to be an illustration of how to draft an informed consent document, not a prescription. Grief counselors wishing to adapt the form for use in their own practices will need to modify its provisions according to their theoretical models, their unique practice styles, and the specific requirements of the agency or setting where they work. We have incorporated all the major elements pertaining to informed consent outlined previously. The language is meant to be easily accessible with a warm, reassuring tone. Clients are often anxious about their first visit to a grief counselor, and use of a form such as this can serve as an extension of the counselor's demeanor in putting clients at ease. At the initiation of the informed consent process, the nexus between good counseling practice and sound ethical practice is evident again. Our goals are to greet clients with an earnest welcome, educate them with requisite information, and, after all their questions have been answered, empower them to make a thoughtful, deliberate decision about whether to elect grief counseling.

CASE VIGNETTE

The following example is an illustration of how the continuous consensual process of informed consent operates in a traditional practice of grief counseling.

Description

A young woman consults a grief counselor with an urban office practice for help dealing with the death of her father. Because she came on her own initiative, she readily embraces the opportunity for consultation. She understands fairly well what grief counseling involves as well as the limits of confidentiality. The remainder of the initial informed consent discussion proceeds fluidly, and she signs the counselor's customized informed consent document.

Later in the first interview, the counselor asks the woman to describe the night her father died. She balks, reluctant to touch off painful emotions of sadness that may overwhelm the poise she has carefully maintained up to this point in the session. The grief counselor responds by acknowledging the client's deep pain and then goes on to gently encourage her to convey the events of her father's death, reassuring the client that sadness is expected and normal. The counselor explains that expressing emotions such as sadness can be cathartic and will relieve some of her inner tension. The counselor further instructs the client that beginning to learn the depth of her sadness will actually help her build a better sense of control and mastery over such raw emotion.

Still somewhat hesitant, the client begins to describe her father's deathbed scene but then breaks into wracking sobs while burying her face in her hands. The counselor next takes a soothing, steady approach using empathic affirmations—for example, "I can see that losing your father was really painful"—to help the client manage her emotion while letting the intensity crescendo and then subside. Once the client regains her composure, the counselor asks if she is ready to go further with the inquiry, and she nods agreement, indicating she will be okay.

As they discuss how difficult it was for the client to acknowledge her father's impending death, the counselor asks why it was so hard to tell him goodbye. The client says only, "I guess it was because he was such a tyrant." When the counselor follows up by asking what she meant by the term *tyrant,* the client declares, "I know I'm *not* ready to talk about that yet." Respecting her boundary, the counselor suggests that they can return to that topic at a later point in time and then shifts the discussion to a review of other pertinent family history.

Analysis

This vignette provides an over-the-shoulder look at how the grief counselor progressively and *continuously* guided the young woman through the client role and secured her *consensual* participation in the dialogue throughout the encounter. Well past the formal aspects of initial consent and form signing, there was a *repetitive interplay of permission-seeking by the counselor and permission-granting by the client that honored the client's autonomy at each juncture in the process.* It is much like a physical exam in which an experienced physician systematically identifies the next area of the body to be examined, informs the patient what sensations may be experienced and whether the maneuver may hurt, and then elicits cooperative consent before proceeding (cf. Ritter, Reis, & Rascoe, 2007).

In the example of the bereft daughter, the grief counselor systematically probes important areas related to the client's loss of her father. In the case of asking about his actual death, the counselor notes the client's hesitation and then uses reassurance and education to persuade her of the importance of exploring this aspect of her story. In effect, she consents to give a verbal description of his death. Yet when the subject of her father's tyranny was broached, the client refused to go forward and declared the topic off-limits, at least for the time being. In short, consent was refused, so the counselor proceeded on an alternate track.

In such a case, we anticipate the grief counselor returning later to the subject of the client's relationship with her father. When doing so, the grief counselor may first appraise the client's willingness before pressing the matter further, securing consent by querying, "I wonder if you are ready now to discuss more about your relationship with your father?" Or later the counselor may want to employ a Gestalt technique such as the "empty chair" (Jordan & Neimeyer, 2007; Klass & Walter, 2001; Worden, 2009) to try to recreate symbolically the last moment of leave-taking and recoup the therapeutic value of saying aloud what was left unspoken. With this scenario, the counselor will first explain what the technique involves and secure the client's willingness to try the method, emotional though it may be, in the interest of overcoming the impasse she currently experiences. At each step in the unfolding inquiry, consent is solicited and received in a continuous interplay that is embedded in the counseling dynamic.

INFORMED REFUSAL OR RESISTANCE?

Experienced grief counselors will also recognize in the preceding vignette the possibility that resistance to the counseling process may underlie the client's hesitations, in effect masked by issues pertaining to informed consent. When is the client's reluctance to answer a question or hesitation to discuss certain material an indication that consent is lacking or that the client's psychic defenses, such as denial or avoidance, are impeding a progressive inquiry? Lack of consent, or informed refusal, is a legitimate reason for halting a particular line of questioning, whereas resistance calls for sensitively exploring and probing the conflict material protected by unhealthy psychic mechanisms. The adroit grief counselor can profitably employ what we call colloquially the *shoebox method* in order to discriminate between lack of consent and defensive resistance and so determine a course of action that is both good counseling practice and sound ethical practice.

The shoebox method consists of visualizing the hidden or undisclosed material as if it were inside a closed shoebox. Without opening it, the exterior of the box (i.e., the client's defenses) can be explored in a manner that respects nondisclosure of the box's contents (i.e., the emotionally charged conflict material). For example, in the foregoing case vignette, the counselor could simply comment, "The idea of talking about your father's parenting style must be pretty scary for you." Or the counselor could ask some gently probing questions such as, "What makes it so difficult to talk about your relationship with your father?" or "How will you know when you are ready to address your relationship with your father?" In effect, the counselor and the client are discussing the *prospect* of talking about the client's problematic relationship with her father rather than discussing the actual vicissitudes of the trouble. It is the client's psychic defenses that are being explored without forcing her into a line of inquiry that she is unprepared to handle.

The shoebox method precludes the counselor from overriding a lack of consent from the client while at the same time giving the client an opportunity to thoughtfully consider whether the proposed therapeutic course is acceptable. Generally, one of two outcomes results from using the shoebox method. First, from the discussion of perimeter defenses surrounding the conflict material, the client may come to realize that the subject area *is* approachable—the shoebox can be opened safely and its contents examined in the interest of resolving the problem. Second, the client may be reinforced in the position that it is premature in the counseling to address this particular conflict area. Sometimes clients feel unsure of their own ability to confront strong emotions connected with their loss, or they may not yet feel sufficiently secure in the therapeutic alliance to entrust the counselor with their deeper feelings and fears. In these latter instances, the grief counselor should defer to the client's judgment and, in doing so, honor informed refusal.

INFORMED CONSENT IN EDUCATION AND RESEARCH

Similar logic governs consent by students and trainees when participating in educational curricula designed to prompt self-disclosure, self-awareness, personal development and growth, or affective learning. The ADEC Code of Ethics spells out the necessity for a consent process between faculty trainers and students before undertaking such curricula.

> When a program or learning experience has a focus upon self-disclosure, self-understanding or growth, members ensure that potential students are made aware of this fact before they enter the program or begin the experience. (ADEC Code of Ethics, DE-I. Responsibility to Others, C)

In short, students need to understand sufficiently what is involved in the contemplated learning experience (i.e., full disclosure by the faculty trainer as to what will occur) before they can consent freely to participate. Especially in experiential exercises, consent as a continuous, consensual process applies. At each step, students and trainees must be free to choose their level of participation in experiential learning without coercion.

Suppose a faculty educator was using psychodrama techniques to teach concepts about emotions activated at the end of life. In reenacting a deathbed scene where there is tension around leave taking, a student may play the main role of protagonist, play a supporting role as an auxiliary ego, or simply remain part of the observing audience (Dayton, 1994). A student may be invited, but not forced, to assume a particular role in the drama. Similarly, in the postdrama discussion intended to enable students to assimilate key learning objectives, students must be free to determine the extent of their self-disclosure of thoughts, feelings, associations, or memories. Students tend to be remarkably open about sharing their affective responses and personal reactions when an appropriate atmosphere of trust exists and curiosity is encouraged. Nonetheless, the ADEC Code of Ethics requires a nonjudgmental stance from faculty trainers regarding the nature and extent of students' self-disclosures.

> When a student is expected to disclose relatively intimate or personal information about themselves as part of their learning experience, educators and supervisors shall not evaluate the student based upon such self-disclosure. The degree of self-disclosure will be respected without coercion or punitive measures. (ADEC Code of Ethics, DE-I. Responsibility to Others, E)

In all such educational endeavors, informed consent between faculty and students operates in a fashion parallel to how grief counselors obtain informed consent with clients.

The process of obtaining informed consent from prospective research participants is a highly formalized one. Institutional review boards (IRBs) that approve research with human subjects follow federally mandated guidelines designed to protect the rights and dignity of participants (U.S. Department of Health and Human Services, 2005). Prospective participants must have sufficient opportunity to deliberate about whether to participate without any sort of undue pressure or coercion. All information about the research study must be presented in understandable language. According to federal guidelines, informed consent documents for research participation must include the following essential elements: explanation of the study's purpose with a description of the procedures to be used; warning of any adverse risks; description of potential benefits to the subject or others; alternatives to participation; confidentiality of data collected; explanation of any compensation or treatment available, if more than minimal risk is present; information on whom to contact with questions or complaints; and a statement assuring that participation is voluntary, that there is no penalty for refusal, and that the person may terminate participation at any time without reprisal.

These standards are largely incorporated into the ADEC Code of Ethics, which sets forth for research investigators their responsibilities to research participants regarding informed consent.

> When obtaining informed consent, members inform participants about the purpose of the research, expected duration, and procedures; and about their right to decline to participate and to withdraw from the research study without penalty. (ADEC Code of Ethics, RT-II. Responsibility to Research Participants, A)

> When members conduct research with clients/patients, students, or subordinates as participants, members take steps to protect the prospective participants from adverse consequences of declining or withdrawing from participation. (ADEC Code of Ethics, RT-II. Responsibility to Research Participants, B)

> When research participation is a course requirement or an opportunity for extra credit, the prospective participant is given the choice of equitable alternative activities. (ADEC Code of Ethics, RT-II. Responsibility to Research Participants, C)

> Members may dispense with informed consent only (1) where research would not reasonably be assumed to create distress or harm and involves (a) the study of normal educational practices, curricula, or classroom

> management methods conducted in educational settings; (b) the use of anonymous questionnaires, naturalistic observations, or archival research for which disclosure of responses would not place participants at risk of criminal or civil liability or damage their financial standing, employability, or reputation, and confidentiality is protected; or (c) the study of factors related to job or organization effectiveness conducted in organizational settings for which there is no risk to participants' employability, and confidentiality is protected or (2) where otherwise permitted by law or federal or institutional regulations. (ADEC Code of Ethics, RT-II. Responsibility to Research Participants, D)

Perspicacious readers will recognize that federal prescriptions for informed consent in research settings, now in force for more than 2 decades, have penetrated and influenced informed consent practices in clinical settings. Several elements of these mandates have made their way into the standard forms used by grief counselors when securing informed consent from clients (see appendix D). In particular, the provisions for describing potential risks and benefits, how confidentiality is guarded, where to direct complaints, and freedom to discontinue participation at any time have become standard provisions of informed consent. This is a good example of how cross-fertilization between professional endeavors of research and counseling enhances not only counseling technique but also ethical sensitivity.

SUMMARY

Informed consent is a continuous consensual process between grief counselor and client that rests on twin pillars: (1) full disclosure of information the client needs to make a reasoned decision about participation and (2) free choice established at the beginning of counseling and reestablished periodically throughout the cycle of care. In addition to oral explanations of what grief counseling entails using descriptions that meet the subjective standard for client comprehension, it is recommended that grief counselors also use a written form to ensure that all applicable conditions influencing a client's consent, including exceptions to counselor–client confidentiality, are understood at the outset. A similar consent process is required in educational curricula and research protocols. Because professional confidentiality is so central to informed consent, these two topics are truly inseparable. Therefore, confidentiality is the subject of the next chapter.

5 Confidentiality

Confidentiality is a sine qua non of grief counseling. Traced back to its origin with the oath of Hippocrates sworn by physicians (Adams, 2005), professional confidentiality is a sacred trust upon which the counselor–client relationship rests. Indeed, confidentiality is one of the fundamental reasons clients consult counselors, along with seeking the benefit of a counselor's expert knowledge and opinions. Clients trust that whatever information they convey in the counseling context will not be revealed to any other party. This assurance of confidentiality allows clients to express more openly their deepest personal thoughts and feelings, thus imbuing the counseling relationship with its unique healing properties. In short, confidentiality is a core aspect of the ethical principle of fidelity.

Given the primacy of confidentiality in grief counseling, one may wonder why ethical dilemmas related to confidentiality are those most frequently reported by practicing psychologists, both in the United States (Pope & Vetter, 1992) and in Europe (Pettifor, 2004). How can something as categorical, unambiguous, and ironclad as professional confidentiality pose problems to practicing grief counselors? Unfortunately, even licensed mental health professionals and health care providers sometimes misunderstand or disregard their ethical obligation of confidentiality. Sometimes agencies, organizations, or businesses with whom grief counselors work unwittingly promote breaches in confidentiality.

Bersoff (2003a) commented on the irony that confidentiality may be better known by violations of the ethical obligation it imposes than by honoring it. Quite clearly, maintaining confidentiality in grief counseling requires both vigilant self-monitoring by the counselor and unflagging enforcement of its boundaries.

THREE DEFINITIONS

Understanding what is involved in a grief counselor's ethical obligation of confidentiality demands clear definitions of three related terms: privacy, confidentiality, and privilege.

Privacy is a right of individuals to their personhood and to ownership of their personally determined thoughts, attitudes, feelings, and behaviors. In the United States, a person's privacy is understood to be guaranteed by the Bill of Rights, specifically the Fourth Amendment outlawing unreasonable searches and seizures and the Ninth Amendment precluding abrogation of rights not specified in the Constitution, often taken to include privacy. Although an individual's right to privacy may be augmented or diminished by a variety of court rulings that attempt to define its recognizable limits, privacy against unwanted intrusions by others or by the government is the purview of free citizens. Thus, individuals have control over *when* to disclose *what* personal information to *which* persons. Choosing to confide private information to a grief counselor is one example of a citizen's prerogative.

Confidentiality refers to the ethical duty of grief counselors, mental health professionals, and health care providers to protect the identity of clients and the information they disclose during the provision of care. This means not revealing counseling information to any other party, in effect, a professional pledge of secrecy regarding what is discussed during grief counseling. Confidentiality is the counselor's obligation to honor the client's trust by voluntarily refraining from any disclosure of the contents of the counseling.

Privilege refers to a legal concept wherein clients can choose not to disclose personal information sought by parties in a legal proceeding or by a court of law. Ordinary rules of evidence require citizens with knowledge pertaining to a matter in dispute to testify in order that the court may discover the truth about the matter and render justice. The privilege *not* to testify is an exception to this common law. It is important to remember that *privilege belongs to the client.* As with doctor–patient, husband–wife, attorney–client, and priest–penitent communications, privilege extends to psychotherapist–client communications. By refusing to disclose counseling information to parties in a legal proceeding, the grief counselor is protecting the client's privilege. However, if a client waives the protections of privilege, there is no independent right on the part of the grief counselor to refuse to disclose pertinent information.

Shuman and Foote (1999) asserted that privilege in a psychotherapy relationship is a relatively porous barrier even in the best of circumstances. This is because privilege depends on statutory law to sustain it, and state courts primarily have jurisdiction in such cases. Although the U.S. Supreme Court decision in *Jaffee v. Redmond* (1996) privileged therapist–client communication from judicially compelled disclosure for cases tried in federal courts governed by Federal Rules of Evidence (1975), states vary in whether and how they recognize privilege for confidential communications between mental health professionals and their clients. For example, all 50 states and the District of Columbia make provision for some level of privilege for psychologists' relationships with clients (Glosoff, Herlihy, Herlihy, & Spence, 1997), whereas clients' communications with licensed professional counselors are privileged in 44 states and the District of Columbia (Glosoff, Herlihy, & Spence, 2000).

Because providers from diverse professional disciplines practice grief counseling, it behooves grief counselors to know the state laws governing privilege for their respective professional group. This may involve consulting with an attorney knowledgeable in matters pertaining to confidentiality and privilege in the jurisdiction where the grief counselor practices. Also helpful is consulting jurisdiction-specific reference works, such as the American Psychological Association's book series on mental health law in various states (cf. Shuman, 2004).

The interrelationship between privacy, confidentiality, and privilege is well-described by Zuckerman (2003), who wrote, "A Venn diagram would show three concentric circles—the largest being privacy, the middle confidentiality, and the smallest privilege" (p. 364). He reminds counselors and therapists that although all privileged communications are confidential, not all confidential communications are necessarily privileged. This is because many exceptions to confidentiality exist. In light of these challenges, Shuman and Foote (1999) described confidentiality in a counseling relationship as a "fragile and perishable commodity" (p. 483). It is the grief counselor's responsibility to guard and protect confidentiality as the cornerstone of trust on which the counseling relationship is built (Glosoff et al., 1997).

ADEC STANDARDS

The ADEC Code of Ethics is clear and comprehensive on the subject of confidentiality. It covers a variety of contingencies that grief counselors need to consider in the course of maintaining and preserving confidentiality. References to confidentiality in five distinct sections of the ADEC Code of Ethics underscore the importance of this ethical obligation. However, because there is some redundancy in the various sections that mention confidentiality, a simple listing of these provisions is inadequate for achieving a full understanding of the subject. Instead, the ADEC code's provisions are embedded in the subsequent discussion of key issues regarding confidentiality. Most important is establishing the primacy of confidentiality.

> Members regard as confidential all information arising in the course of the professional relationship. Consideration for the client welfare is an abiding concern of members. (ADEC Code of Ethics, VIII. Confidentiality and Privacy, A)

LIMITS TO CONFIDENTIALITY

The grief counselor's obligation to make clients aware of the limits of confidentiality links the two cardinal concepts of informed consent and confidentiality. Only when clients understand thoroughly that there are limits to confidentiality can they make a truly informed decision consenting to counseling. The ADEC Code of Ethics calls for this to be explained both orally and in writing.

> Members inform clients about the limits of confidentiality in a given situation. (ADEC Code of Ethics, VIII. Confidentiality and Privacy, B)
>
> Clients/legal guardians are informed verbally and in writing at the time of the first interview about the limits of confidentiality as stipulated by law, regulation, or organizational process. (ADEC Code of Ethics, GC-I. Responsibility to Those Served, D)

It is fallacy for grief counselors to take a laissez-faire, reactive approach to informing clients about limits to confidentiality, such as thinking they can deal with it when situations demand. Waiting to inform clients that material they have disclosed cannot be kept confidential for various reasons "is like closing the proverbial barn door after the horse has escaped" (Welfel, 2006, p. 119). Like so many aspects of ethical practice of grief counseling, such contingencies need to be anticipated and dealt with in advance to preclude compromising dilemmas later.

Such was the case with the grief counselor treating the bereaved sister of a man who had been brutally murdered. Because the counselor did not regularly discuss informed consent or limits to confidentiality before starting the first interview, the client assumed mistakenly that anything she said would be kept completely private by the counselor. Thus, only *after* the client revealed that her rage about the brother's killing was so great that she had been hitting her own children did the grief counselor notify her that the matter must be reported to proper authorities. The client was shocked to find that she had no privacy in confiding her problem behavior to the counselor and feared that, should child protective services investigate, she could lose her children just as she had lost her treasured brother. Needless to say, all efforts at maintaining therapeutic rapport failed, and the client, so in need of grief counseling, dropped out after the first session.

The case of third-party evaluations or treatment is another illustration of the importance of giving clients advance notice of confidentiality limits. Sometimes a third party, such as a court or an employer, requires clients to be evaluated by a grief counselor or undergo counseling for a bereavement-related problem. In general, such situations occur less frequently in grief counseling than in other types of counseling (e.g., substance abuse, impulse control problems, or child custody evaluations). Nonetheless, when a third party mandates such services, communication from the grief counselor back to the third party regarding the outcome of the evaluation or the progress of counseling is often stipulated as a condition, especially when the costs incurred are covered by the third party. It is incumbent upon the grief counselor to clarify anticipated disclosures of counseling information, including whether the counselor will provide no information, minimal information (e.g., dates of counseling appointments, type of service such as individual or family counseling, and diagnosis), some information (e.g., a summary of the evaluation or counseling sessions), or complete information (e.g., a photocopy of the full evaluation report or counseling progress notes). With third-party consultations, it is advisable to have clients sign an appropriate authorization to release information specifying their agreement *before* services start.

> When members agree to provide services to clients at the requests of third parties, the nature of each of the relationships of the involved parties is clarified, accepted by all, and documented as such. Any limitations to confidentiality will be noted as well. (ADEC Code of Ethics, GC-I. Responsibility to Those Served, G)

A related question is what to do in more routine situations where another professional has referred a client for grief counseling. For purposes of building a practice and strengthening a referral network, most grief counselors wish to acknowledge to referral sources that they have completed the initial evaluation and recommended a course of action. Although such professional courtesy is commonplace, clients should be apprised of such customary contacts before services start and their consent is obtained. Rarely do clients object, but when they do, their preferences should be honored.

EXCEPTIONS TO CONFIDENTIALITY

Perhaps no aspect of confidentiality is more studied than those occasions when confidentiality may be breached in service to what society perceives as an even greater good. Considering the august nature of the confidentiality obligation, no exception should be made lightly. "Confidential until proven otherwise" would be a good working model for grief counselors faced with dilemmas about disclosure of confidential counseling information. However, there are instances when breaking confidentiality is the right and lawful thing to do. Ethical practice means the grief counselor is well prepared with thorough knowledge of those circumstances or conditions that require breaching confidentiality rather than protecting it.

Although statutory laws vary in different states and jurisdictions, there are eight principal contingencies that require or permit the grief counselor to disclose confidential counseling information: client-authorized releases of information; danger to self; danger to others; neglect or abuse of children or vulnerable adults; complaints or litigation against the counselor; litigation claiming emotional pain and suffering; court-ordered or statutory requirements to disclose; and requirements of third-party payers. Each reason is addressed in some detail in this chapter because the burden on the grief counselor to understand each of these eight circumstances is so great.

1. Client-Authorized Release of Information

Harkening back to the principle of autonomy, clients retain the right to disclose the contents of their grief counseling to whomever they choose. Most often, such requests are for transmission of counseling information to other professionals, such as a physician, or to another mental health professional. Disclosure may be needed for coordinating care (e.g., to a psychiatrist who is treating the client with psychoactive medicines or to a marriage counselor when grief issues impact relationship conflicts), transferring care to a new counselor (e.g., when a geographic move necessitates a change in provider), or communicating with the professional who referred the client.

The written consent form on which the client authorizes release of counseling information should include a description of what material is to be disclosed, to whom, and for what expressed purpose. Table 5.1 contains recommended elements to include in authorizations for release of confidential counseling information. Typically, clinics, agencies, hospitals, and established organizations use a standard form for such instances

Table 5.1

RECOMMENDED ELEMENTS OF AUTHORIZATION FORMS FOR RELEASE OF CONFIDENTIAL COUNSELING INFORMATION

- Client's name and demographic information
- Grief counselor's name and contact information
- Name and contact information of third party to whom the information is released
- Indication if information is only to be *sent* to the third party, or if the grief counselor is authorized to *talk with* the third party, or both
- Dates of service to which the authorization applies
- Delineation of what information is to be released (e.g., copies of confidential records or a summary only)
- Purpose(s) for which information is being released (e.g., transfer of care, second opinion, insurance, legal, educational, personal)
- Stipulation that released information must not be forwarded to any other party without the written consent of the client
- Request that information be destroyed immediately in the event that it is accidentally received by any party other than the one for whom it is intended
- Waiver of responsibility on the part of the grief counselor if the released information is misused, misinterpreted, or in any way mishandled by the receiving party
- Signature block, with date, for the client (or legal guardian)
- Signature block, with date, for witness

of client-authorized release of information. For grief counselors in private practice or just entering the field, templates for how to construct such forms may be found in Zuckerman (2003). When creating such a form for use in independent practice, review by the attorney advising the grief counselor on practice matters is strongly suggested.

Forms should indicate that released information is not to be forwarded to any other person or agency without the written consent of the client. Likewise, grief counselors should not forward to anyone else client reports received from other professionals. However, where germane, a synopsis of such information from other sources may be incorporated into the grief counselor's ongoing record of the client's sessions.

> Client information received in confidence by one agent or agency is not forwarded to another without the client's written consent. (ADEC Code of Ethics, VIII. Confidentiality and Privacy, J)

In all cases, the grief counselor discloses only information pertinent to the matter motivating the client's request and avoids disclosing other contextual information that is nonessential to the issue at hand.

2. Danger to Self

When clients pose a clear and imminent danger to their own lives because of suicidal behavior, grief counselors have an ethical obligation to help protect suicidal clients from themselves. This means that the counselor may breach confidentiality to notify law enforcement authorities, family or friends, or others who may be in a position to intervene with the client. This duty is based on the ethical principle of beneficence—advocating for the client's welfare and working to produce a positive outcome. In so many instances of suicidal behavior, the potential victim is ambivalent. That is, many suicidal clients are not completely committed to ending their life. Most suicidal people choose to live another day when given an opportunity to reevaluate and reconsider their decision, frequently with the help of compassionate professionals and loving family and friends. Giving suicidal clients that second chance to rethink their decision is the greater good that justifies breaching confidentiality in these situations.

This ethical obligation toward suicidal clients is stated clearly in the ADEC Code of Ethics.

> When members believe that a client's or student's condition indicates that there is a foreseeable, serious, and imminent danger to the client, to the

> student, or to others, members take immediate, reasonable, and prudent action and/or inform appropriate authorities in accordance with applicable legal mandates. Consultation with other knowledgeable professionals is highly encouraged. (ADEC Code of Ethics, III. Responsibilities to Those Served, B)
>
> Members are free to consult with other professionals about clients and/or students provided that the consultation does not place the consultant in a position of conflict of interest and providing that all concerns of privacy, informed consent, and confidentiality are met appropriately. (ADEC Code of Ethics, III. Responsibilities to Those Served, C)
>
> Members shall disclose confidential information when members believe there is clear and imminent danger to the client or to others, and that the danger can be alleviated or avoided by disclosing the information. In such circumstances, members are encouraged to consult with other knowledgeable professionals. (ADEC Code of Ethics, III. Responsibilities to Those Served, D)
>
> When members disclose confidential information without client consent, they do so only with appropriate others and only for compelling reasons. (ADEC Code of Ethics, III. Responsibilities to Those Served, E)
>
> In those rare instances when members may disclose information, they disclose only that which is relevant within the context of the incident. (ADEC Code of Ethics, III. Responsibilities to Those Served, G)

Note that the ADEC code reiterates the advisability of consulting with colleagues as a reasonable check when contemplating a breach of confidentiality in the interest of averting a potential suicide. Certainly such an emergency meets the "compelling reasons" criteria for disclosing confidential client information.

In grief counseling, suicidal behavior in clients is often linked to the loss they are grieving. An elderly widower may no longer be motivated to keep living without the comforting presence of his beloved wife of so many years. A bereaved mother may be so aggrieved over the untimely and unexpected death of her child that she believes the only option for reestablishing a parental bond with the child is dying herself. A middle-age client who has reached a point of dejection and despair may decide to follow the path of the parent who committed suicide decades before as the way out of disillusionment and meaninglessness. The scenarios are countless, and the attentive grief counselor remains ever attuned to indicators of suicide potential. Asking clients about suicidal tendencies should be a standard aspect of every intake interview. Yet because suicidal inclinations among the bereaved are relatively common, how does the grief counselor distinguish between suicidal thinking that is more musing or fleeting and suicidal behavior that presents clear and imminent danger?

The prudent counselor incorporates literature-based risk profiles and state-of-the-art practices for assessing danger to self. Scholarly reviews document the demographic, psychosocial, and clinical factors most clearly associated with suicide risk in adults (Barnett & Johnson, 2008; Jacobs, Brewer, & Klein-Benheim, 1999; Rudd, 2006). These factors are listed below.

- Male gender
- Single, especially separated, divorced, or widowed
- White or Native American
- Age over 60
- Lack of social support, especially not having young children in the home
- Unemployment
- Decline in socioeconomic status or financial problems
- History of abuse (sexual, physical, or emotional)
- Presence of a psychiatric condition, particularly mood disorder
- Recent discharge (up to 1 year) from inpatient psychiatric treatment
- Medical illness
- Family history of suicide, especially first-degree relatives
- History of previous suicide attempt
- Psychological turmoil (e.g., "suicidogenic" relationships or hopelessness)
- Alcohol use or abuse
- Presence of firearms

For adolescents, occurrence of a "mini-epidemic" in the community, such as a series of peer suicides, constitutes an additional risk factor because of a modeling effect.

Age is an important epidemiological factor, with the highest rate of suicide found among the elderly population (Chan, Draper, & Banerjee, 2007; Erlangsen, Bille-Brahe, & Jeune, 2003; Friedmann & Kohn, 2008; Moscicki, 1997; Stillion & McDowell, 1996). The risk increases with age, especially after 65 years, and the oldest elderly, those age 75 and older, have the highest suicide rates of all. When risk factors are considered in concert, elderly White men who are divorced or widowed, and who are ill or destitute, make up a highly vulnerable group (cf. Osterweis, Solomon, & Green, 1984).

The occurrence of "psychological turmoil" denoted by Jacobs et al. (1999) could refer to any number of life problems. For example, turmoil could be interpersonal. Maris (1997) coined the phrase "suicidogenic relationships" to describe those relations generating high levels of anger and conflict that could be especially vexatious to suicide-prone individuals. Alternately, turmoil could refer to an individual's cognitive processes. Rudd, Joiner, and Rajab (2001) characterized the belief system of suicidal individuals as one marked by a pervasive conviction of hopelessness. Three core beliefs underpin suicidal hopelessness: unlovability (e.g., "I don't deserve to live"); helplessness (e.g., "I can't solve this"); and poor stress tolerance (e.g., "I can't stand this pain anymore").

Another important consideration is evaluating a client's suicide plan for its specificity, intent, and lethality. Suicide plans that carry higher risk are those with greater specificity about how they will be executed, those with more urgency as to the client's intent, and those employing the most lethal means, such as firearms or hanging.

It is important to remember that risk factor models for assessing danger to self are only guidelines and not foolproof. In the final analysis, each grief counselor must account for assessing whether a client's suicide threat constitutes a clear and imminent danger serious enough to breach confidentiality. Ideally, the grief counselor's judgment of a client's suicide potential should integrate the risk factor models described together with any individual factors pertaining to the client as a unique person. Sometimes suicidal behavior can be countermanded by genuine reasons for living.

3. Danger to Others

Although the obligation to intervene with suicidal clients who pose a threat to themselves may seem intuitively obvious, the obligations of the grief counselor when clients present a real and immediate danger to someone else are more controversial and less straightforward. Generally referred to as the *duty to warn,* a mental health professional's obligation to breach confidentiality for purposes of warning and protecting the intended victim(s) of a homicidally violent client who confides the plan in therapy owes its existence to the famous case *Tarasoff v. The Regents of the University of California* (1976). Grief counselors need to understand the origin of the duty-to-warn imperative, what requirements it imposes on their practices, and the importance of up-to-date knowledge about how duty to warn applies in their state or jurisdiction.

Descriptive summaries of the *Tarasoff* case (Everstine et al., 1980; Herbert, 2002) and the text of the original court opinion (Gostin, 2002) are available for those readers interested in its history. For purposes of our discussion of duty to warn and protect, we recount only the essential facts of the *Tarasoff* case. Psychologists and psychiatrists treating the assailant in a voluntary, outpatient university clinic knew of his self-admitted plan to murder a young woman and judged him to be dangerous. They notified campus police but never gave warning to the intended victim or her parents. The assailant later murdered the woman. Subsequently, her family sued the professional caregivers and the police. The California Supreme Court found the mental health care team liable for failure to warn the intended victim. The court's decision inaugurated a new ethical obligation for psychotherapists—a duty to warn and protect targeted victims of violent clients. Thus, breaking confidentiality is mandated in these instances, based on the court's logic.

> We conclude that the public policy favoring protection of the confidential character of patient-psychotherapist communications must yield to the extent to which disclosure is essential to avert danger to others. The protective privilege ends where the public peril begins. (Gostin, 2002, p. 10)

As a result of the *Tarasoff* ruling, the ADEC Code of Ethics calls for grief counselors to disclose confidential counseling information "when members believe there is clear and imminent danger to the client *or to others* [italics added]" (ADEC Code of Ethics, VIII. Confidentiality and Privacy, D). Counselors should "take immediate, reasonable and prudent action and/or inform appropriate authorities in accordance with applicable legal mandates" (ADEC Code of Ethics, III. Responsibilities to Those Served, B). In practice, discharging this ethical responsibility involves both assessing dangerousness and taking effective action when indicated.

Homicidal violence among nonhospitalized, ambulatory clients in mental health settings is a relatively rare event. As a result, predicting client dangerousness is notoriously difficult for mental health professionals as a whole, and grief counselors are no exception. In our experience, grief counselors are most likely to encounter potentially violent impulses when clients' loved ones either were murdered or died a wrongful death as a result of someone's negligence or recklessness. Even then, homicidal ideation presents primarily as a manifestation of righteous anger rather than genuine intent to harm a third party. Nonetheless, screening for two main risk factors—previous history of violent behavior toward people or animals and possession of a firearm—is required.

Monahan (1993) and colleagues (Monahan et al., 2001) provide a detailed framework for violence risk assessment and intervention. They emphasize that counselors need to gather appropriate information about the client in order to estimate risk. Accordingly, counselors need to investigate past mental health records and current treatment records, such as hospital charts, for evidence of violent behavior. They urge questioning clients directly about violent tendencies, such as "What is the most violent thing you've ever done?" or "Do you ever worry that you might physically hurt somebody?" In the absence of archival information, or with a client who is an unreliable informant, asking significant others about any previous or current violent behavior, or threats of the same, can help.

Once convinced of a client's violence potential, grief counselors are well advised to consult with colleagues before implementing actions designed to hospitalize the client, notify authorities, or warn and protect potential victims. Knowing clearly the extent of a counselor's obligation to break confidentiality and warn others of a violent threat is a daunting proposition because the *Tarasoff* decision has been controversial from the start, and some think it goes too far in eroding counselor–client privilege in favor of an ambiguous responsibility to society at large (Bersoff, 2002). Furthermore, the *Tarasoff* ruling has spawned a patchwork of legislation across the United States with the result that some states impose an actual duty to warn, some only grant permission to warn, and others are silent on the issue (Herbert, 2002). It is absolutely vital that grief counselors receive adequate education from their state associations and licensing boards on the jurisdictional status of duty to warn and protect. Also advisable is consulting with a knowledgeable attorney familiar with state law on the subject of duty to warn.

As in all ethical matters, the judgment of the counselor is the final guiding step. Where there remains no clear-cut answer on the question of duty to warn and protect, it is sometimes helpful to mentally submit the situation to a hypothetical jury by asking oneself, "How would a jury of peers view the steps I am taking, or not taking, in response to this potential threat? Would my explanation of the rationale for my decision satisfy a jury that I had discharged any applicable professional responsibility?"

4. Neglect or Abuse of Children or Vulnerable Adults

Another well-known exception to client confidentiality is the obligation to notify appropriate protective and regulatory agencies in cases of reported or suspected abuse of children or vulnerable adults. Because so many emotional problems are linked to a developmental history of abuse, neglect, or exploitation, discussion of such topics is a high-frequency event in mental health counseling in general and in grief counseling in particular. The presence of a conflicted, ambivalent, or otherwise troubled relationship between decedent and mourner is a well-known risk factor for complicated mourning (Gamino et al., 1998; Rando, 1993; Worden, 2009). Mistreatment such as abuse and neglect, often rooted in alcoholism or drug dependence, is a major cause of such conflicted relationships. Additionally, grievers with high distress levels associated with complicated mourning are those most likely to seek grief counseling (Gamino et al., 2008) and most likely to benefit from it (Schut, Stroebe, van der Bout, & Terheggen, 2001). Thus, grief counselors can expect to encounter problem dynamics related to abuse and neglect with some regularity.

When adults describe a developmental history of abuse or neglect from childhood, there is no reporting obligation for the grief counselor. However, in cases where abuse of children is still occurring, or even suspected, the grief counselor has a moral and legal obligation to notify authorities who can properly investigate the situation and, if necessary, remove children from harmful situations to protect them from further abuse. This is consistent with the duty of all citizens to ensure the safety of minor children who cannot adequately protect themselves. In the United States, human service professionals, such as grief counselors, are required to report known or suspected child maltreatment in all 50 states (Kalichman, 1999), and in some states (e.g. Texas) all citizens must report.

The ethical obligation for grief counselors to report suspected abuse or neglect is in force regardless of whether the perpetrator, or suspected perpetrator, is the client in counseling or someone else identified by the client. Sometimes clients object to such mandated reporting, even when given full notice of such mechanisms during the informed consent process, because so many of these cases involve a family member or friend as the perpetrator. When this is the case, the client may be reluctant to be the whistleblower. Although such sympathies are understandable, they are, nevertheless, misplaced when considering the greater good of society's humane duty to protect minor children from mistreatment.

Besides minor children, the reporting obligation extends to situations involving abuse, neglect, or exploitation of vulnerable adults. This includes elderly or disabled people who, like minor children, are compromised in their ability to defend themselves from perpetration of abuse or neglect. Grief counselors who work with special needs populations—clients in nursing homes, those on hospice care, developmentally disabled adults in group homes or residential facilities—should constantly be vigilant to indications of abuse, neglect, or exploitation. Because so many of these vulnerable adults have communication impairments and cannot adequately express themselves in verbal language, it is quite important to heed observational indicators of abuse or neglect, such as bruises, burns, or untended medical and hygiene problems, as well as behavioral signs of abuse or neglect, such as flinching, crying, or clinging.

Grief counselors should not hesitate to break confidentiality and report cases of suspected abuse or neglect concerning children or vulnerable adults because they are legally required and ethically bound to do so. Counselors who make such reports in good faith are immune from any civil or criminal liability for such reporting, even if later investigation proves the suspicions unfounded or exonerates suspected perpetrators (Kalichman, 1999).

5. Complaints or Litigation Against the Counselor

Should a disgruntled client file an ethics complaint against the grief counselor with either a licensing board or the ethics committee of a state or national professional association, that client surrenders the privilege to keep the counseling information confidential. Typically, licensing boards or ethics committees require the complainant to sign an authorization to release information as a condition of investigating the complaint. Counseling records are then available to investigators, and the grief counselor is free to explain or defend opinions given and actions taken or not taken. From a risk-management perspective, such situations are a very strong argument for keeping thorough records that denote the contents not only of each counseling session but also of any other client contacts such as telephone calls, letters, faxes, or e-mails.

Similarly, should a client initiate legal action against the grief counselor for malpractice, for example, it is not reasonable to expect that records of the counseling can remain confidential (Koocher & Keith-Spiegel, 2008). Grief counselors sued by their clients have a right to self-defense or to their "day in court" in an effort to exonerate themselves of the charges brought against them. In such cases, grief counselors may freely discuss the course of a client's counseling with their defense attorney and may testify about the particulars of the counseling during depositions and court proceedings. In other words, confidential counseling information cannot be used both to attack the counselor for malpractice and, at the same time, to defend against disclosure to third parties by invoking confidentiality. Clients who complain against or sue their grief counselor give up their rights to keep counseling information private if that very information is the basis of their claim.

6. Litigation Claiming Pain and Suffering

Consider the case of the bereaved couple whose young daughter drowned in the swimming pool of a private day care. The pool's enclosure had a faulty gate. Because of inattention by the designated child care worker, the toddler wandered into the pool area, apparently pushed open the broken gate, and was found underwater several minutes later. Resuscitation attempts failed. In the pursuant criminal trial, the child care worker was convicted of negligence but given only a probated sentence.

The bereaved couple considered the outcome of the criminal case to be a travesty in light of their only daughter's death, so they sued in civil court for compensatory damages, including consideration for psychological pain and suffering. Because the couple had consulted a grief counselor, the records of that counseling were necessarily opened for purposes of the court discovering the truth about the extent of their pain and suffering as documented by the grief counselor. Initially, the bereaved couple was reluctant to have confidential counseling information disclosed because some of their sessions had focused on marital conflict. This conflict had its origin years before the death of their daughter but had intensified as a result of their loss. However, the counseling records were germane to their legal claim of pain and suffering, and in order to go forward with the suit, they had to agree for the record to be made available to attorneys on both sides. Otherwise, if privacy was of paramount concern to the couple, they could have dropped their claim. Thus, when disclosure of confidential counseling information is of legal consequence to a party's claim or defense, the protective privilege granted to communications in the counselor–client relationship is suspended.

7. Court-Ordered or Statutory Requirements to Disclose

The client privilege to refrain from disclosing confidential counseling information is not an impermeable barrier. Despite the U.S. Supreme Court's ruling in *Jaffee v. Redmond* (1996) protecting counselor–client communication from judicially compelled disclosure for cases tried in federal courts, there are instances when courts of law can compel testimony from counselors even when the client has not authorized it. Criminal cases are a prime example. Depending on state laws, counselor–client privilege may not apply in criminal proceedings. Also, when the court requires a counselor to testify as an expert witness, invoking privilege on behalf of the client may not be an option (see Chapter 12, "Grief Counselor as Expert Witness").

Certainly, when grief counselors conduct court-ordered evaluations of litigants regarding mental competency or level of psychological distress suffered as a result of trauma or loss, the contents of the counselor–client interchange are not confidential in the traditional sense. As in other types of third-party evaluations, either the person being evaluated has waived privilege, effectively consenting to disclosure, or the court never recognized such a right to exist because the evaluation is compulsory rather than elective.

In some states or jurisdictions, statutory law may require mental health professionals to disclose confidential counseling information. Examples of such situations, besides criminal cases, are lawsuits pertaining to the parent–child relationship such as custody disputes, civil commitment proceedings to determine whether an individual requires involuntary psychiatric hospitalization, or litigation of abuse or neglect claims. Clearly, some sophistication on the part of the grief counselor is needed to deal with various kinds of court-related disclosures in a manner that comports with state laws but also upholds the sacred trust of confidentiality to the greatest extent possible.

Being served with a subpoena can create confusion if the grief counselor is inexperienced or uncertain how to respond. Attorneys, as officers of the court, can issue a subpoena (literally, "under penalty"), which is a legal command to appear to provide testimony. A *subpoena duces tecum* additionally directs the professional to bring along specific documents, such as counseling records or progress notes, pertaining to the case in question. Even facing a subpoena, the grief counselor still has a responsibility to protect the client's confidentiality unless the client has specifically waived privilege, a legal exception to privilege exists as in statutory requirements to disclose, or the court orders the counselor to testify. Thus, a subpoena requires a timely response from the grief counselor, but that response is not necessarily one of disclosing confidential counseling information (Koocher & Keith-Spiegel, 2008). So how does a responsible grief counselor proceed when a subpoena is served?

The Committee on Legal Issues of the American Psychological Association (2006) outlined a six-step strategy for dealing with subpoenas. First, with the help of legal counsel, determine whether the subpoena is legally valid and thus requires a formal response to the attorney or the court. Second, contact the client, who may choose to authorize disclosure or waive privilege. Remember, in states with statutory privilege for counselor–client communication, counselors are enjoined from disclosing confidential counseling information, even if subpoenaed by an attorney, without client consent (Welfel, 2006). Third, if the client does not consent, negotiate with the requesting party about alternatives to wholesale disclosure. Fourth, if negotiation fails, appeal to the court for a ruling on whether the requested disclosure is required. HIPAA (1996) privacy regulations may shield psychotherapy notes from disclosure, thus limiting the information that may be conveyed. Fifth, through their attorneys, clients sometimes file a motion with the court to quash, or nullify, the subpoena or seek a protective order to limit disclosure of sensitive client information. Sometimes, a judge will hear sensitive testimony in camera, or in closed chambers, in order to find out the truth about the case at hand while also respecting the privacy concerns of the client. Sixth, when the court compels the counselor to testify, having one's own attorney at the deposition or court proceeding to provide guidance is advisable.

Ultimately, the judge will decide whether confidential counseling information must be disclosed in the interest of adjudicating a legal dispute. At all times, however, the grief counselor should follow the practice of disclosing only the minimum information necessary to address the matter before the court. Pragmatically, this means answering only the questions asked and limiting the disclosure of contextual information whenever possible. This is consistent with the ADEC Code of Ethics on confidentiality.

> When members disclose confidential information without client consent, they do so only with appropriate others and only for compelling reasons. (ADEC Code of Ethics, VIII. Confidentiality and Privacy, E)
>
> In those rare instances when members may disclose information, they disclose only that which is relevant within the context of the incident. (ADEC Code of Ethics, VIII. Confidentiality and Privacy, G)

Additionally, the ACA Code of Ethics (ACA, 2005a) is more specific on the issue of court-ordered disclosures.

> When subpoenaed to release confidential or privileged information without a client's permission, counselors obtain written, informed consent from the client or take steps to prohibit the disclosure or have it limited as narrowly as possible due to potential harm to the client or counseling relationship. (ACA Code of Ethics, B.2.c.)

8. Requirements of Third-Party Payers

Grief counselors with appropriate training, licensure, and professional credentials expect to be paid for counseling services. Although the legitimacy of charging professional fees is understood almost universally, explanation of the fee-for-service arrangement during the informed consent process is good ethical practice, good counseling practice, and good business practice. Many clients carry health insurance that underwrites some or all of the costs of professional grief counseling. Clients with insurance deserve the benefits they paid for, and third-party payers are entitled to valid claims against those policies. Grief counselors and their billing staffs are responsible for verifying the claim information submitted to insurers by policy-holding clients.

Obviously, for grief counselors to provide the verification third-party payers need, some confidential counseling information must be disclosed. The commerce of third-party insurers reimbursing claims for mental health services is not controversial, but just how much confidential information grief counselors disclose in order to be paid, or for clients to be reimbursed, is unsettled. The minimum necessary information required to document a claim usually includes the client's name, identifying demographic data, dates of service, type of service rendered (e.g., individual, family, or group counseling), duration of sessions (e.g., 60 or 90 minutes), and the associated professional charges. However, the controversies begin when additional information is requested, such as clients' diagnoses, symptom presentation, and case summaries. Many third-party payers have multiple tiers of mental health benefits, with complex decision rules in place to determine which claims will be reimbursed and at what level of coverage. This is especially true of managed care companies, which are often involved in monitoring the type of counseling provided, and its progress, as a prerequisite for continuing authorization of services.

For example, the severity of the client's diagnosis may make a tremendous difference in applicable coverage. A grieving client diagnosed as having a major depressive disorder may merit considerable reimbursement, whereas a client diagnosed descriptively with "bereavement" as a focus of care may be deemed ineligible for any coverage on the rationale that simple grieving is not a mental health problem warranting professional counseling. The ethical questions generated by controversies over diagnosis and access to care are addressed in Chapter 10, "Ethical Controversies in Grief Counseling." The question here is how much confidential information should the grief counselor disclose in order to justify reimbursement? Will information about diagnosis, symptoms, or complicating factors be protected by third-party payers, or will it be used to prejudice future claims or bias eligibility for future coverage? Will disclosure of preexisting problems (e.g., a mood disorder with onset prior to the loss), or of concomitant problems (e.g., ongoing substance abuse), disqualify or limit the client's health care coverage as it pertains to the grief-related episode?

In light of these uncertainties, the most prudent course of action for grief counselors is to exercise the ethical principle of fidelity. Grief counselors disclose the minimum necessary confidential information to third-party payers in order to validate claims for services. When completing written forms that explain services rendered or talking over the telephone with a managed care overseer, grief counselors reveal only information relevant to the matter under discussion. Similar to disclosures during court testimony, contextual information is provided only on an as-needed basis. This is a situation where the Golden Rule applies—protect the client's confidential counseling information the same way you would want the counselor to protect your information if you were the client.

Another ethical dilemma can arise when making disclosures to third-party payers. Because more comprehensive coverage may be available if a client's diagnosis is more severe, there may be a temptation to exaggerate the client's level of distress so as to justify assigning a more severe diagnosis. Sometimes called *up-coding* (Welfel, 2006), such a practice is fraudulent and should be studiously avoided. Up-coding justified as promoting client welfare—better financial benefits for the client, lower out-of-pocket expenses, or greater latitude in number of counseling sessions allowed—is rationalization. These practices likely benefit the counselor's compensation and confound the issue of just whose welfare is being served. Ethical practice of grief counseling in dealing with third-party payers means not only rendering the minimum necessary information needed for reimbursement but also providing an objectively determined assessment of the client's condition and projected need for service.

HIPAA

The Health Insurance Portability and Accountability Act (1996), or Public Law 104–191, set a federal standard for privacy protections in health and mental health settings that became effective in 2003. Because many state laws are even more stringent in protecting privacy, HIPAA regulations can be thought of as the minimum necessary requirements for handling clients' protected health information. Protected health information includes individually identifiable data such as name, address, zip code, phone numbers, Social Security number, date of birth, insurance policy numbers, agency-assigned case numbers, and the like.

HIPAA (1996) governs how such health information is protected in maintenance of records, payment transactions, electronic transmissions, and communications with individuals or entities beyond a provider's office staff or an agency's workforce. For example, when records are kept electronically in a computerized system, particularly one connected to the Internet, the grief counselor should employ a sufficient series of firewalls, virus protections, passwords, and encryption programs to ensure confidentiality from hackers. When client information is stored on collateral devices such as an external hard drive, CD, or flash drive, these devices need to be stored safely and their information protected by password, encryption, or both. When data are sent to a third-party payer, such as an insurance company or managed care organization, special precautions must be taken to guarantee the confidentiality of that information, particularly faxes and electronic transmissions (see Chapter 9 on Internet counseling). Once information leaves the counselor's purview, there is no way to guarantee its proper disposition by others. Thus, counseling clients are required to sign an authorization to release information when the grief counselor is sending written documents to someone outside the office or agency where the grief counseling is provided.

The first step in HIPAA (1996) compliance is to provide clients with a notice of privacy practices. Such a notice outlines plainly how clients' confidential counseling information will be safeguarded, and what they should do if they want to review their protected health information or, when necessary, request that it be amended. Clients' consent is secured at the outset of counseling to use their protected health information to provide treatment, bill for services, and otherwise maintain operational practices within the office or agency where the counseling is conducted. Consent authorizes office staff and subordinates to access, use, or transmit confidential counseling information. Support staff are agents of the professional, and the grief counselor holds administrative responsibility for workers honoring the confidentiality of client information.

It is optimal to maintain client records so that case material could be reviewed, for audits or research efforts, without revealing client identities or compromising protected health information. De-identifying records for research purposes means denuding them of protected health information and cataloging them according to a research-based numerical system independent of counseling case numbers. Generally, text information such as narrative reports and progress notes is not a problem unless it contains specific references that could provide a "crosswalk" back to the client's identity. For example, if the client is described as "CEO of Quarry Stone Mining Company in Hardrock, Nevada" or "4th grade teacher at George Washington Elementary School in Cherrytown, Maryland," then it may be possible for a reader to trace back and discover the client's identity. The safest practice is to refer to clients in the body of reports as "client" instead of using their names and to describe information on employment or civic positions in generic terms. In the previous example, the clients' identities could be disguised easily with descriptions such as "an executive with a local manufacturing company" or "an elementary educator in a suburban school district" and still convey the essential demographic features.

CONFIDENTIALITY IN RECORD KEEPING

Keeping adequate records is a professional responsibility, and keeping records confidential is an ethical responsibility. Our discussions of consent and confidentiality should have convinced readers of the importance of maintaining thorough records of counseling activities and client contacts, including documentation of any exceptions made to counselor–client confidentiality and the rationale for such action. Grief counselors need to maintain client records with the utmost care, so that untoward breaches of confidentiality resulting from mishandled case records do not occur. It is much like guarding against errant verbal disclosures. The ADEC Code of Ethics specifies several key points of the grief counselor's obligation to ensure confidentiality of clients' counseling records.

> Members safeguard written and recorded information about clients and are alert to potential threats to confidentiality in duplications processes, in use of computer equipment, and in electronic mail and facsimile transmission. (ADEC Code of Ethics, VIII. Confidentiality and Privacy, F)

> Members clarify and establish interpersonal relations and working agreements with supervisors and subordinates especially in matters of professional relationships, confidentiality, distinctions between public and private material, maintenance and use of recorded information, and work load accountability. (ADEC Code of Ethics, V. Responsibility to Employers, A)

Of special significance here is the grief counselor's responsibility to train and supervise subordinates in how to protect clients' confidentiality, especially when dealing with client records. Record keeping begins with the first phone call placed by the client or the referring professional when seeking an appointment. It continues through the informed consent process, taking of payment or insurance information, and receiving information about the client from other professionals. Logs of phone calls, letters, e-mails, or other communications from clients are also part of the counseling records. Of course, the evaluation reports or progress notes of consultation sessions generated by the grief counselor make up the heart of client records. But even these are often seen and handled by subordinates. Staff should be trained so that their handling of client records when performing clerical tasks is an extension of the careful stewardship exercised by the grief counselor. Any misstep by a subordinate not only reflects badly on the grief counselor's professional reputation but also creates potential professional liability.

Counseling records may be kept in either paper or electronic format, or both. Many offices and agencies maintain records in both formats in order to achieve a backup function. Regardless of whether the paper format, such as charts and folders, or the computerized system is considered the primary one, both must be safeguarded. Filing cabinets or storage areas where clients' paper records are kept need to be locked securely and access restricted only to personnel with a direct need to retrieve them. Records in electronic formats must be protected in accordance with HIPAA guidelines explained in the previous section of this chapter. When electronic records are the primary format, and the backup consists of information transferred to collateral devices such as an external hard drive, access to these devices must be protected by password or encryption, and the physical device must be stored securely in the same manner as paper records.

Although these measures offer reasonable protection against breaches of confidentiality from criminal break-ins or computer hackers, carelessness by grief counselors and office staff may be the biggest culprit when records are not kept confidential. For instance, how often are client charts left on countertops, desks, or work areas where other clients or visitors may observe names and other personal client information? In offices with electronic records, how often are paper copies made for use in everyday practice but then not shredded or properly safeguarded? How often are laptop computers loaded with client files, taken home after office hours, and put to use in other ways, either by the grief counselor or by other family members? Do counselors view, edit, or write client entries on laptops during commutes on planes or trains where strangers seated nearby can view confidential material? In trying to use time efficiently, how often do busy grief counselors carry paper records with them to review while waiting at the barber shop, hairdresser, or pharmacy where they inadvertently expose confidential material to others? How often are paper records or laptop computers transported in the grief counselor's personal vehicle, which others may enter or exit, affording an unanticipated opportunity for prying or outright loss of confidential material? How often are laptop computers put at risk of theft by imprudent handling in taxis, hotels, airports, or public restrooms? (cf. Zur & Barnett, 2008). Unfortunately, this list of hypothetical scenarios where confidential records are exposed is inexhaustible.

To combat carelessness and keep proper boundaries around counseling records, whether paper or electronic, we suggest treating records with a "bricks-and-mortar" mentality. Simply put, this means thinking of the practice's counseling records as part and parcel of the office or agency's physical structure. Records of the professional practice belong at the practice location, not in the grief counselor's briefcase, handbag, car, home, or personal computer. Operating with a bricks-and-mortar mentality can prevent many of the confidential breaches just mentioned. Although this type of boundary enforcement is ideal, it may not be practical in all circumstances. Sometimes computers must travel with the counselor, or records must be reviewed away from the office. Some practitioners travel to multiple office locations, and carrying client records on a laptop or flash drive is the only practical solution. Even in these instances, fostering an acute awareness that records belong with the practice makes the grief counselor a more conscientious custodian of confidential client records and heightens vigilance to potentially compromising situations. Zur and Barnett (2008) warn that "psychotherapists who carry patient records with them are at risk for security violations and may be held legally and ethically accountable for security and privacy breaches" (p. 22). They suggest treating one's laptop computer like the cash in one's wallet and never leaving it unattended.

Two additional points concern the perpetuity of keeping records confidential. First, states and jurisdictions have specific laws regarding how long client records must be maintained after the last client contact. Again, knowing these statutory regulations and abiding by them are crucial for the ethical practice of grief counseling, as contained in a specific directive to this effect in the ADEC Code of Ethics.

> Members keep records and other information related to clients confidential for at least the number of years determined by laws in the member's state, province or country of practice. (ADEC Code of Ethics, GC-I. Responsibility to Those Served, H)

However, keep in mind that statutory laws generally govern the *minimum* time period that counseling records must be maintained. Yet for many grief counselors, once a professional relationship is inaugurated with a client, that client is eligible to return at any point in the future for continuing care, even if a mutually agreed termination is enacted at some point in time. Such an open door policy is most common among counselors who view an individual's development as a continuously unfolding process throughout the life cycle and who recognize that various life transitions, including loss in all its forms, may necessitate additional consultation. Some refer to this philosophy as, "Once a client, always a client." When adhering to this philosophy, it is logical for grief counselors to maintain records indefinitely in the event that clients request additional counseling services in the future.

A mindset of maintaining records indefinitely leads to a second point regarding perpetuity. What happens to confidential records when grief counselors move, retire, or close their practices? Chapter 13, "Moving or Closing a Practice," deals extensively with this question and provides detailed guidance for the many issues involved. In short, when grief counselors work for agencies or institutions with multiple professionals on staff, there are usually established provisions for how client records are maintained beyond the tenure of any individual provider. Or grief counselors in private or solo practice make arrangements with a local colleague to provide maintenance of confidential records. Likewise, as described in Chapter 3, a Professional Will provides for similar contingencies should a grief counselor become incapacitated or die unexpectedly. In Chapter 4, we also urged declaring such arrangements in informed consent documents.

CONFIDENTIALITY AND HIV/AIDS

Despite advances in treatment of human immunodeficiency virus (HIV) and acquired immune deficiency syndrome (AIDS), HIV is still a potentially life-threatening illness (Kalichman, 2003). Farber and McDaniel (1999) elucidated how newer, highly active antiretroviral therapies have supplanted previous expectations of dying with hope that HIV can be managed as a chronic, rather than a terminal, condition. HIV is contagious through unprotected sexual contact or needle sharing during injection-drug use. Contracting HIV disease presents serious health risks that can be fatal.

Although some grief counselors work exclusively with individuals suffering with HIV/AIDS, every grief counselor needs to be prepared to deal with cases from the HIV health epidemic. The existential issues raised by living with HIV/AIDS are ones that grief counselors are ideally suited to address with clients affected by this disease. At the same time, there are confidentiality concerns involved in the care of persons with HIV/AIDS. Grief counselors should be aware of these and know what is lawfully required in their state or jurisdiction.

Because HIV is a communicable, potentially life-threatening disease, most states require physicians and laboratory workers involved in the diagnosis of this condition to report positive test results to state health departments (Kalichman, 2003). This information is sometimes passed on to federal oversight agencies, such as the Centers for Disease

Control and Prevention. Otherwise, information on HIV status is confidential, just like any other private medical information. Typically, a mental health professional or a grief counselor does not carry any routine reporting obligation should clients disclose that they have HIV/AIDS, unless that counselor works as part of a multidisciplinary team in a treatment center that does diagnostic testing. Most frequently, clients who reveal to a grief counselor their positive HIV status have already been tested, and any attendant reporting obligation has been accomplished by the diagnosing physician or testing laboratory. Should clients suspect possible exposure to HIV, the responsible grief counselor urges them to seek diagnostic testing immediately, both for the sake of starting early, postexposure treatment, if needed, and for the sake of not spreading the virus unwittingly should they test positive.

Confidentiality dilemmas posed by clients with HIV/AIDS pertain to whether the grief counselor has a *Tarasoff*-type duty to warn and protect third parties from HIV exposure when a client knowingly engages in risky sexual or drug-use practices that could spread the disease without regard for the safety of other individuals involved. In a cogent exposition of such dilemmas, Chenneville (2000) described how breaching confidentiality with HIV-positive clients may erode the solvency of the therapeutic relationship and thus potentially harm the client's overall well-being. Likewise, Driscoll (1992) argued that, because psychotherapeutic relationships have a covenant quality involving a high level of fidelity, breaching confidence with HIV-positive clients violates the primary bond of trust and interferes with the therapeutic endeavor toward client insight and behavioral change. Yet keeping strict therapeutic confidentiality may result in harm to third parties through exposure to a potentially lethal virus. How does the grief counselor negotiate the resulting double bind?

Unfortunately, the ADEC Code of Ethics does not address directly the ethical issues involved when working with the potential dangers of HIV/AIDS beyond a general statement about how the grief counselor "strives to improve the health and well-being of the individual and society" (ADEC Code of Ethics, Basic Tenets, 4). However, the ACA Code of Ethics (ACA, 2005a) does address the limits of confidentiality with individuals with life-threatening, contagious diseases.

> When clients disclose that they have a disease commonly known to be both communicable and life threatening, counselors may be justified in disclosing information to identifiable third parties, if they are known to be

> at demonstrable and high risk of contracting the disease. Prior to making a disclosure, counselors confirm that there is such a diagnosis and assess the intent of clients to inform the third parties about their disease or to engage in any behaviors that may be harmful to an identifiable third party. (ACA Code of Ethics, B.2.b.)

The first line of defense against the spread of HIV/AIDS is for HIV-positive individuals to inform their sexual partners or drug-use associates. Accordingly, counselors working with HIV-positive clients should first urge responsible disclosure by clients to anyone they may put at risk of infection. When clients are unwilling to disclose their HIV status, or their reliability in doing so is questionable and cannot be verified, then the counselor's duty to protect comes into play. Counselors convinced of their need to breach confidentiality in order to protect third parties at risk do so only after notifying clients of their plan. Of course, the counselor should document carefully the procedures used and steps taken when exercising duty to protect with HIV/AIDS, so that the rationale for the counselor's actions is clear in the event of a later liability claim by the client.

Chenneville (2000) proposed a decision-making model for providers facing the prospect of disclosing confidential counseling information to protect a third party from HIV-related danger. Two pivotal elements in the decision are *foreseeability* of harm and *identifiability* of victims. Several variables influence foreseeability of harm. The level of risk inherent in the client's sexual or drug-use practices matters, such as whether condoms are used or whether needles are cleaned. Also the number of sexual partners should be considered and whether these contacts are more casual or more intimate. Personality variables such as impulsivity or aggressiveness, as well as submissiveness or shyness, can increase risk. Concomitant substance abuse also increases risk by decreasing inhibitions and planfulness. Identifiability of the victim refers to knowing that a specific person is at risk of exposure, such as a spouse or lover, whose identity is easily attainable. Also, risk to a specific group or class of persons, such as members of a certain social club or residents of a particular boarding house, constitutes a higher level of identifiability.

A grief counselor's knowledge of specific laws governing HIV/AIDS disclosure in the state or jurisdiction in which they practice is crucial. Some states have partner identification programs that allow mental health professionals to disclose to the health department confidential information about clients engaging in behavior that is high risk for HIV contagion. In turn, the health departments handle notification of potential victims without revealing the identity of the person by whom they may have been exposed to HIV. This allows for maximum confidentiality to be retained by the client while still serving the public welfare by reasonably protecting at-risk third parties. Some states with partner notification programs *permit* counselors the option of relying on these programs to fulfill any duty to protect, whereas other states *require* such notification. Grief counselors must stay current on statutory and case law that determine their legal obligation.

A final note is in order on disclosures involving clients with HIV/AIDS. HIV and its sources of transmission (e.g., risky sexual behavior and indiscriminate needle-sharing during injection drug use) can incite polarized and prejudicial responses in people. Grief counselors are not immune to this. Countertransference feelings based on moral positions, spiritual beliefs, or political views can stir judgmental reactions in the grief counselor that interfere with therapeutic neutrality. When working with clients who have HIV/AIDS, grief counselors need to ensure that any actions taken to warn and protect third parties, whether directly or through partner notification programs, are not discriminatory or punitive in nature (Koocher & Keith-Spiegel, 2008). Instead, decisions to breach confidentiality in cases of HIV/AIDS, where there is a foreseeable danger to an identifiable person or persons, should be made with reasoned consideration of the potential danger involved and should strike a balance between the client's right to privacy and the rights of third parties at risk (Welfel, 2006).

POSTMORTEM DISCLOSURE

An ethical dilemma faced more frequently by grief counselors than most other health care professionals is that of postmortem disclosure. Because grief counselors work specifically with the dying and the bereaved, questions may be raised by family and associates of the decedent about the cause of death, health conditions antecedent to the person's demise, coroner's reports, or autopsy findings. In handling such situations, it is of paramount importance to recognize that *a deceased person's right to confidentiality does not expire at death.* As articulated by Kottow (1986), "Death does not cancel the obligation of confidentiality which remains of import to all survivors within the radius of interests of the deceased" (p. 119). Legally, the prerogative for allowing postmortem disclosure of the decedent's confidential health information rests with the personal representative—ordinarily, the next of kin, or sometimes the executor of the estate. Whether the decedent's private medical or counseling records are released to anyone is determined by that personal representative. However, competing agendas and mixed motivations can easily complicate this seemingly clear-cut rule, as illustrated by the complexity of the following extended case example.

Case Example

A remarried, White woman in her 70s sought counseling to assist with recurrent major depression as well as problems with two of three adult children—an estranged son and a querulous daughter. After the second counseling session, the client got into a heated telephone argument with the difficult daughter. Abruptly, she completed suicide by shooting herself in the chest. A few months later, the other daughter, with whom she had been on good terms, found an appointment card with the grief counselor's name and deduced correctly that her mother had been in counseling. She contacted the counselor, asking to talk about her mother's state of mind prior to her suicide.

Although the grief counselor was sympathetic to the daughter's request—for compassionate reasons of wanting to aid the surviving daughter's adjustment—it was not immediately clear whether this daughter had a legal right to access her mother's confidential counseling information. Consultation with a knowledgeable attorney revealed that, in the state where the mother had resided, the executor of the mother's estate was considered the personal representative for decision making about postmortem disclosure of health care information, rather than the mother's second husband as next of kin. The executor was the estranged son. It was necessary for the inquiring daughter to get her brother's written permission to be able to discuss with the grief counselor anything about her mother's psychological and emotional state in the weeks preceding her suicide. The daughter did so.

Once it was established that the daughter could legally talk with the grief counselor, a meeting took place. However, when taking the mother's developmental history, the grief counselor had discovered that the mother had had a teenage pregnancy out of wedlock and had adopted out the baby. Her three children from her first marriage were never told. Part of the grief counselor's dilemma was whether to disclose this information.

Several considerations influenced the grief counselor's decision. By principle, any disclosures of confidential information should be directly related to the matter at hand. Protecting the client's confidentiality, even postmortem, requires discretion in relaying contextual information. The pregnancy and adoption decades ago may not have been directly relevant to the mother's suicide, or were they? Then again, the adoption episode was documented in the mother's counseling records that the inquiring daughter would be entitled legally to read, if she requested. The mother's suicide appeared to have a high degree of impulsivity and was not anticipated; she had denied suicidal ideation or intent on the initial evaluation interview. So there had never been any direct discussion with the grief counselor about the mother's wishes regarding postmortem disclosure of her confidential health information. How did the grief counselor balance these various considerations when meeting with the daughter?

During the meeting, the daughter expressed gratitude to the grief counselor for the attempt to help her mother. They discussed the mother's recent conflict with the sister as well as her extensive history with lifelong depression, including previous suicidal behavior, psychiatric hospitalizations, and electroconvulsive therapy. The daughter was attempting to understand her mother's mindset and also gauge what this "family history of suicide" meant for her and her children's mental health. When the direction of the discussion led the daughter to observe, "I think my mother was an unhappy person her whole life," the grief counselor chose to reveal the history of the pregnancy and adoption as relevant contextual information for helping the daughter come to a conceptual understanding of her mother's suicide. The meeting ended amicably. The daughter asked if she could be seen as a client by the grief counselor in the future should she find that she was having trouble dealing with her mother's death.

Analysis With the Five P Model

This case example raises at least as many questions as it answers about postmortem disclosure of confidential counseling information. How would one apply the Five P Model of ethical reasoning in this situation?

Person

First, the client is a deceased person to whom the grief counselor still owes professional loyalty and whose welfare the counselor has an obligation to promote. The client's privacy rights do not end with her death. Unfortunately, her preferences for how to handle her personal health information after her death are not known. Extrapolating from the client's age cohort and from the fact that she chose not to tell her children about the teenage pregnancy, it could be assumed that her sense of privacy might be fairly strong and that certain personal information would never be conveyed even to an adult child. Yet this remains conjecture.

Although the surviving daughter is a protagonist in the scenario, her agenda does not necessarily supersede the client's privacy rights. However, the fact that the client had a good relationship with the inquiring daughter may be a consideration in gauging how extensively disclosures are made.

Problem

Second, the problem is defined as one of protecting posthumously the client's confidential counseling information from unnecessary disclosures. This requires determining not only *to whom* information can be conveyed legally and ethically, but also *how much* information is disclosed to a third party. With the executor brother's permission, the daughter has a legal right to access her mother's personal counseling information, but the grief counselor still exercises some discretion in judging exactly what to disclose. Because the client never told any of her children, including the inquiring daughter, about her teenage pregnancy, does this mean the client would *not* have wanted this information to be disclosed?

Place

Third, the relevance of place in this discussion revolves around the mother's counseling in a health care setting so that HIPAA (1996) guidelines apply, in concert with any state statutes or privacy laws. These regulations are intended to ensure the privacy of the mother's protected health information, even after death. If the HIPAA regulations are more stringent in protecting privacy than are state laws in the jurisdiction where the mother resided, then the federal code takes precedence. Conversely, if state laws are stricter than HIPAA guidelines, state law prevails.

Principles

Fidelity is the chief ethical principle, the fourth aspect of the Five P Model, that applies in this case. Fidelity, which is the basis for confidentiality and loyalty to the client, operates here in that the client's privilege does not end with death. Rather, privilege continues under the auspices of the client's personal representative who holds legal authority over archived health information. There is a parallel to how an executor handles disposition of a deceased person's estate. Instead of death creating open season for claims on the deceased person's effects and possessions, the executor has power to allocate such assets in accord with the deceased person's intentions, not the preferences of the potential beneficiaries. In this case, the brother exercised his discretion by permitting his sister to talk with the mother's grief counselor. But would he have done the same for the querulous daughter with whom the client was arguing immediately before the client shot herself?

Fidelity demands that confidentiality be maintained out of loyalty to the client unless there is a compelling reason to disclose information. Even when disclosure is required, the professional grief counselor is still bound to reveal only that information needed for addressing a particular matter. The question of how much information is enough is quite pertinent in this case, particularly as it pertains to the client's history of teenage pregnancy and adoption. Is it a violation of the client's privacy to disclose this to the daughter? Or is such information part and parcel of understanding the client's apparent lifelong depression and unhappiness? Does disclosing this information sully the mother's reputation in the daughter's eyes (violating the principle of nonmaleficence)? Or, does disclosing it bolster the daughter's chances of constructing an understandable explanation for why the mother killed herself (accomplishing a good outcome and so achieving beneficence)? Could the latter explanation aid the daughter's adjustment as a suicide survivor and potentially offset the increased risk of suicide on the part of the children and grandchildren brought about by introducing the permanent variable of positive family history of suicide? Reasoning that disclosure may potentially help several other family members is based on the utilitarian theory of ethics—the greatest good for the greatest number.

Guidance from ethics codes and legal sources also constitutes important information about the principles involved in resolving a case such as this one. Although the ADEC Code of Ethics is silent on the specific topic of postmortem disclosure, the ACA Code of Ethics (2005a) directly addresses the topic of confidentiality for deceased clients.

> Counselors protect the confidentiality of deceased clients, consistent with legal requirements and agency or setting policies. (ACA Code of Ethics, B.3.f.)

However, no further guidelines are provided on how to handle difficult dilemmas such as those posed by this case example.

The American Medical Association (AMA) Council on Ethical and Judicial Affairs (2000) studied the topic of postmortem confidentiality and proposed that all information within a deceased person's medical record should be kept confidential to the greatest possible degree. They declared that confidentiality protections after death should be equal to those in force during the person's life. When disclosure is considered, several questions arise. What is the likelihood of imminent harm to any identifiable persons or to the public health? Conversely, is there a potential benefit to at-risk individuals or to the general public, such as a communicable or inherited disease being prevented or treated? Did the deceased person make any verifiable statements or leave any specific directives regarding postmortem release of personal health information? How might disclosure of confidential information impact the reputation of the deceased? Finally, the AMA council warned professionals to consider carefully whether the prospect of personal gain, such as releasing private health information of celebrity clients for purposes of publication or other self-enhancing or profit-driven endeavors, would unduly influence their ethical obligation to preserve confidentiality.

Other scholars have written on the subject of postmortem disclosure of confidential health information. Werth, Burke, and Bardash (2002) acknowledged grudgingly that grief counselors and other health care professionals comply narrowly with the letter of the law when releasing confidential counseling data to the deceased client's legal representative. Yet they questioned whether the spirit of the law is fulfilled by perfunctory adherence to legal obligations. They suggested greater weight be given to whether it is in the client's best interest for records to be released. Additionally, Burke (1995) asked about the impact on counseling when active clients recognize that the information they confide to their counselor may be disclosed after their deaths, possibly to the very persons who may figure prominently in their conflicts and concerns, such as family members. Will clients still reveal their deepest fears, concerns, and vulnerabilities?

In a similar vein, Berg (2001) found the most compelling argument justifying postmortem disclosure is when surviving individuals stand to realize potentially helpful health benefits from disclosure. This might be family members seeking information important to their own health profiles, public health authorities attempting disease control or prevention, or even biomedical researchers developing cures. The weakest argument for disclosure is what Berg termed "general interest," such as the curiosity of members of the media or biographers. Berg advocated balancing the need for disclosure against the need for confidentiality. Applying that logic to this case example shows how sound ethical practice involves not just knowing the law, but also considering thoughtfully how one's ethical principles can be discharged faithfully in situations where there are no easy answers.

Process

The process of settling what to do in this case, the fifth aspect of the Five P Model, involved several steps in order to respond appropriately. The grief counselor first consulted a knowledgeable attorney to determine the legal status of the daughter's request and to establish whether there was a legitimate basis for communicating with the daughter. Next the counselor consulted the collateral sources mentioned above for guidance on how much confidential counseling information to disclose postmortem while still maintaining fidelity to the client even after death.

In the end, the discussion with the daughter was quite comprehensive and covered all the major historical factors in the client's life, including her previous suicide attempts and psychiatric hospitalizations as well as her teenage pregnancy and adoption out of the daughter's half-sibling. In attempting to strike a balance between competing considerations of privacy protection for the deceased client and possible health benefits for the survivors, the grief counselor reasoned that neutralizing or minimizing any increased risk for suicide or mood disorder among the surviving family members warranted such a comprehensive discussion of the client's mental health problems.

Because the daughter's attitude toward the client was compassionate rather than critical, it seemed that disclosure of the teenage pregnancy and adoption would not sully the client's reputation. On the other hand, disclosure seemed to contribute to a fuller appreciation of the client's lifelong depression. At a practical level, the counselor could see that the daughter was intent on understanding what had happened to her mother and, if she was not satisfied with the discussion with the counselor, could elect to view the entire medical record. Therefore, the counselor elected to disclose the pregnancy and adoption when its significance could be discussed with the surviving daughter rather than omitting this important history only to have it be potentially discovered later by the daughter.

CONFIDENTIALITY IN EDUCATION AND RESEARCH

Grief counselors engaged in education and research incur additional responsibilities for preserving confidentiality. These responsibilities apply when case examples are used for teaching purposes, when students or trainees divulge personal information during educational endeavors, and when handling data collected from research participants.

Case Examples

Seasoned educators know that case examples are the spice that brings counseling theory and research findings to life. When students and trainees can see how ideas and concepts apply in the actual practice of grief counseling, they more often consolidate the lessons to be learned. Yet how do grief counselors incorporate case material into their lectures and presentations without violating the confidentiality pledged to the clients and families whom they counsel?

When describing counseling cases in class, displaying clients' artistic and creative products, or reviewing verbatim transcripts, the task of preserving client confidentiality is relatively straightforward. As required by HIPAA (1996), these descriptions need to be stripped of any specific identifying information such as names, positions, titles, and so forth. Another helpful device is to alter contextual aspects of the client's history by "scrambling" the facts sufficiently so as to disguise the actual clients involved. For example, switching the gender of the main character, substituting a different terminal illness, or modifying the individual's loss history camouflages the identity of the original client who inspired the vignette. These same strategies generally apply to written case summaries published in journal articles or books. As long as the client's anonymity is maintained, these uses of client information do not violate the spirit of confidentiality. The ADEC Code of Ethics uses anonymity as the standard for permitting such disclosures.

> Members adequately disguise clinical and other material they use in teaching, writing, and public speaking in order to preserve client anonymity; an alternative is to obtain adequate prior client consent. (ADEC Code of Ethics, VIII. Confidentiality and Privacy, H)

Sometimes grief counselors are asked to present public lectures or address self-help groups in their communities, such as the Compassionate Friends or Survivors of Suicide. In these instances, greater caution is warranted in using case examples (see Chapter 11, "Potential Pitfalls of Public Service"). The best policy is to ask clients' permission for such specific uses of their case material. Many clients are pleased to contribute their story to a legitimate educational endeavor that trains professionals to be more sensitive to loss-related issues or that may help other grieving persons to know they are not alone. Still, some may prefer not to have their story retold, and when clients feel this way, their preference should be respected. When in doubt about the client's sensibilities, it is better to err on the side of caution by not using that case as an example in teaching.

Teaching uses of audio recordings, video images, or live observation of actual clients present an additional challenge to confidentiality. Here, the client's persona and unique story are indivisible from the case presentation so that, even though their actual identity may remain private, much confidential counseling information about them is conveyed. The ADEC Code of Ethics addresses this issue.

> Members obtain informed client consent prior to recording or allowing third party observation of their activities. Members inform clients about the purpose of recording/observing, who will have access to the recording and under what conditions, and the disposition of the recording. Client consent for one purpose is not valid for another or different purpose. (ADEC Code of Ethics, VIII. Confidentiality and Privacy, C)

Besides securing client consent for the specific use of recorded or observed sessions, it is important to remember that this consent is not automatically transferable for another purpose. For example, a client treated by a counselor-in-training may consent to videotaping of counseling sessions so that a supervising counselor may review the trainee's work and provide constructive criticism. Those videotapes should not then be used as case examples in the supervisor's graduate course on grief counseling, unless the client has specifically extended permission for that additional use. On the other hand, a grief counselor may show lengthy excerpts from a videotaped interview to hundreds of professionals at an educational conference as long as the client consents to that specific use.

Disclosures by Students or Trainees

The ADEC Code of Ethics speaks clearly on how grief counselors and death educators conduct themselves when students and trainees divulge personal information about themselves in the course of academic work.

> Members who employ exercises and simulations which draw upon participant thoughts, feelings, and memories must ensure that appropriate professional assistance is available to participants during and following those learning experiences. (ADEC Code of Ethics, DE-I. Responsibility to Others, D)
>
> When a student is expected to disclose relatively intimate or personal information about themselves as part of their learning experience, educators and supervisors shall not evaluate the student based upon such self-disclosure. The degree of self-disclosure will be respected without coercion or punitive measures. (ADEC Code of Ethics, DE-I. Responsibility to Others, E)
>
> When a program or learning experience has a focus upon self-disclosure, self-understanding or growth, members ensure the confidentiality and privacy of information shared in this setting. (ADEC Code of Ethics, DE-I. Responsibility to Others, F)

Of special significance here are the personal disclosures elicited from students during experiential learning exercises, such as simulations, psychodrama (Dayton, 1994), family sculpting (Satir, 1972), or Gestalt methods (Melnick, Nevis, & Shub, 2005). Because of the importance of developing the death competence needed for ethical practice of grief counseling, trainees need to confront their own mortality and be comfortable with it. For this reason, experiential learning is emphasized more during graduate training for grief counseling than in many other traditional academic disciplines. The chief operating rule of thumb is that personal disclosures made by trainees during teaching or supervision, especially in the context of experiential exercises, should be honored with the same level of confidentiality accorded to client disclosures during formal grief counseling. Faculty trainers should respect students' privacy by following the principles outlined previously in this chapter for guarding confidentiality, within the limits of bona fide exceptions.

Data From Research Participants

Human research subjects are first and foremost people who deserve basic respect and dignity. Furthermore, in the United States, the rights of research participants and the confidentiality of their research records are protected by law (U.S. Department of Health and Human Services, 2005). See Chapter 2 on ethical decision making for a discussion on international standards to protect the rights of research participants. Also, the ADEC Code of Ethics requires that "confidentiality is protected" for human subjects participating in research (ADEC Code of Ethics, RT-II. Responsibility to Research Participants, D.1.b.).

Handling confidentially the data collected from research participants employs the same guidelines used for de-identifying case material for teaching and protecting disclosures by clients or students. When quantitative researchers compile data for statistical analysis, unique case numbers are assigned that disconnect participants' research data from identifying information such as names, Social Security numbers, or clinical record numbers. Quantitative results are usually presented as aggregates or composites showing group characteristics or differences so that no individual participant is identified. If case examples are used, the same procedures followed when disguising case material for teaching purposes apply.

Qualitative researchers face slightly different challenges to confidentiality because they rely more heavily on biographical or narrative data, yet the same protections against individual identification of participants is in force. Certainly qualitative research data can be gathered, synthesized, and reported without compromising the actual identity of participants. Confidentiality can be maintained through disguises and camouflages similar to those described earlier. When political figures or cultural celebrities are studied as subjects of grief research, any reputable information available in the public domain can be disclosed as long as an attitude of respect is maintained in how descriptions are crafted. When qualitative researchers investigate prominent individuals by interviewing relatives or exploring family archives, such information should be treated confidentially and disclosed to others only with the consent of the individual under study or, when the study subject is deceased, the family.

CLIENTS' EXPECTATIONS OF CONFIDENTIALITY

Having reviewed the ethical mandates for confidentiality, the situations in which exceptions to confidentiality operate, and special challenges to confidentiality posed by HIV/AIDS, postmortem disclosure, and educational or research endeavors, we now turn our attention to consumers' expectations of confidentiality. What do clients expect of the grief counselors to whom they have entrusted highly sensitive personal information about their thoughts, feelings, perceptions, and experiences? How well do counselors keep the trust they have been given? These questions go to the very heart of ethical principles of fidelity and respect—the core values underlying confidentiality in the counselor–client relationship.

All grief counselors are human, and that humanity is a two-edged sword. It is humanity that enables the grief counselor to truly empathize with clients and care enough to counsel effectively (Gamble, 2002). However, that same humanity carries with it natural inclinations to talk about the work and share with others the burdens and triumphs of a counseling career. Welfel (2006) commented astutely on the challenge to confidentiality posed by counselors' all-too-human tendencies to disclose client information to others.

> Honoring confidentiality requires integrity precisely because it can be difficult—the human tendency to want to share experiences does not bypass mental health professionals simply because they have a credential, nor does the desire to discuss important or difficult issues that arise at work end with entrance into this profession. (p. 67)

Woody (1999) used his experience as an attorney advising and defending mental health practitioners to offer a sobering assessment of the numerous ways in which professionals inadvertently lower their guard and inappropriately reveal confidential information to family members and others. According to Woody, these "domestic violations" of confidentiality come about chiefly because practitioners do not clearly separate their professional and personal lives. Grief counselors who believe they are doing a good job maintaining and preserving confidentiality are urged to review Woody's inventory of potentially compromising scenarios—ones that too often become the Achilles' heel of otherwise well-intentioned efforts at keeping client information confidential. Arrangements such as an office in the home or a shared family computer can result in breaches of confidentiality. Habits such as discussing cases at the family dinner table, even anonymously, or confiding in a spouse, who is unprepared or ill-equipped to honor clients' confidentiality, can result in violations.

As a conclusion to this chapter on confidentiality, we offer readers an opportunity to take a self-assessment test of their own proclivities and practices where professional confidentiality is concerned. Reading this chapter should acquaint newcomers to the field of grief counseling with the basic information needed to protect confidentiality and provide mature grief counselors a reflective refresher on the topic. This is an ideal opportunity to ponder just how well each of us does in honoring the privacy of information clients confide to us. We propose examining the subject from the perspective of the consumer—clients in grief counseling who view confidentiality through a lay person's lens, not a professional one.

In suggesting this person-in-the-client-chair approach, we borrow from the work of Weiss, Senf, Carter, and Rothe (1986), who conducted an empirical survey of the confidentiality expectations of patients in university teaching hospitals and private medical offices. Even though this study was done over 2 decades ago, before HIPAA (1996), and targeted only physician providers in medical settings, it yielded intriguing and provocative results. The researchers simply asked whether patients thought it was "common practice" for the doctor to discuss their confidential health information in several different hypothetical situations. The results may surprise readers, particularly when consumers' perceptions and providers' actual practices diverge.

The structure of Weiss et al.'s (1986) study lends itself readily to adaptation for grief counselors and mental health professionals. Instead of "physician(s)," we have substituted "grief counselor" or "colleagues" to extrapolate a similar meaning for the domain of grief counseling. We suggest that readers consider each of the following questions and ask themselves, "How often do I do this?" In parentheses following each question are the percentages of medical patients who indicated that they thought this was common practice for their doctors. For each question, two values are shown. The first percentage is from patients in university teaching hospitals, where expectations of anonymity are generally higher. The second percentage is from patients in private medical offices, where expectations of some information sharing among staff members are slightly more normative.

Is it common practice for your grief counselor to

1. Discuss your case informally with 1–2 colleagues for purposes of getting a second opinion? (teaching hospital = 92%; private office = 94%)
2. Discuss your case at a large professional meeting because it illustrates an important teaching point? (teaching hospital = 83%; private office = 87%)
3. Discuss your case with office staff? (teaching hospital = 67%; private office = 78%)

4. Submit your case to a professional journal because it is interesting? (teaching hospital = 67%; private office = 61%)
5. Describe your case anonymously as an interesting story at a party with professional colleagues? (teaching hospital = 45%; private office = 44%)
6. Discuss your case with his/her spouse or partner? (teaching hospital = 39%; private office = 42%)
7. Describe your case anonymously as an interesting story at a party with nonprofessional friends? (teaching hospital = 35%; private office = 33%)

Our conclusion is that honoring confidentiality starts with the grief counselor's integrity in handling client information and requires follow-through with sound office practices, secure record keeping, and appropriate staff training. Grief counselors should guard constantly against inadvertent domestic violations or careless indiscretions that jeopardize a client's privacy. Only then will conscientious grief counselors live up to that sacred trust placed in them by their clients.

6 Ethical Dilemmas at End of Life

End-of-life decisions have changed dramatically in the modern era (Pence, 2004). At the beginning of the 20th century, only the poor and those without families went to a hospital to die. Today more than 80% of those who die in the United States die in hospitals. Before passage of the 1914 Harrison Narcotics Tax Act, Americans could legally purchase heroin and other opiates in order to medicate themselves from the pain of cancer and other illnesses. Opiates were standard ingredients in various patent medicines. Before World War II, most people died of acute illnesses such as pneumonia and cholera. However, "today, most people live longer and die more slowly from emphysema, diabetes, cardiomyopathy, cancer, and coronary artery disease" (Pence, 2004, p. 64). Pence says that these chronic illnesses and protracted, often painful dying periods have contributed to increased interest in end-of-life issues, such as when to transition from curative treatment to comfort care, how best to involve families in medical decisions, and how to protect the rights of the dying person.

Ethical decision making at the end of life can be extraordinarily complex and difficult. Today's grief counselors must be well versed in the many issues involved with end-of-life care of the dying and the bereaved in order to perform the pivotal educational and therapeutic roles for which they are uniquely suited. This work entails an enormous professional and ethical responsibility. In order to prepare grief counselors to meet this challenge, we address in this chapter several major areas pertaining to ethical dilemmas at end of life: planning ahead with advance directives, withdrawing or withholding treatment, artificial nutrition and hydration, terminal sedation and physician-assisted suicide, capacity for medical decision making, surrogates, children's roles in decision making, and organ donation and transplantation.

PLANNING AHEAD

"Prevention is the best medicine" certainly applies to ethical dilemmas at end of life. Anticipating how one's health could deteriorate with any of the chronic illnesses mentioned earlier, making decisions in advance about what level of medical treatment to accept or reject based on one's personal value system, and signing appropriate documents verifying one's wishes are optimal ways to prevent problems later. However, even under the best of circumstances, things can go wrong. Consider the complications that developed in the following case.

Case Example: Melissa

Melissa is a 75-year-old mother of three middle-aged adult children. Melissa finished high school and, at age 19, married Harry, 24, who was a college graduate. Harry was a successful businessman, and Melissa was a stay-at-home mother. She reared the children while Harry worked hard to get ahead in his career. The two older children are both sons, and the youngest is a daughter. As the only girl, the youngest was the family princess. She and Melissa shopped together and enjoyed one another's company. The two sons liked their sister but sometimes felt she "got away with things" with their parents.

When the daughter was a young adult, she attended a seminar on health care for seniors and became convinced that her parents needed to make decisions about end-of-life care. She had a friend whose mother had died of cancer and had witnessed how difficult it was for the friend to try to make those determinations for her mother. At first, Melissa and Harry did not see any pressing need to formalize end-of-life plans. However, at the daughter's insistence, Melissa followed through and signed a durable power of attorney for health care so that her beloved daughter could make decisions in case of Melissa's incapacity.

Some time later, Melissa and her daughter had a serious breach in their relationship. The daughter married a man who abused her. Melissa wanted the daughter to divorce him, but she refused. Neither of the sons liked their brother-in-law, and they told their sister she could only come to family events without him. Subsequently, the daughter moved away with her abusive husband and had very little contact with the family.

About 30 years into Melissa and Harry's marriage, when he was 54 and she was 49, he decided he did not want to be married anymore. Going through some kind of midlife crisis, Harry told Melissa he was not "happy" and felt "restricted" in the marriage. Harry filed for divorce and basically removed himself from the family, leaving Melissa alone. Melissa was devastated, emotionally and financially. Not only had she lost the relationship with their beloved daughter, but now she had lost the love of her husband too. In addition, she had to go to work for the first time to support herself. The two sons tried to help Melissa all they could.

However, throughout the divorce, Harry stayed in contact with his daughter, the "apple of Daddy's eye." As painful as the divorce was for all of them, the daughter sided with Harry and said she knew what he was going through. She understood his feelings of being restricted, and she now believed Melissa had been too strict on her growing up. This unhappy situation left the family divided—Melissa and her sons were on one side; Harry and his daughter were on the other. There was very little communication between the two groups. At age 78, Harry died of a heart attack while vacationing in Alaska with his second wife. His funeral was the last time Melissa and her children were together.

Two years after Harry's death, the daughter received a phone call from one of her brothers. The brother told her that Melissa had lung cancer and was in terrible pain. The brothers debated about even informing their sister, given that she had treated her mother so terribly during the divorce and then had barely spoken to her at their father's funeral. The brother told her that they were just trying to keep Mom comfortable and that the end was near.

To the brothers' surprise, their sister immediately made plane reservations and flew home. When she arrived, they met her at the airport and told her they were glad she had come. She informed them she had arranged to be gone from work for up to 10 days. They updated her on the palliative care decisions they had made and told her that Melissa was barely able to speak because of the pain. They told her once again that they had instructed the doctors to just keep Mom "comfortable." They said that Mom would be moved to hospice care in the next few weeks.

The daughter was furious and demanded to know why she had not been contacted sooner. The brothers were very confused, and they told her they were not sure what she wanted to know. There had been no communication from her during the 2 years since Harry's funeral, and that is why they did not call her sooner.

Upon arriving at the hospital, the daughter demanded to see the doctor. The attending physician was a middle-aged, female oncologist who told the daughter that her mother was a courageous woman. She said Melissa had fought hard to survive, but the cancer had been too aggressive for any treatment to have much of an impact. The doctor explained to the daughter that Melissa was "in and out" of consciousness and was now unable to make clear decisions. They were just trying to keep her comfortable. The doctor tried to assure the daughter that all decisions had been made with her two brothers, and they were all in agreement that no further treatments, other than comfort care, should be given.

At that point, the daughter opened her purse and showed the doctor the durable power of attorney for health care that her mother had signed years before, indicating that the daughter was to be the surrogate decision maker. The daughter informed the doctor that her brothers had no business making those health care decisions for their mother. She then told the doctor not to give up, but to do "whatever is necessary for my mother to be better. I did not come here just to watch my mother die, while you and my brothers stand by and do nothing. How would you feel if your children just abandoned you when you were dying?" She wanted her mother moved to an intensive care unit.

The sister then turned to her brothers and told them that they had no right to make the decisions about Melissa's care. She said bluntly, "I may not have been a perfect daughter, but I will not abandon my mother when she's dying. Just because you do not like my husband is no reason for you to think you can just push me out of this family."

Necessity for Planning Ahead

In the case of Melissa, even advance planning did not avert decision-making dilemmas at the end of her life. Later in this chapter, we offer an analysis of Melissa's case using the Five P Model for ethical decision making. First, it is important for the reader to know the rationale behind planning ahead for end-of-life care and to understand the meaning of some basic concepts.

A working familiarity with the lexicon of end-of-life care is de rigueur for grief counselors who want to stand ready to help clients and their families who face difficult dilemmas. Table 6.1 contains the definitions of terms and concepts frequently encountered in end-of-life dilemmas. Knowing the language enables the mental health practitioner to enter a medical setting more easily, participate readily as a peer with other health care professionals, and, when needed, translate accurately for clients and families grappling with end-of-life decisions.

Sometimes people are hesitant to talk about dying and death because it seems so "improper." General social etiquette discourages any conversation that may be negative or uncomfortable. May (1981) and Becker (1973) argued that denial of death is ubiquitous in many Western societies, particularly the United States. Because death is not an easy or comfortable topic of discussion, many people die without having any conversation with friends or family about what they want for their care at the end of life. However, death is universal. It is important for people to think ahead about their preferences for end-of-life care before the time of need actually arrives and the necessity of circumstances forces a decision.

Rocker and Curtis (2003) report that, in the United States, among patients with chronic diseases who die in the hospital, approximately one-half are cared for in an intensive care unit within 3 days of their death. In addition, about one-third spend at least 10 days of their life in intensive care during their final hospitalization. Intensive care, therefore, involves difficult decisions about the use of life-sustaining treatments for critically ill patients who do not respond to critical care therapies. Rocker and Curtis assert that an important goal is to achieve the best possible death and the most compassionate care possible for families. Meyer (1998) calls this dying "a good death," and Byock (1997) calls it "dying well."

A provocative study by Jacobs et al. (2008) posed hypothetical questions about intensive care units and end-of-life care both to members of the public and to health care professionals. The clear majority in both groups (72% and 77%, respectively) indicated that, if the intensive care unit were full, patients expected to die should be transferred to make room for others with a greater chance of survival. However, the public much more frequently endorsed beliefs that someone in a persistent vegetative state could be saved by a miracle (61% public; 20% professionals) and that divine intervention by God could save a family member even if the treating doctors said medical futility had been reached (57%

Table 6.1

DEFINITIONS OF TERMS AND CONCEPTS FREQUENTLY ENCOUNTERED IN END-OF-LIFE DILEMMAS

LEGAL TERMS

- *Advance directive*—An umbrella term that refers to the instructions given by competent people so that they can influence their own treatment in the event of serious illness or loss of mental abilities (e.g., whether or under what conditions to use various forms of artificial life support). An advance directive may be written (i.e., a living will) or may be accomplished by appointing a proxy to make the health care decisions.
- *Living will*—An advance directive document, sometimes called "directive to physicians" or "medical directive," in which a mentally competent adult formally expresses preferences regarding medical treatment in the event of future incapacitation or incompetence to make medical decisions. A living will is essentially a statement of a person's preferences regarding resuscitation efforts or artificial life support. It is statutorily binding in most U.S. states.
- *Durable power of attorney for health care*—An advance directive document, sometimes called "medical power of attorney," that allows people to appoint a substitute decision maker to implement their preferences regarding continued life support in the event of incapacitation.
- *Capacity*—A person's mental ability to comprehend information, weigh alternatives, and make a reasoned decision about health care treatment. Sometimes the term *capacity* is confused with *competence.* Competence is the legal determination of capacity. In actual practice, the two terms are used interchangeably.
- *Proxy* or *surrogate decision maker*—The individual who is chosen to make decisions for another person in case of the incapacity to make one's own decisions, using substituted judgment. Sometimes known as the *health care agent* or an *attorney in fact.*
- *Substituted judgment*—When the proxy or surrogate represents the desires of the patient if the patient is not capable of making medical decisions. It is *not* what is in the best interest of the patient from the surrogate's point of view. Rather, it is a substituted judgment representing the actual desires of the patient. Accordingly, the proxy or surrogate should be someone who knows well the patient's desires regarding end-of-life treatment.

MEDICAL TERMS

- *Cardiopulmonary resuscitation (CPR)*—Activities performed in order to revive a person whose heart and lungs have stopped functioning adequately to sustain life. CPR involves a variety of maneuvers designed primarily to restore circulation. These actions may include external heart defibrillation (i.e., shocking a quivering or irregularly beating heart so it restarts in a normal rhythm), applying chest compressions, or injecting medicines intravenously to aid the heart. Breathing may be maintained by inserting a tube into the trachea (windpipe) and using a ventilator to force air into the lungs.
- *Artificial life support*—Use of machines and technology to keep alive a person who would not be able to sustain life otherwise. May include use of

Table 6.1

DEFINITIONS OF TERMS AND CONCEPTS FREQUENTLY ENCOUNTERED IN END-OF-LIFE DILEMMAS *(continued)*

a ventilator to breathe, devices such as pacers or pumps to assist the heart, dialysis, and tubes for supplying nutrition and fluids.

- *Artificial nutrition and hydration*—Placing a tube into a person's vein, stomach, or upper intestine to carry nutrients and fluids directly into the body when a person cannot eat or drink. Commonly known as "tube feeding."
- *Do not resuscitate (DNR)*—An order written into a patient chart that explicitly and unequivocally states that CPR should not be initiated if the patient is found in cardiac arrest. DNR is generally understood to mean *not* using a defibrillator, compressing the chest, or inserting a throat tube for artificial respiration.
- *Non-hospital DNR*—An advance directive document specifying that a patient who is not hospitalized, such as a hospice patient at home, does not want CPR. Otherwise, if 911 is called, emergency personnel will immediately begin whatever lifesaving procedures are deemed necessary by the circumstances, including CPR. To be effective, these out-of-hospital documents must be immediately available and verifiable when emergency personnel arrive. Wherever the patient goes, the documents must go also.
- *Allow natural death (AND)*—A contemporary term gaining wider acceptance in medicine that attempts to state the DNR concept in a positive manner. AND means that only comfort measures are provided to a terminally ill patient, allowing the dying process to occur naturally rather than prolonging it through treatments such as putting the patient on a ventilator or inserting a feeding tube.
- *Minimally conscious* or *semiconscious*—The person shows occasional moments of awareness. The person may be seen as trying to communicate, either through speech or by writing. However, the person does not come to full consciousness to a degree that these activities of attempted communication are actually accomplished or sustained.
- *Persistent vegetative state (PVS)*—Refers to cognitive death. It includes a persistent loss of upper cortical function. In PVS, the person is completely bedridden, nutritional support is completely passive (e.g., feeding tube), and the person is incontinent. PVS patients do not require respiratory support or circulatory assistance for survival. They are in a state of chronic wakefulness without awareness, which may feature spontaneous eye opening, brief smiles, or sporadic movement of facial muscles and limbs. Behavior is non-intentional. Recovery is rare.
- *Coma*—A deep, almost sleep-like state from which the person cannot be aroused. The eyes remain closed, and there are no emotional responses, no responses to surrounding environmental noises, and no responses to direct stimulation, except sometimes a reflex reaction to painful stimulation.
- *Palliative care*—Any treatment of a terminally ill patient intended to alleviate pain and suffering. In providing palliative care, the medical team recognizes the incurable nature of the disease. Sometimes treatments, such as surgery

(continued)

Table 6.1

DEFINITIONS OF TERMS AND CONCEPTS FREQUENTLY ENCOUNTERED IN END-OF-LIFE DILEMMAS *(continued)*

or radiation therapy, are used to reduce or shrink tumor masses compressing vital structures in order to achieve a better quality of life during the patient's remaining time. In hospice settings, the connotation of palliative care is pain control achieved through medicine, only without palliative chemotherapy, surgery, or radiation.

- *Comfort care*—Similar to palliative care but without any surgery or radiation therapy and without artificial nutrition or hydration. Actions may include medicine for pain control, breathing problems, or depression. Other actions provide tender loving care through emotional support, environmental manipulation (e.g., lighting, music), ensuring the patient is clean and dry, and comforting the family.

Definitions adapted from *The dictionary of modern medicine: Illustrated,* by J. C. Segen, 1992, Park Ridge, NJ: Parthenon, and *The guide to living wills and health care proxies: How to protect your right to make crucial health care decisions,* by Harvard Medical School, 2008, Boston: Harvard Health.

public; 20% professionals). Clearly, decision making at the end of life can be complicated by differences in belief systems and personal values.

When options for curative treatment are exhausted, the American College of Physicians recommended the following five practice guidelines for improving palliative care at the end of life (Qaseem et al., 2008):

1. Any treatment should be assessed regularly to be sure it is providing benefit to the patient for end-of-life pain, dyspnea (i.e., trouble breathing), and depression.
2. Nonsteroidal anti-inflammatory drugs as well as opioids are effective for patients with cancer-related pain. In addition, bisphosphonates are recommended for bone pain.
3. Use morphine, oral or nebulized (i.e., inhaled mist), and oxygen to treat dyspnea.
4. Treat depression in cancer patients with medication and/or psychosocial interventions. Treating pain alone does not treat depression; they are two different disorders.
5. Advance care planning should occur as early as possible in the course of serious illness.

Grief counselors may play an important role in facilitating such advance planning as members of a multidisciplinary health care team.

Consider that Sulmasy, Sood, and Ury (2008) found that physicians and resident doctors in training were more comfortable discussing consent for a medical procedure with patients and surrogate decision makers than they were discussing a do-not-resuscitate order. Interestingly, male physicians were more comfortable than female physicians in discussing end-of-life issues, and staff physicians were more comfortable than resident doctors. Also, there is a role for grief counselors and mental health professionals when staff and family confer in order to clarify goals when managing end-of-life medical decisions for patients in intensive care units. Several medical specialists have recommended making available counselors and pastoral ministers during the course of the patient's illness and at the time of death (Abbott, Sago, Breen, Abernethy, & Tulsky, 2001; Curtis & Rubenfeld, 2005; Truog et al., 2008).

McCullough (2008) decries the practice of subjecting elderly, chronically ill patients to what some have called "death by intensive care." Sedated and unable to communicate, they endure impersonal medical protocols in strange, disorienting surroundings. Or they are stranded in limbo on life-support machines while families hover in waiting rooms, uncertain how to help. Instead, McCullough champions the concept of "slow medicine," which replaces the exhaustive regimen of a medicalized end of life with a more deliberate, family-centered, hands-on form of conservative medicine combined with liberal doses of love, kindness, and companionship for elderly patients.

The more careful consideration a person gives to end-of-life decisions, the better the outcome will be when that time arrives, when so many significant decisions must be made, often within a very short time. The two ethical principles of beneficence and autonomy are particularly relevant. The goal is for an individual to make known in a clear way what is believed will be good care based on one's own values. In addition, such decisions should be made freely without any coercion from family, friends, or medical staff, although one's end-of-life decisions may be made in consultation with all of these people.

It is important to understand that the person is making decisions regarding various *treatment* options at the end of life. There should never be a decision to end *care* for a person at the end of life. The various decisions that are decided beforehand and recorded in a living will are for the *health care* team (not the *illness treatment* team) to know what treatments are desired or refused by the patient. It is a description of what treatment that person feels will constitute good care at the end of life. Regardless of preferences for or against specific treatments, patients at the end of life will always receive care from those around them

(Truog et al., 2008). Providing *care* is doing good (i.e., beneficence), whereas choosing or declining *treatment* is a matter of personal choice (i.e., autonomy).

Methods for Planning Ahead

Many hospitals have preprinted forms readily available for making advance directives to physicians and designating a power of attorney for health care. These can be filled out, signed, and witnessed at any time, whether or not the person is ill and whether or not the person is a patient of that particular hospital. Durable power of attorney for health care decisions can also be executed with the help of a knowledgeable attorney.

The organization Aging With Dignity (2007) has produced a 12-page booklet titled *Five Wishes. Five Wishes* guides the reader through a series of documents and helps the person think about various medical, personal, emotional, and spiritual options for care at the end of life. Forms are provided for the signatures and witnesses necessary for the wishes to be legally valid, which they are in 40 states in the United States. Basically, *Five Wishes* doubles as a living will and a designation of a proxy for making health care decisions if the person becomes incapacitated. *Five Wishes* is for individuals 18 and older who are mentally and physically capable of making health care decisions for themselves. For example, someone who has Alzheimer's or some other dementia-related disease cannot legally complete the forms or be coerced into making end-of-life decisions.

Wish 1

The first wish is to select a person to make health care decisions as a proxy when the patient can no longer make those decisions independently. The person should be someone who knows the patient well, in whom the patient has confidence, and who can make difficult decisions for the patient, if necessary.

Wish 2

The second wish is for what kind of medical treatment the individual wants, or does not want, at the end of life. Options to consider include extraordinary treatment, such as CPR and life support, or limited treatments, such as palliative care, comfort care, DNR, or AND.

Wish 3

The third wish is to be made as comfortable as possible. Although this wish includes pain control, it also includes care for breathing problems, depression, nausea, or other acute symptoms that need to be treated in order for the patient to be comfortable. This wish also includes desires for the general environment, such as being with family and friends, playing one's favorite music, and keeping the bed and the patient clean and dry.

Wish 4

The fourth wish is the patient's desire for how to be treated by others at the end of life. For example, does the patient want someone to stay at the bedside, hold a hand, massage with oil, sing, pray, or read sacred texts? This applies even if the patient appears unconscious. This wish may include wanting to die at home, if possible.

Wish 5

The fifth wish is more personal—what the patient wants loved ones to know. Often, this involves communication of love, gratitude and forgiveness as well as reassuring loved ones that the patient is not afraid to die. In addition, the patient can list preferred ways to be remembered and what type of memorial or funeral service is desired. Wishes regarding disposition of the body—for example, earth burial or cremation—and organ or tissue donation can be expressed.

One of the major advantages of *Five Wishes* is people *writing* down their preferences for end-of-life care. The more formal and clear the written guidelines, the easier the decision-making process will be for a proxy or surrogate, should that need occur.

Another helpful booklet for discussing end-of-life issues is *A Guide to Living Wills and Health Care Proxies: How to Protect Your Right to Make Crucial Health Care Decisions,* published by Harvard Medical School (2008). It contains explanations and definitions about end-of-life care options as well as forms for designating a health care proxy and making a living will. In addition, these forms can be downloaded from the Harvard Web site at http://www.health.harvard.edu/downloads/LW forms.pdf.

The American Association of Retired Persons (AARP; 2005) recommends a durable power of attorney for health care decisions in addition to a living will. Because the end of life is not known when the document is executed, the actual situation in which decisions need to be made may not be addressed. Thus, although the patient can make individual preferences known in writing through an advance directive like a living will or *Five Wishes*, if unanticipated circumstances occur at the end of life, then a surrogate, designated by a durable power of attorney for health care, can address the situation for the person.

Sometimes people have a concern that if they designate someone as a health care proxy or surrogate, HIPAA (1996) rules will prevent their proxy from having access to the private medical information necessary for decision making at the end of life. However, HIPAA rules do not affect a health care proxy. Most signed living wills grant the proxy permission to access medical records and discuss the patient's condition with medical providers.

Case of Melissa: Analysis With the Five P Model

Unfortunately, cases such as Melissa's happen all too often. Those who believe they have the patient's best interest at heart also believe they are the primary decision makers. Melissa's sons have cared for her and watched her deteriorate, and nothing has seemed to help. In consultation with the oncologist, they have made the best decisions possible for their mother's care, given the circumstances. They are now taken aback by their sister's refusal to go along with palliative care. They did not know their sister had any real interest in the situation until she got to the hospital. They were unaware of the durable power of attorney designating their sister as the decision maker. Now they are confused.

The case raises ethical difficulties for the doctor as well. A plan of care has been made by working closely with the sons over the last 2 months. Now the estranged sister wants to change the medical plan. Does the sister have the right to overrule the decisions of her two brothers? Who is the legal representative for Melissa? Is the durable power of attorney for health care decisions valid?

Person

The person of interest in this case is Melissa, a 75-year-old woman with terminal lung cancer. She has struggled, emotionally and economically, since her divorce. She has two supportive sons and one estranged daughter. Because her lung cancer has progressed to the point where she is in and out of conscious alertness, her sons have been making decisions for her in concert with the attending oncologist. She does not demonstrate the capacity to determine for herself the plan of care.

Problem

The problem is that Melissa's two sons want her to receive comfort care during her advanced stage of cancer. Her daughter, who has been estranged from the family, has durable power of attorney for health care and wants the doctor to "do everything" for her mother. The brothers view the problem as one created by their sister and her unrealistic goals for Melissa's treatment. The daughter views it as her brothers' lack of concern for their mother. The disagreement is over comfort care versus more aggressive medical treatment. The brothers view comfort care as doing good, beneficence, and needlessly aggressive care as doing harm, maleficence. The sister is of just the opposite opinion. She views intensive care as doing good, beneficence, and comfort care as giving up on Melissa, maleficence. The oncologist is also involved in the decision.

Place

The location of the dilemma is a hospital. Melissa is gravely ill and cannot go home without the support of hospice and family members. Because her children are in disagreement about a course of action, hospice care cannot be instituted until the conflict is resolved. Also, by virtue of being in a hospital, the medical staff and their code of ethics are relevant to the dilemma. Hospital staff cannot be compelled to provide treatment that is medically futile, in their estimation.

Principles

The ethical principles of doing good, beneficence, and avoiding harm, nonmaleficence, are especially relevant to the case of Melissa. There is also the question of Melissa's autonomy, that is, her ability to direct her own health care decisions. State law comes into play in that the daughter has a legal document, durable power of attorney for health care, that designates her as the agent to make decisions for Melissa. In other words, she has the legal authority to exercise substituted judgment for Melissa. The daughter is the advocate for Melissa's autonomous wishes (i.e., what Melissa would want for herself, as best she understands it).

The ethical principle of justice also enters the picture. Emotionally speaking, the two loyal sons believe that, because of their closeness to

Melissa, they grasp what she would have wanted for herself under these conditions of an excruciatingly painful terminal illness. They believe the sister is acting out of guilt or regret for the estrangement and is trying to "hold on" to allow for some kind of reconciliation before Melissa dies. In their opinion, the sister is making it "about her" when it is really "about Mom," which they view as a miscarriage of justice. However, their subjective sense of justice is contradicted by justice in the legal sense because the daughter is the decision maker of record.

Justice also applies to the doctor's position. In terms of allocating resources fairly, is it ethically defensible to put a terminally ill cancer patient in the intensive care unit when there is no hope of reversing her condition, and when the only medically indicated treatment is palliative care through hospice? Can the physician justify, literally, the cost associated with intensive care treatment or placing Melissa in a bed that may best serve someone with a legitimate hope of recovery?

Process

There are three main voices of interest: the brothers, the sister, and the doctor. The time limitations are pressing but not immediate—intensive care treatment can be started soon, or the mother can be moved to hospice. There is also the possible limitation that the daughter will be in town only for 10 days.

What ethical theory will be used? The sons seem to be using both principle-based reasoning and rule deontological ethics. They believe that doing good, beneficence, is helping their mother to be comfortable at the end of her life, not subjecting her to unnecessary medical measures with all their attendant discomforts and annoyances, that is, avoiding harm or nonmaleficence. They also believe that comfort care is "doing the right thing," both for Melissa in particular and for patients like her with terminal cancer (i.e., Kant's categorical imperative).

The daughter seems to have unresolved issues with her mother. She appears to be embracing a virtue ethics approach, in other words, wanting to be viewed as a daughter who supports her mother. As such, she does not want to be seen as abandoning Melissa in her hour of need because of how it would reflect on her as a daughter. Yet the question remains whether she is acting out of remorse for her past actions and, in effect, putting self-interest first by demanding intensive care for Melissa.

The oncologist seems to be using a combination of utilitarian ethics and principle-based ethics. All too familiar with such end-of-life scenarios, the doctor looks at what is the greatest good for everyone involved. Melissa is terminally ill and will die, with or without intensive care treatment. From the doctor's perspective as a physician and non–family member, quality care is comfort care. Comfort care affords Melissa the pain control and dignity she deserves at the end of her life. It gives the family the opportunity to say farewell in a supportive atmosphere. Comfort care also serves the ethical principle of justice—giving Melissa the best possible care for her terminal condition while allocating intensive care treatment to those who can most benefit from its technological sophistication.

To further the decision-making process, the oncologist needs to spend more time with the family, particularly the daughter. The focus needs to shift away from what the daughter wants for her mother to a more accurate understanding of substituted judgment, that is, what would Melissa want for herself under these conditions if she could make her wishes known (cf. Curtis & Rubenfeld, 2005)? The doctor will continually bring the conversation back to this point: "What would Melissa want, if she could tell us? There is no medical treatment that will improve her condition. The best we can offer, and my medical recommendation, is comfort care." Ultimately, the daughter has the legal right to decide, even though her brothers may disagree. At this point in the process, a grief counselor may be consulted to work more intensively with the family to help mediate the impasse.

The grief counselor may inquire about the daughter's insistence on intensive care for Melissa. What is her understanding of the diagnosis? What does she hope to accomplish through intensive care treatment? What would she want to say to her mother if Melissa were suddenly lucid and communicative? In the event that the daughter acknowledges unfinished business with Melissa, the grief counselor can gently point out that there is still time for the daughter to *talk to* her mother about any heaviness of heart that she is carrying. The counselor could recommend Byock's (2004) notions of the most important things to say to a dying person regarding forgiveness, love, gratitude, and goodbye and could offer to help with this conversation, if needed. The daughter may require some time to absorb all the recommendations of the medical staff and the grief counselor. Even though comfort care seems to be the best choice, it should not be an unnecessarily hurried decision or one that feels forced. The grief counselor can remain available to her.

Also, it is strategic for the grief counselor to try to defuse the family conflict by talking with the brothers as well and enlisting their cooperation to give their sister time to reconsider her position. As an ombudsman, the grief counselor keeps the staff apprised of the progress of the family's negotiation and works to keep the oncologist involved because most families single out the attending physician as the preferred source of information and reassurance (Abbott et al., 2001).

These collective efforts on the part of the grief counselor are consistent with the ADEC Code of Ethics, which "envisions a world in which dying, death, and bereavement are recognized as fundamental and significant aspects of the human experience" (ADEC Code of Ethics, Preface). Additional provisions also apply to the grief counselor's actions in the case of Melissa.

> The member serves in an advocacy role to assist the individual or society to cope with death-related issues. (ADEC Code of Ethics, Basic Tenets, 5)
>
> The member strives to present various views of a death-related question, indicating the member's own values if appropriate, and respecting the student's or client's choice among alternatives. (ADEC Code of Ethics, Basic Tenets, 6)
>
> The member works to promote greater understanding among lay persons and professionals of dying and death so that each member of society can achieve a more satisfying life and personal acceptance of death. (ADEC Code of Ethics, Basic Tenets, 9)

CONTROVERSIAL END-OF-LIFE SITUATIONS

Additional controversies compound the complexity involved in making end-of-life decisions. Grief counselors should bear in mind that they do not work alone in medical settings when end-of-life decisions are contemplated. Besides the medical staff, most hospitals have bioethics committees with whom to consult when decisions are not clear-cut. Grief counselors bring to the table their communication skills and dexterity with interpersonal relationships to ease decision making by the patient or proxy in conjunction with the family and the health care team.

Withholding or Withdrawing Treatment

In bioethics, a distinction can be made between withholding treatment and withdrawing treatment. Some ethicists view withholding treatment as a passive decision, whereas withdrawing treatment is an instrumental action. It is one thing not to start treatment at all, in which case the decision to withdraw never occurs. It is quite another thing to begin treatment and then decide to stop it. For example, with CPR, it is one thing not to begin emergency resuscitation and just let the person die. It is quite another thing to decide, after starting emergency resuscitation, to stop the lifesaving efforts.

Regardless of whether one withholds or withdraws treatment, the end result is the same—at some point, the patient is not treated. Legally, withholding or withdrawing treatment is viewed the same way (Truog et al., 2008). A health care proxy sometimes agrees to begin treatment because it seems to be the "right thing to do at the time" (i.e., rule deontological reasoning). "Doing something" may exonerate the proxy from any accusation of neglect or inaction toward the patient. Also, beginning treatment may be an indirect way of deferring difficult questions about what to do in the event of treatment futility. However, stopping treatment after it is started is very often a more agonizing decision than not beginning treatment at all. Proxies may believe they are "killing" the patient by agreeing to discontinue life support and therefore feel guilty. Disheartened family members may accuse the proxy of abusing the patient by stopping treatment.

Two famous legal cases in the United States have influenced the controversy over withholding or withdrawing treatment at the end of life. Karen Ann Quinlan was 21 years old in 1975 when she lapsed into a persistent vegetative state after coming home from a party. At the hospital, she was placed on a respirator to breathe and supplied with nutrition and fluids through a feeding tube. With no hope for Karen's recovery, her parents decided to have the respirator turned off. However, the hospital refused. After a legal battle, the New Jersey Supreme Court ruled her parents could have the respirator turned off. Over several days, Karen was slowly weaned off the respirator. To everyone's surprise, Karen continued to breathe on her own. Her parents did not seek to withdraw nutrition and hydration. She was moved to a nursing home where she died of pneumonia in 1986, never having regained consciousness (Lamers, 2007b; Pence, 2004).

Nancy Cruzan was 24 years old in 1983 when she lost control of her car, crashed, and was ejected. Her heart stopped for about 15 minutes but was restarted by paramedics. However, she never regained consciousness and was left in a persistent vegetative state. Although able to breathe on her own, a feeding tube enabled her to receive food and fluids. She remained this way for 7 years. Nancy's parents waged a 3-year legal battle to have the feeding tube removed. The U.S. Supreme Court recognized a constitutional right to die but supported the State of

Missouri to set reasonable standards to guide the exercise of that right. Ultimately, a local court ordered that the feeding tube could be removed, and Nancy died in 1990 (Lamers, 2007a; Pence, 2004).

In both of these legal cases, one side argued for withdrawing treatment. The Quinlan case focused on the withdrawal of the respirator, whereas Cruzan's parents sought permission for removal of the feeding tube. Now in the United States, all 50 states have some kind of natural death law empowering patients to choose a natural death when they could not otherwise survive without life-sustaining medical technology (Lens, 2007b). In addition, there is a federal law, the Patient Self-Determination Act (Omnibus Budget Reconciliation Act of 1990), encouraging patients to exercise their rights by completing advance directives (Lens, 2007a).

The resolution of these cases introduced a distinction between medical care that is *extraordinary,* or disproportionate, and *ordinary,* or proportionate. In the Quinlan case, her parents were Roman Catholic. They argued that Catholic moral theology does not require that extraordinary means be employed in preserving a patient's life (cf. Sacred Congregation for the Doctrine of the Faith, 1980). *Extraordinary* means are any procedures that offer no reasonable hope of benefit; that place undue burden on the patient, the family, or others; and that go beyond the basic care required to sustain life. By contrast, *ordinary* means include basic essentials such as food, water, air, and hygiene. A patient can refuse extraordinary means of medical treatment, even if this will hasten natural death. As guardians, Quinlan's parents used this principle in appealing successfully to the New Jersey Supreme Court that the respirator constituted extraordinary means (Pence, 2004).

Unfortunately, there are shortcomings to the process of health care proxies or surrogates exercising substituted judgment in making end-of-life decisions for incapacitated patients. Research shows that proxies are accurate in predicting patient preferences about two-thirds of the time when it comes to electing specific treatments such as intensive care, intubation, CPR, tube feeding, and dialysis (Sulmasy, Haller, & Terry, 1994). Writing from a perspective of feminist ethics, Powell (1999) made two key points regarding psychological aspects of surrogate decision making. First, proxies themselves are nearly always grieving over the compromised state of their loved ones when asked to make decisive and frightening choices on behalf of those loved ones. Acute grief and shock can render decision making very difficult. Second, Powell argues it is fiction to believe proxies will have no self-interest in the outcome of their decision or that they can merely act as alternative voices for incapacitated patients. Inevitably, their decisions will be influenced by who the patient was in relation to them and will not necessarily duplicate either the patient's would-be decisions or the decisions of a different proxy.

Adding further to the debate, Curtis (2005) documented considerable variability among intensive care unit physicians in agreeing to withhold or withdraw end-of-life treatments, variability that appeared to be driven by physicians' attitudes and biases. For example, physicians with more years of practice experience and fewer beds in their intensive care units showed an increased willingness to withdraw treatment. Thus, pure pragmatism may play a role. Also, Christakis and Asch (1995) reported that physicians who were younger, who were specialty-trained, and who spent a greater percentage of time in clinical practice were more willing to withdraw life support. Interestingly, Roman Catholic and Jewish physicians were less willing to accommodate withdrawal of life support.

Annas (1991) pleaded with medical professionals to use living wills and powers of attorney as opportunities to increase communication between medical providers and patients about preferences for end-of-life care and, in so doing, ensure patient autonomy. When a health care proxy decides to withhold or withdraw treatment, it is very important that the process and the decision be documented accurately in the patient's medical record. For example, "Mr. Smith, the legal health care proxy for Mrs. Jones, in consultation with Drs. Green, Brown, and Black, and Mrs. Jones's family, as well as the hospice social worker, Ms. Atwood, decided to withdraw life support for Mrs. Jones at 7:50 A.M. on Friday, October 24, 2008."

Artificial Nutrition and Hydration

The reader is challenged to compare and contrast the following two accounts of deaths involving decisions about artificial nutrition and hydration.

Ruth Graham, the wife of well-known evangelist Billy Graham, died peacefully at their home in Montreat, North Carolina (Associated Press, 2007). The news article noted that Mrs. Graham died while surrounded by her husband and all five of their children. The family spokesman reported that, at Mrs. Graham's request and in consultation with her family, she had stopped receiving tube feedings for the previous few days. In other words, it was a "good death" (cf. Meyer, 1998), and all were supportive of it.

Terri Schiavo was age 26 in 1990 when she collapsed from cardiac and respiratory arrest. She remained in a permanent vegetative state until her death in 2005. In this highly publicized case, arguments raged for years contesting who was the legal guardian for Terri and whether her feeding tube could be removed. Her family maintained that Terri would not want to go against her Roman Catholic faith and supported continued nutrition and hydration as ordinary means of "food and water." Her husband countered that Terri had indicated on several occasions that she never wanted to live as a vegetable. Terri's parents posted on a Web site a brief video of Terri appearing to respond to human interaction. This family feud incited an international debate about her life. Extensive legal wrangling, which included all three branches of the U.S. government, resulted in Terri's feeding tube being removed and reinserted twice during a 30-month period before it was removed for the third and last time. Terri died 13 days later (Welie, 2008).

Does artificial nutrition and hydration constitute extraordinary, disproportionate medical treatment that can be declined, or is it humane provision of "food and water" that is ordinary, proportionate care of a dying person or of someone who is in a persistent vegetative state or irreversible coma?

Sheehan (2008) reported on the Roman Catholic perspective on artificial nutrition and hydration with the permanently unconscious patient. The position of John Paul II (2004), from a pontifical address to participants in an international congress on life-sustaining treatments and the vegetative state, unequivocally asserted that administering food and water, even artificially, is a natural means of preserving life, not a medical act. Based on this reasoning, withdrawal of artificial nutrition and hydration is seen as a moral violation that does harm by starving the patient to death rather than honoring basic human dignity by feeding one who needs food.

Others disagree. Casarett, Kapo, and Caplan (2005) explained how a patient in a persistent vegetative state can live for 10 or more years receiving artificial nutrition and hydration, as was the case with Terri Schiavo, but will die within days or weeks if it is withdrawn, as was the case with Ruth Graham. Arguing from a medical rather than a moral perspective, Casarett et al. made three main points. First, artificial nutrition and hydration is *not* the same thing as giving someone food to eat. In fact, it is often administered because the patient cannot eat food or drink liquids. It is a medical intervention that requires the technical skills of specially trained practitioners to insert tubes for feeding and hydration. In this respect, artificial nutrition and hydration has more in common with other medical procedures than it does with the simple act of feeding, a point endorsed also by a Lutheran perspective (Holst, 1991). Second, unlike the basic provision of comfort via shelter or warmth, Casarett and colleagues argued that artificial nutrition and hydration carries considerable risks and discomfort, as well as uncertain benefits. Third, artificial nutrition and hydration is not intended for the purpose of making the patient more comfortable—"in fact, during the administration of high-quality palliative care, symptoms of hunger or thirst generally resolve in a short time" (p. 2608).

Whether artificial nutrition and hydration is a moral or a medical issue remains a polarized debate, deeply rooted in cultural and religious beliefs (cf. Casarett et al., 2005). From either position, it is sobering to realize that, in the United States, there are approximately 10,000 patients in a permanent vegetative state, and withdrawing artificial nutrition and hydration can be a very anguishing decision. For example, of the 41 states that recognized living wills as legal documents in 1991, half of them prohibited the withdrawal of artificial nutrition and hydration, even if an advance directive specified such withdrawal (Holst, 1991). A more recent study by Sieger, Arnold, and Ahronheim (2002) showed that 20 states in the United States have explicit statutory provisions delineating separate and more stringent standards for refusing artificial nutrition and hydration than for refusing other medical treatments when patients lack decision-making capacity. Because these are not easy decisions, grief counselors must exercise great sensitivity when participating in end-of-life discussions about the possibility of withdrawing artificial nutrition and hydration.

Life Insurance

A concern that sometimes arises during end-of-life treatment decisions is how a person's life insurance carrier will view the cause of death. Many life insurance policies enact some payment limitations when death is caused by suicide. If a person refuses life-support measures at the end of life, or a health care proxy refuses life support based on knowledge of the patient's wishes, can this decision be viewed as the intentional taking of one's own life?

Consider the case of the elderly patient with intractable cancer who declined palliative treatment with radiation therapy intended to improve the quality of remaining life—that is, shrink the tumors to reduce pain and immobility. As the disease progressed unchecked, the patient's deteriorating condition required hospital care. However, life support was refused for subsequent breathing problems, although morphine was used to ease the struggle to breathe. When the patient died, the cause of death was clear. It was the cancer.

The refusal of treatment at the end of life does not mean the patient is enacting suicide. When a patient with terminal illness dies, the actual cause of death is the medical disease, not the voluntary act of refusing treatment (Harvard Medical School, 2008; Holst, 1991). It is similar to a physician recommending the discontinuation of life-support treatment based on medical futility, that is, where there is no hope for recovery or even improvement. Should the proxy or surrogate agree that discontinuing life support is what the patient would have wanted, turning off the life-support apparatus is not viewed as murdering the patient or even as a mercy killing. Instead, it is a medical decision to let the disease take its natural course and allow the patient to die (Truog, 2007; Truog et al., 2008). Some may argue that, technically speaking, removal of life support is the *proximate,* or immediate, cause of death. However, the *distal,* or underlying, cause of death is the disease. In other words, the patient dies from the disease, not from the decision to forego life support.

Terminal Sedation and Physician-Assisted Suicide

Terminal sedation means giving sufficient medication for the patient to remain unconscious until death in order to relieve suffering from otherwise uncontrollable end-of-life symptoms such as intractable pain, breathing problems, seizures, or delirium (Quill & Byock, 2000; Quill, Lee, & Nunn, 2000). Usually, this means that other life-sustaining treatments have been stopped, such as mechanical ventilation or artificial nutrition and hydration. For example, terminal sedation may be used to prevent suffocating sensations when patients discontinue mechanical ventilation. The sedation is "terminal" in that it occurs at the end of life, not because it causes death. However, many palliative care specialists acknowledge that there is a fine line between medication sufficient to sedate the patient and a level that would suppress breathing and lead to imminent death. Here the doctrine of "double effect" operates, that is, the medicine given for sedation purposes or pain control may have the foreseen but *unintended* consequence of hastening death (Truog et al., 2008). It is the *intent* of the doctor's action—alleviation of pain—that makes it acceptable palliative care, reasoning based on rule deontological ethics.

Some ethicists argue that terminal sedation is really a form of euthanasia, "comfort killing" rather than "comfort dying." The term *euthanasia,* whose Greek roots mean "easy" or "good" death, has come to refer to the practice of killing hopelessly sick or injured individuals or animals for reasons of mercy—to avert continued or increased suffering. Withholding or withdrawing life-sustaining treatment may be considered by some to be a passive form of euthanasia, although without the intent to end the person's life. In contrast, active euthanasia is a deliberate act of commission in which the intent of the course of action is the death of the patient (Welie, 2008). The legal system and public opinion in the United States have been more tolerant of passive euthanasia than active euthanasia, or physician-assisted suicide (Walker, 2003).

Physician-assisted suicide, wherein doctors provide the medicine for terminally ill people to end their lives electively, is highly controversial. Physician-assisted suicide is legal in the Netherlands, Belgium, and certain areas of Switzerland, albeit with strict medical guidelines (Humphry, 2007). It is illegal in every U.S. state except Oregon (Ardelt, 2003; Hedlund, 2005). The controversy over physician-assisted suicide became more heated as a result of two events in the 1990s. In a 1991 article in the *New England Journal of Medicine,* Dr. Timothy Quill reported his participation in the "rational suicide" of a female patient, "Diane," suffering from acute myelomonocytic leukemia (Quill, 1991). Then, in 1998, came the publicly broadcast video of Dr. Jack Kevorkian "assisting" a patient with advanced amyotrophic lateral sclerosis (Lou Gehrig's disease) to die by lethal injection (Walker, 2003).

Those opposing physician-assisted suicide believe that when a doctor helps an individual to complete suicide, that physician is complicit in the death of another person, a clear violation of the ethical principle of nonmaleficence, "First, do no harm." According to Ardelt (2003), the case against physician-assisted suicide rests on traditional moral and spiritual values: the identity of the doctor as healer, not an agent of death; the sacredness of life as a gift from God, not something to be ended by human action; the importance of compassion for the sick and the dying; and viewing the end of life as an opportunity for both the dying patient and the caregivers to attain spiritual growth or develop a deeper understanding of life (cf. Byock, 2004; Clarke, 1999). Opponents also worry about a slippery slope effect wherein legalization of physician-assisted suicide for the terminally ill might lead to its acceptance for other marginalized populations: the chronically ill, the disabled, the mentally ill, or the poor (Ardelt, 2003; Roos, 2005).

Those in favor of physician-assisted suicide for individuals with a terminal or incurable illness usually cite as the chief arguments the right of self-determination and control and relief from suffering (Ardelt, 2003). Self-determination, based on the ethical principle of autonomy, means mentally competent, terminally ill patients should be permitted to make noncoerced decisions to end their lives. The physician who prescribes the medicine dose sufficient for death is carrying out the wishes of the patient and remaining involved as a pledge of nonabandonment (Quill, 1991, 1993; Quill et al., 2000). Arguments based on alleviation of suffering may be challenged by those who point out that suffering has multiple layers, including not only physical pathology but also emotional and spiritual components. It is difficult to reduce a person's subjective experience of pain only to physical parameters.

Doctors disagree on the subject of physician-assisted suicide. Curlin, Nwodim, Vance, Chin, and Lantos (2008) reported that 69% of U.S. physicians are opposed to physician-assisted suicide. Highly religious physicians are more likely to object (84%) than less religious physicians (59%). Regarding the practice of terminal sedation, 25% of highly religious physicians objected, compared to only 12% of less religious ones. However, only 5% of U.S. physicians surveyed objected to withdrawal of life support. Higher rates of objection to physician-assisted suicide and terminal sedation were found among doctors of Asian ethnicity or Hindu affiliation. Also, physicians who have more experience working with the dying are more likely to object to physician-assisted suicide while endorsing withdrawal of life support as an alternative.

Although controversy continues about the merits and liabilities of physician-assisted suicide, readers desiring a more detailed analysis of the arguments on both sides can consult several available texts (Dyck, 2002; Kaplan, 2000; Quill, 2001).

It is more important than ever for grief counselors to possess the death competence needed to face, without fear or denial, these highly charged end-of-life issues such as withholding or withdrawing treatment, artificial nutrition and hydration, terminal sedation, and physician-assisted suicide. Grief counselors can be an important resource to hospital staff, intensive care units, the patients who die there, and the families who grieve.

CAPACITY FOR MEDICAL DECISION MAKING

In making end-of-life medical decisions, it is important to know that the decision maker has the mental *capacity* to make responsible decisions about treatment. Various physical and mental conditions, some temporary and some permanent, can compromise decision-making capacity. For example, permanent conditions that limit capacity include brain injury or mental retardation. For these individuals, it is hoped their lack of capacity to make independent decisions about their health care has already been addressed through appointment of a guardian or designation of a durable power of attorney for health care. Temporary conditions that may impede capacity include delirium or depression, which often subside with treatment and time.

Health care professionals, as well as family and loved ones, may question whether a patient has the capacity to make end-of-life decisions, such as declining curative treatment or authorizing DNR. Similar to the determination of competence for giving informed consent discussed in Chapter 4, lucid adults of reasonable intelligence are considered to have the capacity to exercise autonomy and make medical decisions for themselves, unless demonstrated otherwise. If a person's capacity for making health care decisions is unclear or disputed, a legal determination of competency can be made only by a judge or court of law. Typically, input from medical and mental health professionals who have examined the patient for the purpose of evaluating decision-making capacity figure prominently in a court's determination of competence.

An evaluation of capacity for medical decision making is specific to medical decisions. The patient needs to be able to understand the diagnosis and prognosis for the disease, what options for treatment are available, which particular treatment is being recommended, and the probable consequences of accepting or declining any or all of the recommended treatments. Capacity for medical decision making is not a determination of capacity for making business decisions or handling personal finances. Those are separate evaluations. In addition, having mental illness does not mean a person is incapable of medical decision making. For example, individuals with depression or schizophrenia may still be capable of making end-of-life medical decisions, such as understanding that without an emergency appendectomy, they will die.

When a patient's capacity for medical decision making is in doubt, a physician or a mental health professional may be consulted to conduct an evaluation. The provider explains the medical information to the patient in plain, clear language (i.e., the subjective standard) and then asks the patient to summarize what has been presented. Does the patient understand the information? Can the patient articulate the treatment options? Does the patient comprehend the consequences of accepting or declining treatment? Is the patient making a noncoerced, independent decision? Evaluating capacity for medical decision making parallels the continuous, consensual process of informed consent. It is an interactive process between the provider and the patient of explaining and clarifying and then listening and documenting the patient's capacity for medical decision making. The intent is respecting patients' rights to self-determination, if they are capable.

Generally, evaluators will favor open-ended questions to gauge patients' capacity to comprehend their condition and treatment options. For example, "How do you understand what I've told you about your condition?" or "What is your preference about the choices for treatment that I've explained?" The evaluator listens carefully for any gaps in understanding and provides clarification, if needed. Closed-ended questions designed to yield only a "yes" or "no" answer, such as, "Do you understand what I have said to you?" are generally avoided because they reveal less about the patient's true capacity. The best use of such closed-ended questions is for final verification of the patient's wishes once a thorough discussion has taken place—for example, "So, I understand that you do not want the radiation therapy we are recommending, even though it could ease some of your pain and mobility problems, because you do not want any more treatment, is that correct?"

Family Influence and Capacity Judgments

Most people know when they are seriously ill, and most also know when they are going to die. An honest conversation with the patient is an important part of evaluating capacity and providing end-of-life counseling. Sometimes family members want to shield the dying person from the medical conversation, feeling that any talk of possible death is detrimental to the patient's hope for recovery. However, hope is not destroyed or compromised by the truth. If the patient is capable of making decisions about end-of-life treatment, then the health care team must include the patient in the conversation.

Sometimes family members or friends believe they know what is best and what needs to be done for the patient. Sometimes these voices are quite insistent, even though the patient is trying to object and overrule the suggested decisions. An elderly parent may be protesting, "I don't want any more surgery," while an adult son insists, "He doesn't really mean that. He wants to be well again."

Questions sometimes arise about whether family members, or other interested parties, should be present during the interview to evaluate capacity. If too many people are present, it can be confusing and distracting. Or the presence of others may keep the patient from feeling totally free to express an honest opinion. On the other hand, the presence of one or two family members may provide assurance to the family that their loved one does understand the medical situation and has the capacity to make a reasoned decision. Hopefully, their presence will enhance their support for accepting the patient's preferences.

If there is family conflict over the patient's treatment, then having a representative present from both sides during the evaluation of capacity may be helpful. Or having no family members present may be the best solution. In the latter case, the provider will conduct an evaluation of the patient's capacity for medical decision making and then report the results to the conflicting parties. If it is determined that the patient is capable of medical decision making, then respect for the patient's autonomy takes precedence over the conflicting views of the family members.

If the patient is not capable, then decision making shifts to application of advance directives, such as a living will or a durable power of attorney for health care. However, despite the encouragement of the Patient Self-Determination Act of 1990, most people still do not complete advance directives (Lens, 2007a). Without the benefit of an advance directive or designation of a proxy, decision making is assigned according to an established hierarchy of surrogates—spouse, adult child(ren), parent(s), and so on—according to state law (cf. Sulmasy et al., 1994). When family members are in disagreement over a course of action, a grief counselor may become involved in mediation or resolution of the dispute. In extreme situations, such as the legal battles in the Quinlan, Cruzan, and Schiavo cases, the disputes can be settled only in a court of law.

Case Example

The following is an innovative case example of a clinician conducting an evaluation of capacity for medical decision making with a patient who presents communication impediments.

The patient is an elderly man in the intensive care unit following a major heart attack. He is unable to speak or write. His eyes are open, and he appears alert and responsive. The ethical question centers on his capacity for medical decision making in regard to resuscitation. No family or loved ones are available to help. In this case, closed-ended questions are necessary as the only alternative for communicating. Carefully, the evaluator asks a series of questions to determine if "yes" or "no" answers are adequate to assess the patient's comprehension of his condition and his preferences about end-of-life treatment. It is a form of mental status exam based on a limited response—an eye blink.

First, the evaluator establishes with the patient that one blink will mean "yes," and two blinks will mean "no." Then, the evaluator asks the following questions:

"Sir, are you Mr. Jones?" The patient blinks twice, for "no."

"Are you Mr. Smith?" The patient blinks once for "yes."

"Mr. Smith, are you at home?" The patient blinks twice for "no."

"Are you in the car?" The patient again blinks twice for "no."

"Are you in the hospital?" The patient blinks once for "yes."

"Mr. Smith, is the current year 1957?" The patient blinks twice for "no."

"Is it 2009?" He blinks once for "yes."

"Is it spring time, right now?" He blinks once for "yes."

"Is John Kennedy the current president of the United States?" He blinks twice for "no."

"Is the current president Bill Clinton?" He blinks twice for "no."

"Am I your accountant?" He blinks twice for "no."

"Am I a medical doctor in the intensive care unit?" He blinks once for "yes."

From this exchange, the evaluator establishes that, even though the patient is not verbal, he is alert, oriented, and cognizant of his surroundings. The evaluator then proceeds to explain the medical nature of the patient's condition—telling him that he has had a major heart attack and explaining the possibilities for full or partial recovery. He describes the recommended treatment and the consequences of choosing no treatment. At each step, the evaluator carefully words the questions so that the "yes" or "no" answers can be accepted as reliable regarding the patient's understanding of his physical condition and the treatment options. At the conclusion of the examination, the evaluator judges that the patient is capable of the cognitive reasoning necessary for medical decision making.

MINORS AND CAPACITY FOR MEDICAL DECISION MAKING

Children, by legal definition and precedent, do not have the capacity for making medical decisions, except in certain circumstances. At times, older children are given some degree of say in decisions that impact their own health. Children under age 18 may be declared no longer to have minority status, based on conditions such as marrying, becoming a parent, serving in the military, seeking treatment for substance abuse or sexually transmitted disease, or obtaining a declaration of emancipation from a judge. Emancipation to majority status means the child is fully independent and self-sufficient and not receiving educational, physical, financial, or emotional support from the parents. If emancipated from minority status, the child is now an adult, by law, and considered capable of making medical decisions.

According to Diekema (2006), parenting is a form of applied beneficence, promoting good for one's children by supervising and training them. It is also applied nonmaleficence, avoiding neglect and preventing harm where possible. Even though minor children do not have the capacity for making medical decisions, they deserve respect as persons. However, sometimes force is necessary in making decisions and seeing that minors get the medical care they need. For example, a 6-year-old child with a dirty laceration from a bicycle accident may be crying in pain and resisting any medical treatment because of fearing more pain. However, a physician, with parental consent, will proceed to clean and suture the wound, even as the child cries loudly and objects. This 6-year-old does not make the medical decision but is due respect, dignity, and compassion.

Rule of Sevens and Mature Minors

Children develop emotionally and cognitively at different rates, so health care providers who treat children must always consider a minor child's developmental level and capacity for understanding when approaching a medical procedure. Even though parents have the legal right of decision making, the child's understanding must be taken into account and respected during explanations of the diagnosis and discussion of treatment alternatives.

The Rule of Sevens, based on English common law, gives parents and health care providers an operating guideline for assessing a minor child's capacity to participate in medical decision making (Newman, 2001). Through age 7, it is understood that the child is an immature minor and has no capacity for medical decision making, as in the previous example of the 6-year-old with an accidental injury. For ages 7–14, it is possible that the child may object to a medical procedure, and there may be reasons for rebutting a claim of the child's *in*capacity. Children in this age group are moving toward possible status as mature minors, and their increasing cognitive capacities need to be honored. Finally, during ages 14–21, the child's views are considered more carefully, as if the child has capacity for medical decision making. These older children are considered mature minors who have capacity (Hickey, 2007), even though there may be reasons for rebutting a claim of capacity to override their wishes (Diekema, 2006). The greater the harm that could occur as a result of following the child's wishes, the stronger is the argument for overriding them (Strong, 1995).

Consent and Assent

How do parents and health care providers appropriately involve children of different ages in medical decision making? Allow them to express a reasonable preference about treatment and, where possible, adhere to their wishes? Although the legal right of *consent* for treating children remains with the parent, health care providers and grief counselors should work to secure a child's *assent,* or agreement with the proposed treatment or procedure. Even though the child's assent does not carry full legal status, it encourages the child's cooperation with and personal investment in the treatment process. With mature minors, their assent increasingly resembles the consent an autonomous adult would give, but it still cannot be equated legally with consent.

Diekema (2003) proposed that assent is more about beneficence than about autonomy. He cited several reasons that it is a good thing to seek assent from school-age children and mature minors for activities that involve them. Securing assent reminds parents and caregivers that children should be treated with dignity and respect. Permitting children a shared role in decision making benefits their development as autonomous individuals. Also, the process of assent affords children the opportunity to learn the meaning of respect for others, asking someone if it is okay before attempting to do something to that person. Even though Diekema was writing about children's assent for involvement in research, his ideas transfer well to health care settings.

Even so, Koocher (2005) offers a word of caution about assent. Namely, in soliciting a child's assent, the parent or health care provider may give the child the impression of having more say in the decision than the child actually has. If the child does not assent to the recommended treatment, but the parent proceeds to overrule the child's objection, the child may feel somewhat betrayed by the parent and the provider. Thus, any discussion with a minor child to seek assent must be done carefully and respectfully, without misleading the child about how much decision-making authority the child actually has.

Grief counselors who work with children and families need to be familiar with parents' legal rights as decision makers for their children, the Rule of Sevens, and the concept of assent. Frequently, when grief counselors become involved in decision making about end-of-life treatments for minors, it is because there is some dissention between the child and the parents or caregivers over the proposed treatment. In situations where mature minors want a different decision about their medical treatment than that being chosen by the parents, courts often invoke the 50% Risk Rule in addition to the Rule of Sevens (Diekema, 2006). If the mature minor is refusing treatment, and the various risks of not receiving the treatment are less than 50%, then the court will generally rule in favor of the mature minor. On the other hand, if the risks to the child of no treatment are greater than 50%, then the courts will generally rule in favor of the parents to proceed with a decision for treatment.

Grief counselors and health care professionals should recognize that there are legal limits to the authority that parents have over their own children. For example, a parent may be legally determined by a court to be incompetent as a parent for reasons of abuse, neglect, or exploitation and replaced by a guardian or representative of the state with decision-making responsibility for the children's medical treatment. If a parent acts contrary to the best interests of a child's health or well-being or puts the child's life in jeopardy, the state may intervene. In medical decision making, such intervention by the state is most likely to occur when the child is suffering from a serious and potentially life-threatening illness or injury that can be readily managed with medical treatment, except for the parents' objections. Diekema (2004) advocates using the *harm principle* to guide health care professionals and courts in deciding when to intervene over parental authority. The harm principle applies if the decision made by the parents to refuse medical treatment places their child at significant risk of serious harm.

Case Example

A 14-year-old boy, who is a Jehovah's Witness, lacerates his leg in a lawnmower accident while mowing the grass at his home. His parents wrap towels around the leg and rush him to the hospital emergency room. Upon entering, they identify themselves as Jehovah's Witnesses and tell the emergency personnel they do not want their son to have any blood transfusions. The physicians assess the boy and inform the parents that he needs emergency surgery to save his leg. Also, because of significant blood loss, he will require transfusion in connection with surgery. Without a blood transfusion, the boy will probably die; with surgery and transfused blood, he will probably live. Time is of the essence. A decision must be rendered immediately in order to commence surgery to save the boy's life.

Again, the parents say, "No blood." The boy speaks up and says he wants the surgery and blood transfusion. He does not want to die, and he does not care what the Jehovah's Witnesses believe. Then he says, "It's a stupid rule anyway." Wishing to expedite the surgery, the medical staff calls in the hospital's risk manager and a grief counselor to help mediate the situation.

Analysis of Case Example With the Five P Model

Cases such as this tend to inflame passionate reactions in all parties concerned. Working through the case using the Five P Model can elucidate the many ethical issues involved for the family, the grief counselor, the medical staff, and the hospital.

Person

The patient is a 14-year-old-boy, on the cusp of being considered a mature minor. His input in medical decisions deserves careful consideration. Although he does not have legal standing to consent to a major medical procedure, he has indicated his agreement with the doctors' recommendations. In effect, he has assented to the surgery and transfusion. His parents are directly involved in the deliberation and have medical decision-making power. The medical staff, the grief counselor, and the hospital are all stakeholders in the outcome.

Problem

The problem is how to medically treat a minor who has a life-threatening laceration of the leg. Because of severe blood loss, he probably will not survive without surgery and transfused blood. However, the boy's parents refuse to give consent for the operation and transfusion. The parents are concerned about their son's potential loss of eternal salvation if they consent to a blood transfusion.

Nevertheless, the son is giving his assent for treatment. The patient, who might be considered a mature minor, is at odds with his parents about the decision. This conflict is more than just a family disagreement—limb and life hang in the balance, literally. Part of the problem is, How much weight in the decision should be accorded to the preferences of a mature minor with a life-threatening injury who wants medical treatment to survive?

The medical team members, who are trained for emergencies just as this, see no point in wasting valuable time by bickering over a decision that seems so obvious—treating the boy can save his leg and his life.

Place

The place is the emergency department of a local hospital. Once the injured boy enters the premises, the medical staff has an ethical obligation to diagnose and treat him. Also, the hospital has an interest in protecting itself from a potential lawsuit if it fails to save the life of an injured child when it is within its ability to do so. Thus, the location of the dilemma carries considerable institutional pressure to treat the boy.

Principles

Several ethical principles are evident in this case. The emergency department workers have a duty to the principle of beneficence, doing good by saving the boy. To do so, they recommend surgery and blood transfusion.

However, the boy's parents have different values from the emergency personnel. The parents refuse the blood transfusion in order to uphold the "higher law" of their personal religious faith. In a way, they are heeding the principle of nonmaleficence, albeit with a spiritual interpretation. They believe agreeing to a blood transfusion for their son would be disobeying God's law and would do greater eternal harm than physical death on earth. Taking their obligation as parents and the legal guardians very seriously, they insist on their decision being final.

The son has views different from his parents about the religious restrictions on blood transfusions. He has grown up in the Jehovah's Witnesses church, and he knows its teachings. However, the son does not care what the church teaches, and he wants the surgery and blood transfusion so that he can live. Autonomy—the right to self-determination—is the basis of his position.

Apart from the ethical principles involved, there is case law and precedent that pertain to the problem. Risk management informs the emergency personnel that in *Prince v. Massachusetts* (1944), the U.S. Supreme Court found in favor of the state, overruling the religious objections of the parents who refused treatment for a minor child.

> The right to practice religion freely does not include the liberty to expose the community or child to communicable disease, or the latter to ill health or death (pp. 167–168).... Parents may be free to become martyrs themselves, but it does not follow they are free... to make martyrs of their children. (p. 171)

Additionally, legal precedents generally ignore theological consequences of proposed medical treatments when making a determination of what is in the child's best interest (Diekema, 2004).

Furthermore, both the Rule of Sevens and the concept of a mature minor are pertinent to this case example. At age 14, the boy's *in*capacity for medical decision making can be challenged and his preferences considered, according to his cognitive ability, experience, education, training, and maturity of judgment (Newman, 2001; Strong, 1995). In addition, the 50% rule applies because, by refusing a blood transfusion, the parents are exposing their son to a greater-than-50% risk of harm, namely death. Finally, Diekema's (2004) proposed harm principle applies as well because there is significant risk of serious harm in refusing lifesaving surgery and transfusion.

Process

Part of the process is clarifying who are the decision makers for the boy. The parents assume they will decide. However, based on the Rule of

Sevens, the boy is developing maturity, and his views need to be heard. The process cannot be seen simply as a mature minor defying his parents' directives. The urgency and severity of what is at stake make this a life-or-death emergency, not a commonplace family dispute.

With the information from risk management about case law and legal precedents, the medical staff is empowered to act expeditiously to save the boy's life over the parents' objections. With the boy's assent, they are ready to proceed with the surgery and transfusion. They consider the boy a mature minor who has the capacity to make medical decisions. The decision is made in favor of the boy and against his parents' wishes because the potential benefit of surgery and blood transfusion is saving the boy's life and because there is more than a 50% risk of serious harm (i.e., death) by refusing treatment. Medical ethics and state law compel the staff to treat the son, regardless of the family's faith affiliation. Accompanied by the risk manager and the grief counselor, the medical team informs the parents, who are not happy with the decision. Nevertheless, the hospital staff proceeds with surgery and blood transfusion.

The time urgency and life-threatening nature of this scenario may appear to diminish the role of the grief counselor in the decision-making process. Also, the desire of the risk manager for the grief counselor to spend more time with the parents to soothe their distress may be seen as the grief counselor merely doing the hospital's bidding in trying to explain to the parents that the treatment team is making a medical decision, not a religious one. Yet this case is a good example of the fact that life circumstances do not always permit the luxury of a reflective, unhurried conversation to reach consensus about an ethical dilemma.

After the decision, the grief counselor may be the ideal individual to listen compassionately to the parents' worries for their son and to their anger with the medical system. As someone not directly party to the medical decision, the counselor can empathize with their sense of powerlessness. It may be helpful to affirm that the parents have not betrayed their religious faith by agreeing with their son's wishes, possibly assuaging the guilt they feel about the decision. The decision was made by a third party—the hospital staff. The counselor's work may appear unglamorous compared to the heroic actions of the surgical team, but it is certainly within the province of a well-trained grief counselor and resembles the therapeutic measures used in office settings with traumatized and bereaved survivors who have endured uncontrollable losses. Later, there may also be a therapeutic role for the grief counselor to help heal the emotional divide between the parents and their son.

ORGAN DONATION AND TRANSPLANTATION

Organ donation and transplantation are firmly part of mainstream medicine, but numerous ethical questions need to be answered. When is a person actually dead? When is it appropriate to recover organs for transplant? How do families decide to donate organs? Under what conditions should living donors be accepted? How is the scarce supply of available organs allocated among the many patients who desperately need them?

What Is Death?

Religious tradition has contributed to a contemporary understanding of death and the language used to describe it. In the book of Genesis, or the book of Beginnings in the Hebrew Bible, God created people by breathing into them the "breath of life," and this "breath" (from the Latin root *spiritus*) is synonymous with being alive (Roberts, 2003). *Inspiration* connotes an influx of life force or creative energy. Conversely, when people breathe out their last breath, or *expire,* it is understood that they are no longer alive but dead. Because of the physiological connection between circulatory and respiratory functions, a beating heart is also a time-honored way of determining that a person is alive. Even primitive peoples could detect the presence of a heartbeat or pulse as an indication of life itself. Thus, two notions became joined as a definition of life—breathing lungs and a beating heart. An absence of these two critical life functions means the person is dead.

When a person with a massive brain injury stops breathing, that person may be placed on a mechanical ventilator. In effect, the patient is *respired*—that is, they are provided *respiration* artificially. With a beating heart and mechanically assisted breathing, is this person alive? Consider the newspaper article that reported that a 15-year-old girl "died on February 15...from injuries sustained in an all-terrain vehicle" (Ybarra, 2007, p. 3C). The girl died in an accident on February 15, and she was declared dead on February 16. The article stated, "She was declared *brain dead* the day after the accident, but the family *kept her alive* (italics added) so her organs could be harvested for donation" (p. 3C). So how can the girl be dead if she is being *kept alive*? When is the end of life? This newspaper article shows the limitations of society's language for end-of-life circumstances such as these and the ambiguity associated with the concept of brain death (Truog, 2007).

Currently, in the United States, the legal definition of death can be met by two different sets of criteria (Abt, Fisher, & Singhal, 2006). One criterion is cessation of cardiopulmonary function, meaning that a person's heart has stopped and the person is no longer breathing. When the stoppage is judged irreversible, this is known as *heart-lung death* and meets the traditional definition previously given. The second criterion is cessation of whole brain function, meaning that the patient on life support shows no evidence of higher brain function on electroencephalogram (EEG), fails a series of clinical tests for neurological function, and shows no evidence of brain stem function, which controls respiration. The latter is verified, in part, by the apnea test, which involves removing the patient from the ventilator to determine whether there is any neurological drive to breathe. If no function is detected, the test is typically repeated in 6 to 12 hours. If the findings persist, then the patient is diagnosed with *brain death* (Truog, 2007). The judgment of irreversibility applies to brain death also. These two criteria for pronouncing a patient dead are codified in the Uniform Determination of Death Act (UDDA; National Conference of Commissioners on Uniform State Laws, 1980).

The majority of organs are transplanted from brain dead patients. These "deceased donors are supported by mechanical ventilation and pharmacologic treatment...the donor is brought to the operating room for organ recovery. Organs from deceased donors are perfused by the donor's heart throughout the recovery process" (Abt et al., 2006, p. 208). Sometimes, these situations are referred to in clinical terms as *heart-beating organ donation.* Withdrawing brain-dead patients from the respirator usually results in cardiac arrest shortly thereafter, which would, in effect, meet the criterion of heart-lung death as well. However, the fact that their hearts are still beating at the time of organ removal for transplant raises uncomfortable ethical questions.

In the practice of transplantation, the Dead Donor Rule is a specific prohibition against removing vital organs from patients who are still alive because the recovery of such organs would then become the immediate, or proximate, cause of death (Robertson, 1999). However, if brain death constitutes death by definition, then transplanting organs from these heart-beating donors can be allowed. Because of reservations created by this ambiguity, Truog (2007) has described brain death as a concept "too flawed to endure, too ingrained to abandon" (p. 273).

One safeguard in place to avoid abuse, such as prematurely declaring brain death just so the donated organs can be taken, is strict separation between the medical team managing the clinical care of the patient and the transplant surgery team. One group of physicians assesses the neurological function of the patient, verifies complete loss of brain activity, and makes a declaration of brain death. These same doctors also handle discussions with the family about giving consent for organ donation. Then, a completely different team of doctors assumes responsibility for surgical removal of the organs. No crossover between these two medical teams is permitted (Abt et al., 2006). This mandate was codified in the original 1968 Uniform Anatomical Gift Act (National Conference of Commissioners on Uniform State Laws, 2006).

The Decision to Donate Organs

If health care professionals and bioethicists struggle so mightily with the ambiguities accompanying transplant medicine, what about the families and loved ones of brain-dead patients who are involved in the actual conversations about whether to donate organs? How can grief counselors help with these wrenching end-of-life decisions?

In the case from the newspaper article described earlier, the mother of the brain-dead girl agreed to donate her organs. At first, the mother opposed organ donation, citing her Roman Catholic faith. However, her son convinced her to allow it. The mother later learned that the Roman Catholic Church actually supports organ donation, and so she was very relieved about the decision. Further details provided in the story reported that the person who received the daughter's kidney was doing well with the transplant. The case is a good illustration of how the subject of organ donation and transplantation has become part of the end-of-life decision-making process.

Because donation requires the approval of the patient through an advance directive, like a living will or designation of a health care proxy, some people make the decision about transplant simply by doing nothing. By doing nothing, the person is refusing donation by default. Fewer than 20% of adults in the United States sign forms agreeing to be organ donors (Pence, 2004). Some worry that the sacred value of the dying person will be diminished in order to harvest the organs because they do not trust health care professionals to honor the Dead Donor Rule, or they question whether all reasonable treatment options will be pursued for terminally ill patients who may be seen as potential donors.

Some disability rights advocates suspect that people with disabilities may be devalued or that their lives may be judged wrongly as having less quality in order to justify proxy decisions for withholding or withdrawing treatment at the end of life. Following this logic, people with disabilities could more quickly be declared dead for the purpose of recovering their organs (cf. Werth, 2005). Advocates contend that disability is a condition, not an illness, and that disability is not automatically terminal (Pence, 2004). Consider the case of film actor Christopher Reeve, who starred in the 1978 movie *Superman*. Reeve suffered a spinal cord injury of the neck in 1995, resulting in quadriplegia, or near-total body paralysis, and required a ventilator to breathe but was still very much alive, brain-wise, for 9 more years until his natural death in 2004 (Truog, 2007).

Others refuse organ donation for religious reasons. For example, those who believe in a bodily existence after death may believe that one should not do anything to violate the integrity of the body when it goes into the next life. It is the same reasoning used against cremation. Generally, the three Abrahamic faiths of Judaism, Christianity, and Islam have a view of some form of bodily existence in the next life, and some sects may refuse organ donation or cremation on those grounds. On the other hand, Hindus believe that cremation is the proper way to handle the body after death because, in burning, the soul is released to progress to the next level of incarnation (Rambachan, 2003). It is important to recognize that all major organized religions approve of organ and tissue donation and consider it an act of charity (United Network for Organ Sharing, 2004).

Organ donation should never be compelled, and a prospective donor's autonomy should always be respected. However, many donor families take comfort in knowing that something of their loved ones lives on even after their deaths, as a result of donating their organs and tissue. "Giving the gift of life" to someone in need can bring a degree of consolation to family members whose loved ones die from cardiac arrest or brain death, because of knowing that some good resulted from the loss (cf. Gamino et al., 2000).

Aulisio, DeVita, and Luebke (2007) declare adamantly that any discussions with surrogate decision makers about end-of-life care and withdrawal of life-sustaining treatments for the patient should be kept completely separate from any discussion about organ donation. This is intended to preclude transplant considerations from influencing decisions about withdrawal of treatment and vice versa. Yet even Aulisio et al. acknowledge that ethical decision making at the end of life occurs in context with many value-laden considerations, one of which may be the potentially redeeming value of allowing someone else to live longer or better as a result of donating the deceased patient's organs for transplant.

As a practical matter, discussions about futility of medical treatment, withdrawing care, and potential organ donation often occur in the same time frame (cf. Abt et al., 2006), if not within the same conversation. Inquiry about organ donation is an especially delicate matter when donors die from cardiopulmonary death, sometimes called donation after cardiac death (Aulisio et al., 2007; Bernat et al., 2006). In cases of donation after cardiac death, recovery of donated organs begins immediately following a waiting period of 2–5 minutes after life support has been withdrawn, which is mandated by organ procurement organizations in order to be sure that no cardiopulmonary activity spontaneously restarts. Immediacy of organ recovery for transplant is necessary because vital organs deteriorate so quickly after loss of blood supply and oxygen. Obviously, in these cases, where withdrawal of life support is followed closely by a pronouncement of death and organ recovery begins immediately, the necessary coordination involved cannot occur without prior planning. Even when these events occur in fairly rapid succession, sensitivity should be maintained toward the family members whose loved one has just died and who are saying a final goodbye before releasing the body.

Living Donors

One of the most controversial aspects of organ donation is the increase in the number of living donors, which is now about equal to the number of cadaveric donors (Aulisio et al., 2007). Traditionally, living donors were family members or relatives making a donation directly to the recipient. Over time, the standard was extended to accept nonrelatives such as close friends who shared a relational bond with the recipient.

A restrictive standard was based on ethical concerns about the donors. Because the process of donating a vital organ, such as a kidney or a lung lobe, poses potential health risks to the donor without any appreciable physiologic benefit (Ingelfinger, 2005), it contradicts the ethical principle of nonmaleficence. Without a love connection between the live donor and the recipient, it is difficult to fathom why someone would willingly subject themselves to risk when the potential benefit is only for the organ recipient. Where there *is* a connection, love and caring outweigh whatever violation of nonmaleficence takes place against the voluntary donor. It is an autonomously accepted violation of nonmaleficence for the beneficence of the recipient (cf. Caplan, 2004). Some

Christians view the living donation as a metaphor for the death of Jesus, that is, choosing to suffer for the benefit of another.

With advances in immune suppression making available a broader range of donor–recipient compatibility (Ingelfinger, 2005), some in the transplant community have promulgated extending living donation to all degrees of nonrelative recipients, on a continuum from close friends to total strangers. However, the real move beyond only blood relatives or dear friends donating comes from factors beyond the control of the transplant community. In response to the scarce supply of available organs and lengthy waiting lists, some people attempt to "jump the queue" through direct appeals and public solicitation (Aulisio et al., 2007). For example, some patients advertise their need on a billboard, in the newspaper, or on a personal Web page, hoping a sympathetic person will come forward and make a *directed donation* naming them as the specific recipient (Steinbrook, 2005). Also, commercial Web sites such as MatchingDonors.com attempt to help potential donors and recipients find one another. All of these attempts to procure an organ through directed donation from an anonymous donor are rife with potential for abuse and risk creating a commodities market for human organs and tissue (Aulisio et al., 2007; cf. Delmonico & Graham, 2006; Truog, 2005).

To combat the potential ethical problems presented by direct appeals and solicitations, Aulisio et al. (2007) suggest setting rigorous standards for the presurgical assessment of the decision-making capacity and psychological state of the prospective living donor, together with a detailed informed consent process that unfolds over time and includes significant educational components. They are especially cautious about such direct appeals unwittingly taking advantage of people with psychiatric disorders. Unfortunately, psychiatric patients may come forward for unhealthy reasons, such as grandiosity or believing that their own lives are not worth much.

Beyond the controversies surrounding directed donation of organs is the issue of regulated selling of organs for transplant in order to handle the gap between supply and demand. Caplan (2004) unequivocally rejected any suggestion that society permit direct sale of body parts, such as a kidney, for transplantation. He argued that selling organs for transplant is inherently unethical and exploitative because it violates the supposed autonomy of the economically destitute who may choose such a drastic option only because they have no real alternatives for generating income.

Justice in Organ Allocation

In the 1970s, there was no clear system for evaluating and determining which recipients should have priority for receiving a donated organ. Various regions of the country and various medical centers made their own rules, which were sometimes at odds with one another. The National Organ Transplant Act (1984) created the Organ Procurement and Transplantation Network, which contracts with the United Network for Organ Sharing (UNOS), a nonprofit, scientific and educational organization, to administer a series of regional organ procurement organizations throughout the country. According to the UNOS guidelines and standards, patients waiting for re-transplants are treated the same as those who are waiting for a first transplant. They do not receive any advantage (or disadvantage) because they previously received an organ that their bodies rejected. The urgency of the need for a re-transplant does not push these patients to a place of preference on the organ recipient waiting list (Pence, 2004).

There were approximately 28,000 transplants in the United States in 2006, compared to a wait list of 91,000 who needed organs. This means that approximately 60,000 needy recipients went unmatched that year (Aulisio et al., 2007). Allocating such a scarce resource brings the ethical principle of justice to the forefront. In a country such as the United States that is committed to the sanctity and dignity of every person, who should get priority on the list of recipients waiting for donated organs? A primary objective of UNOS is establishing objective criteria, such as severity of illness, time spent waiting, blood type, and other medical considerations, for rating potential recipients. The goal is a system of allocation that is fair for all concerned and not dependent on social or economic considerations (Delmonico & Graham, 2006). But, does the system always work?

In 1995 the famous New York Yankees baseball player Mickey Mantle was dying from liver failure after 43 years of alcoholism (Munson, 2002). The average time spent waiting for a liver transplant in 1995 was 3 or 4 months; however, Mantle was transplanted the next day after his need was established. He died 3 months later. When Mantle received his liver, others on the list waiting for a liver were passed over so Mantle could receive one. Was this justice? Some contend that Mantle's wealth and notoriety influenced the process; he was a celebrity and could easily afford to pay tens of thousands of dollars for the transplant. Does this mean that Mantle was more deserving of a transplant than someone whose medical bills were paid by government-funded Medicare or by private donations? This episode raises serious ethical questions about justice and the allocation of resources.

Ultimately, a variety of end-of-life ethical concerns relate to donation and transplantation. Many of these concerns pertain to the scarcity of available organs.

> Critical care professionals know the sad reality behind the statistical scarcity of organ supply. . . . They must manage anxious patients and family members who may be waiting for an organ that never comes, triage patients into and out of the intensive care unit, and work through the propriety of shifting goals from cure to comfort when those same patients deteriorate to the point that transplant may no longer be an appropriate medical option or when a transplant fails. Equally significant challenges arise on the donor side, whether it is working through difficult end-of-life decisions, identifying when to call the Organ Procurement Organization, caring for brain-dead patients, managing a potential [candidate for donation after cardiac death], or increasingly, caring for a living donor postoperatively. (Aulisio et al., 2007, p. S95)

There is no doubt that working in the organ donation and transplant field is taxing. Mental health professionals and grief counselors perform an invaluable service when they choose to share their talents and expertise meeting the many demands it imposes. Well-informed, ethically conscious grief counselors can help medical staffs, donors, recipients, and families grapple with the ethical challenges inherent in organ donation and transplantation.

SUMMARY

The best time to plan for the end of life is before the end comes. Various ethical dilemmas and controversies can be avoided with advance planning. Everyone should be encouraged to make decisions about their preferences regarding end-of-life care while they are still fully capable of mental activity. One of the most important considerations is designation of a health care proxy to make decisions should individuals lose the capacity to make end-of-life decisions for themselves. It is important for people to record their wishes in a clear, written document that decreases the possibility of ambiguity or conflict for those whose task it will be to carry out those wishes. End-of-life dilemmas are often the most difficult for patients and families to face, yet they offer many opportunities for grief counselors to educate, mediate, and comfort. Grief counselors are uniquely trained and eminently qualified to assist individuals with their end-of-life planning and decision making.

7 Multiple Relationships in Thanatology

The highly personal nature of grief counseling can lead to ethical conundrums in the arena of multiple relationships (formerly designated "dual" relationships). To the client, a grief counselor may be perceived more like a friend than a professional. Where are the lines of distinction between these two roles? Frequently, the grief counselor must "join" the family system in order to be an effective source of influence or an agent for positive change. So what happens when the client's family considers the counselor to be "family"? What obligations are incumbent upon the grief counselor when the place of service provision moves beyond the traditional consultation office to a patient's hospital bed, the family residence, a funeral home, a place of worship, or an educational setting? Given the level of familiarity that may develop during grief counseling, when is it appropriate to touch or hug a client or family member? In light of such questions, it comes as no surprise that negotiating multiple relationships presents particularly thorny ethical challenges for grief counselors. Indeed, Pope and Vetter (1992) found handling "blurred, dual, or conflictual relationships" (p. 399) to be the second most common ethical dilemma reported by professional psychologists. This chapter is designed to provide a clear framework for addressing the challenges of multiple relationships specific to the ethical practice of grief counseling.

DEFINITIONS

In counseling and psychology, as well as in the ADEC Code of Ethics, the term *multiple relationships* is used to denote instances wherein the professional has more than one association or affiliation with another person. For the grief counselor, this means that there is at least one other professional or personal connection with the client that exists in addition to the counseling relationship. For example, the client may also be one's trainee, employee, colleague, friend, family member, business associate, merchant, and so on. Multiple relationships can include more than one professional relationship (i.e., counselor and professor) or a combination of professional and personal relationships (i.e., counselor and relative). Sometimes multiple relationships occur when the grief counselor has a relationship with someone closely associated with the client, such as when the client's spouse or relative is well-known to the counselor. Multiple relationships can occur concurrently or consecutively (Sonne, 1994, 2005). Consider the following dilemmas:

- A research assistant on a current bereavement study experiences a personal tragedy when the assistant's fiancé completes suicide. The research assistant approaches the faculty investigator and requests grief counseling on the rationale that this investigator has the most expert knowledge on grief and loss of anyone the research assistant knows. Also, the research assistant implicitly trusts the faculty investigator and so prefers confiding in the investigator rather than in another unfamiliar professional. Should the investigator agree to provide grief counseling to the research assistant—concurrent multiple relationships of research supervisor and counselor?
- A grief counselor chooses to shop for a new automobile at the dealership where a former client is a sales representative. The sales agent is thrilled and considers it an honor to do business with the grief counselor who was so helpful during the time of loss. Should the counselor buy a car from the former client—consecutive multiple relationships of counselor, then customer?
- A grief counselor works in a small office practice with two other psychotherapists. A best friend of one of the psychotherapists makes an appointment for grief counseling following a major loss. If the grief counselor agrees to take the fellow therapist's best friend as a client, then concurrent multiple relationships

are created in two ways. First, the grief counselor becomes both counselor and "friend's friend" to the client. Second, the grief counselor becomes both colleague and friend's counselor to the practice partner.

- A grateful former client nominates the grief counselor to serve on the advisory board of a local community center where grief support groups are offered at no cost. The former client is also a board member, so the two end up working together in this volunteer effort. Socializing occurs after many of the functions, and in that context, a friendship develops between the former client and the grief counselor. In this instance, three distinct relationships occur consecutively: counselor, fellow board member, and friend.
- The grief counselor on a hospice staff gets very close to a patient's family, and they are deeply grateful for the counselor's presence and participation in the final days of their loved one's life. After the patient dies, the family invites the counselor to attend the wake service and then come to the family home thereafter, where it is their cultural tradition to drink alcohol and exchange stories about the deceased late into the night before the funeral the next day. To the patient's family, the grief counselor is an honorary family member and thus welcome during their personal time of grief. Should the counselor choose to attend the wake and accept the invitation to the family home—concurrent multiple relationships of counselor and honorary relative?

Myriad examples of such multiple relationships may come to mind even when excluding accidental or incidental extratherapeutic contacts, such as running into a client in a retail setting or at a social event (Pope & Vasquez, 2007).

The ADEC Code of Ethics is consistent with other mental health and medical disciplines in discouraging multiple relationships for two fundamental reasons: potential for impairment of professional objectivity and potential for exploitation of clients.

> Members do not use their professional relationships to further their personal, political, religious, or business interests. (ADEC Code of Ethics, I. General Conduct, E)

> Members refrain from multiple relationships if (1) such relationships could reasonably be expected to impair the objectivity, competence, or effectiveness

> of the member in performing his/her responsibilities; or if (2) such relationships otherwise risk exploitation or harm to the person(s) with whom the professional relationship exists or formerly existed. (ADEC Code of Ethics, I. General Conduct, G)
>
> Members avoid conflicts of interest that interfere with professional discretion and impartial judgment. If a real or potential conflict of interest arises, members take reasonable steps to resolve the issue in a manner that reflects the best interests of the person(s) served. (ADEC Code of Ethics, I. General Conduct, H)

Additionally, the ADEC Code of Ethics addresses ancillary aspects of multiple relationships in guidelines specific to the grief counselor.

> Members make appointments with relatives or collateral[s] of clients only when clients have given their permission, unless an emergent situation requires another course of action. In this case, members consider legal and ethical implications and seek consultation before proceeding. (ADEC Code of Ethics, GC-I., Responsibility to Those Served, F)

It is widely acknowledged that multiple relationships are difficult, if not impossible, to avoid completely (Gottlieb, 1993; Koocher & Keith-Spiegel, 2008; Pope & Vetter, 1992). Particularly in smaller, cohesive communities or rural settings, multiple relationships may be unavoidable and not necessarily undesirable (Barnett & Yutrzenka, 1994; Campbell & Gordon, 2003; Gripton & Valentich, 2004; Schank & Skovholt, 1997; Simon & Williams, 1999). Nor is it universally accepted that all multiple relationships are inherently risky, exploitative, or unethical (Anderson & Kitchener, 1996; Gottlieb, 1993; Lazarus, 1994; Vasquez, 2005).

In determining sound ethical practice when multiple relationships occur, it is important to distinguish between boundary crossings and boundary violations (cf. Welfel, 2006). A boundary *crossing* generally refers to a deliberate decision by the grief counselor to step across a customary division or separation of roles in order to achieve something helpful or beneficial to the client that may not occur otherwise. The motivation lies in the principle of beneficence, striving to accomplish some good for the client and putting the client's welfare above all else.

Take the example of the professor who accepts the research assistant as a client. The rationale may rest on the argument that the faculty investigator is in the best position to expeditiously treat the crisis, whereas if the investigator declines, the research assistant may have trouble finding another counselor knowledgeable in these matters who will offer an appointment in a timely manner. Of course, the conclusion that the professor worked primarily toward the benefit of the research assistant assumes the absence of mitigating factors such as knowing other grief counselors who could competently handle the case, allowing curiosity about an employee's tragedy to cloud professional judgment, or taking the ego-gratifying position that one's own version of grief therapy is peerless. Simon and Williams (1999) note purity of motive is seldom found and insist that practitioners ask themselves, "Am I making this intervention or taking this action for the benefit of the [client's] treatment or for my own personal benefit?" (p. 1441).

A boundary *violation* refers to a more egregious overstepping of customary role divisions where the client may be harmed or the counselor's therapeutic effectiveness compromised by actions taken. In these instances, the resulting negative outcomes could have been avoided if the counselor had thought through consequences more thoroughly or acted altruistically rather than selfishly. Here the ethical breach results from failure to ensure nonmaleficence in favor of furthering self-interest. Inevitably, personal harm to the client occurs, the therapeutic relationship is damaged, and the counselor loses objectivity.

Take the example of the counselor who agrees first to serve on a community board with a former client and then cultivates a personal friendship. First, the counselor's ambition for community involvement or recognition may have played a bigger part in accepting the nomination than genuine compassion or altruism. Second, the counselor is remiss not to consider the former client's motives for the nomination, such as seeking a nonprofessional relationship with the counselor or utilizing the counseling affiliation to enhance the client's status. Third, befriending a former client may involve exploitation, for example, seeking admiration from someone inclined to view the counselor with a halo effect or seeking ascendancy over someone who is easily controlled. Fourth, the friendship alters the relationship in such a way that future provision of counseling is precluded or, worse, if attempted is compromised by the attendant loss of objectivity and neutrality. Of course, these deleterious outcomes assume darker motives on the part of the counselor and a lack of redeeming reasons for pursuing nonprofessional connections with a former client (e.g., creative synergy between two individuals who choose not to let the circumstances of their former counselor–client relationship prevent them from working together for a worthy cause).

SEXUAL INTIMACIES WITH CLIENTS

Much of the literature in the area of multiple relationships concerns boundary violations when counselors engage in sexual intimacies with their clients. Scientific evidence has concluded overwhelmingly that romantic or sexual relationships between professional counselors and their clients or trainees are always destructive and thus clearly unethical (Pope, 1988, 1994, 2001; Pope & Bouhoutsos, 1986). Counselor–client sexual relationships meet both major criteria of a problematic multiple relationship: harm to and exploitation of the client and impairment of the counselor's objectivity and perspective. Because sexualized multiple relationships are so pernicious, the ADEC Code of Ethics, like those of other professional organizations, unequivocally condemns them.

> Sexual relationships with clients, students, and/or their significant others [are] unethical. (ADEC Code of Ethics, I. General Conduct, F)

Instead of this universal proscription, some have argued that sex between counselors and *former* clients may be permissible under certain circumstances, such as sufficient time elapsing between the termination of the counseling relationship and the onset of sexual relations, or when the nature of the counseling was time-limited and focal, or when both parties agree to forgo any future counseling relationship. Generally, those who argue for this loophole in an otherwise blanket prohibition on counselor–client sexual relations do not adhere to the operating principle, "Once a client, always a client" (Anderson & Kitchener, 1996). Yet data from state licensing boards show that the time elapsed between termination of treatment and onset of sexual relations had no influence on perceived culpability of professional psychologists who became sexually involved with former clients (Gottlieb, Sell, & Schoenfeld, 1988). For some, the issue of sexual relationships between counselors and former clients remains a gray zone of ambiguity, whereas others endorse banning counselor–client sexual relationships altogether (Bersoff, 2003b).

For us, such discussion brings to mind the sage advice of a revered training supervisor who explained the injunction against sexual relations between a counselor and former client this way: "You would never take on as a client someone you had dated, so why would you date someone you had seen as a client?" We endorse the more conservative position that sexual relationships between counselors and clients or between counselors and former clients are inherently unethical and expressly verboten.

Similarly, Pope and Vasquez (2007) argue for a fundamental prohibition of counselor–client sex as a *sine qua non* of ethical practice:

> There is . . . a clear prohibition: avoid any sexual involvement with clients. No cause, situation, or condition could ever legitimize such intimacies with any client. . . . The prohibition stands as a fundamental ethical mandate no matter what the rationalizations. (p. 180)

Because for us the ethical mandate prohibiting sexualized multiple relationships is so unambiguous, we refer readers interested in a more detailed treatise on this topic to other texts (Pope & Vasquez, 2007; Welfel, 2006). Accordingly, we devote the remainder of this chapter to exploration of nonsexual multiple relationships in grief counseling.

RECURRING QUESTIONS REGARDING MULTIPLE RELATIONSHIPS

Grief counselors encounter potential multiple relationships in many ways. In part, these relationships are due to the intensely intimate nature of the therapeutic endeavor (i.e., addressing profound existential issues surrounding dying, death, finitude, mortality, afterlife, bereavement, continuing connections, and life after loss). In part, they are due also to the variety of settings in which grief counseling occurs (i.e., offices, hospitals, homes, bedsides, funeral homes, cemeteries, places of worship, or educational environments).

Another reason potential multiple relationships can occur so often for grief counselors is because of the profession's mandate to work actively within one's community as well as broader society to help improve care of the dying and the bereaved.

The ADEC Code of Ethics clearly underscores this societal obligation:

> Members interpret and share with the public their professional expertise regarding issues affecting the welfare of society. (ADEC Code of Ethics, VII. Responsibility to Society, E)

> Grief counselors/therapists are encouraged to offer their expertise in the geographical community in which they live and to take part in collaboration and interdisciplinary teamwork when working in a hospital or school environment. (ADEC Code of Ethics, GC-III. Responsibility to Others, C)

When appropriate, grief counselors are expected to operate beyond the traditional counselor–client dyad or the counselor–family model by sharing their knowledge to benefit those who are aggrieved or traumatized. See Chapter 11, "Potential Pitfalls of Public Service," for an exploration of many ethical issues involved when grief counselors provide public service.

For all of these reasons—intensely intimate therapeutic work, multiplicity of service settings, mandate for public service—grief counselors encounter potentially troublesome multiple relationships with some regularity. In the arena of multiple relationships, there are many parallels between these challenges facing grief counselors and those facing medical and mental health practitioners who work in rural settings and smaller communities. Therefore, we employ some of the findings and recommendations from the literature on rural practice in the following discussion of recurring questions regarding multiple relationships.

What About Power Differentials?

An inherent power differential is embedded in the counselor–client relationship. The very reasons a client consults a counselor are based on a presumption of special knowledge and expertise on the part of the counselor, attributes that afford prestige and power. These elements are crucial to the counselor's ability to persuade the client to consider new concepts, perform rituals, or undertake novel actions that constitute change or healing (Frank & Frank, 1991). Awareness of power differentials and respect for how they operate has much to do with avoiding exploitative or harmful multiple relationships (cf. Ballou et al., 2008; Feminist Therapy Institute, 2000).

Kitchener (1988) incorporated findings from role theory to explore potential conflicts in multiple relationships owing to power differentials. Because social roles carry with them expectations about how a person will behave, grief counselors who simultaneously or sequentially participate in two or more role categories may engender conflicting expectations in themselves and in those with whom they work. Kitchener calls this "role strain." Strain from multiple roles can occur when the grief counselor is confused as to what behavior is appropriate or when others' expectations of the counselor make competing demands. In the example of the hospice counselor who accepts an invitation to the deceased patient's wake, social expectations to swap stories of the deceased may exert strain on therapeutic confidentiality. Kitchener emphasizes how, as the incompatibility of expectations between roles increases, the potential for misunderstanding and harm increases.

According to Kitchener (1988), power differentials are particularly problematic when obligations of one's professional role conflict with one's personal, political, or business interests. Again, as the obligations of different roles diverge more widely, so increases the potential for divided loyalties, diminished respect for the client's welfare, and loss of objectivity by the professional. In the example of the grief counselor who opts to purchase an automobile from a former client, getting a good deal on the car may come at the expense of the client's self-esteem (and income).

Conversely, loss of objectivity on the part of the client can occur as a result of the inequity in prestige and power associated with the role of professional compared with the role of consumer of the professional's services (Kitchener, 1988). As the prestige and power discrepancy increases, so does the potential for exploitation through reduced capacity by clients to remain objective about their own best interests. In the example of the office partner's friend who comes for grief counseling, viewing the counselor not only as an expert professional but also as the good friend of a friend may make it more difficult for the client to evaluate objectively the soundness of the grief counselor's advice or to reject advice when it is not in the client's best interest. Kitchener concludes that as the risk of harm to the client from these power differentials increases, so should the counselor's ethical prohibition against engaging in such multiple relationships.

Gottlieb (1993) devised a decision-making model for professionals contemplating whether to assume a second (or third) association with a client. In considering multiple relationships prospectively, Gottlieb encourages the counselor to assess first the current relationship with the client along three dimensions: degree of power the counselor exerts in relation to the client; duration of relationship, with longer implying more influence; and clarity of termination, referring to the likelihood of the counselor and client having further professional contact. Then these same considerations are applied to the contemplated relationship. When the counselor's power and influence are high, the duration of the relationship has been or will be lengthy, and termination is ambiguous, multiple relationships should be avoided. Power differentials as well as role incompatibilities factor prominently in whether multiple relationships may be harmful or exploitative. Finally, Gottlieb emphasizes that, in order to protect the welfare of the client, multiple relationships need to be assessed *from the standpoint of the client.* Decisions about the advisability of contemplated multiple relationships should be made conservatively, after employing consultation from a colleague and discussing the decision with the client.

Counselor or Friend?

Experienced grief counselors inevitably find that some clients consider their counselors to be like friends, usually based on the confidences divulged during treatment. Many times, the material disclosed to the counselor is something the client has not ventured to share with anyone else. Some clients are isolated and lonely to the point that their counselors may be one of their few outlets, or only outlet, for meaningful interpersonal exchange. It is also the case that some clients are very rewarding to work with, and the "gemütlichkeit" or warm feelings generated by the counseling lead to an air of convivial familiarity that may resemble a conversation between friends. So is the grief counselor a professional consultant or a friend to the client, or both?

Gripton and Valentich (2004) outline four fundamental differences between a professional relationship and a friendship that are helpful to recall when addressing the counselor-versus-friend dilemma. First, friendships are based on the assumption of equality, whereas counselor–client relationships are hierarchical in structure, with the counselor holding special status owing to therapeutic skill and knowledge. Second, friendships are generally open-ended, whereas counseling relationships are more often time-limited, even though some may go on for years or even decades. Third, friendships are built on reciprocal self-disclosure and sharing. By contrast, the counseling relationship involves more one-way self-disclosure by the client, so that counselor and client contribute differently to the relationship. Fourth, confidences are mutual in friendships, whereas in counseling the onus for confidentiality rests with the counselor. Thus, these differences suggest that the roles of counselor and friend are incompatible in many ways.

Certainly, an earnest, friendly demeanor on the part of the grief counselor can facilitate client comfort and help establish rapport. Interpersonal warmth and unconditional valuing of the client have been well established as fundamental counselor attitudes necessary for enabling constructive change (Rogers, 1957). Especially for clients from cultures that value warmth and welcoming, a friendly style is important (Vasquez, 2005). However, friendliness as therapeutic role behavior should not be confused with license to relate as friends with the client.

Even when the client feels like the grief counselor has become a friend, these feelings are best understood in the context of positive transference, that is, a tendency by the client to view the counselor in an idealized manner. The phenomenon of positive transference, as understood from a psychodynamic perspective (Bauer & Kobos, 1987), is a byproduct of the counselor–client dynamic wherein the client responds with admiration and appreciation to being heard, understood, valued, and helped by the counselor. It is important to acknowledge positive transference as a natural response from a grateful client to appropriate role behavior by the counselor, rather than viewing it as an endorsement or confirmation of the counselor as a special person.

Often it is easier for counselors, especially novices, to manage negative transference from clients (e.g., hostile feelings) than it is to manage positive transference. When managing negative transference, counselors more readily understand clients' negative attributions toward them as reactions to role behavior or displacement of feelings more appropriately directed toward someone else in the client's life, rather than as an accurate reflection of the counselor as a person. Yet positive transference can be more seductive because counselors who are not self-aware may take to heart such attributions in order to gratify their own ego needs for recognition and adulation or to satisfy an exaggerated need to be important in the client's life. Such unexamined countertransference feelings on the part of the grief counselor can lead to risky blurring of the boundary between counselor and friend.

The principles of beneficence and fidelity come into play when answering the question of whether the grief counselor is professional or friend. Beneficence dictates that the welfare of the client is paramount. Thus, cultivating a cozy friendship with a client in order to meet one's own needs is inconsistent with acting in the best interest of the client. Likewise, the client's emotional vulnerability entrusted to the grief counselor demands a good-faith response by the counselor to honor that trust. It is the counselor's expertise and guidance that is sought by the client. Pursuit of a friendship, either by the client or the counselor, is merely a disguised social transaction. It is not grief counseling, and it is not ethical practice.

In summary, friendly role behavior on the grief counselor's part is not the same thing as having a friendship with the client. Friendliness is encouraged; friendship is discouraged. Nonetheless, the complexity of this issue will become even more apparent in subsequent sections of this chapter devoted to specific venues in which grief counseling is conducted.

Is Nonsexual Touching Permissible?

In the psychoanalytic tradition, psychotherapy and counseling are conducted according to the principle of *abstinence,* meaning the professional should abstain from obtaining personal gratification at the expense of the patient beyond the professional satisfaction gained in helping the client and the material benefit realized from the fee rendered (Simon, 1995; Simon & Williams, 1999). This concept can be traced back to Sigmund Freud. Recommended boundaries include counselor neutrality and anonymity, an effort to foster the psychological separateness of the client, and verbal interaction rather than physical contact. When this traditional model of therapy is practiced in a contemporary climate charged with risk-management concerns, any physical contact between grief counselor and client beyond a perfunctory handshake could represent a potential boundary violation. Certainly, this model is closely aligned with the European cultural roots of its developers and thus represents one end of a continuum.

At the other end of the continuum are models based on multicultural or feminist perspectives wherein there is a much more fluid approach to the question of nonsexual touch (Vasquez, 2005). Along these lines, many grief counselors would have little hesitation extending a gentle, noncoercive touch of the hand, arm, or shoulder to a frightened client who is dying. Likewise, a warm, nonsexual hug may be a very appropriate way of communicating care, comfort, and compassion to a newly bereaved family member. So how does the grief counselor dedicated to ethical practice determine what is permissible regarding nonsexual touching of clients?

As a caution, some scholars (Gutheil & Gabbard, 1993; Simon, 1995) warn of the slippery slope regarding nonsexual touching where serious boundary violations such as sexual intimacies with clients start with a series of seemingly innocuous boundary crossings. In these scenarios, the counseling relationship moves from formality to familiarity by using first names, allowing social conversation to intrude on counseling work, permitting increased self-disclosure by the therapist, and progressively engaging in some body contact. The regular frequency with which counselors experience sexual fantasies about clients (Bernsen, Tabachnick, & Pope, 1994; Pope, Keith-Spiegel, & Tabachnick, 1986) requires the ethical practitioner to scrutinize whether nonsexual touch occurs in the service of the therapeutic agenda, rather than for either self-interest or gratification of inappropriately seductive, regressive, or self-debasing strivings by the client.

In addition to whether there is a clear therapeutic imperative to touch the client, there are a number of other questions to be asked when evaluating the appropriateness of nonsexual touch in grief counseling. Is the counselor personally comfortable with touch? Does the counselor's therapeutic style or methods (e.g., some Gestalt exercises, psychodrama, family sculpting) regularly involve touch? If so, can the client expect therapeutic use of touch, and is there opportunity for the client to decline (i.e., informed refusal)? Does the client's cultural and ethnic background permit or prohibit touch in a counseling context? Do the client's history (e.g., trauma, abuse) and personal sensibilities render any form of touch uncomfortable or problematic? Answering these questions involves self-awareness on the grief counselor's part as well as continuous monitoring of the client's reactions.

In attempting to discern the appropriate boundary between problematic ways of touching clients and acceptable forms of physical contact such as a pat on the back, a touch of the arm, or even a hug, we recommend the "living room test." That is, asking oneself the following question: "Is what I am saying to the client or doing with the client something I would be comfortable saying or doing in my own living room with a family member present as a silent observer?" If the answer to this self-appraisal question is affirmative, then the private behavior of the counseling relationship is more than likely appropriate. In these cases, there really is no multiple relationship dilemma because the nonsexual touch is an extension of the therapeutic process between counselor and client.

However, if the answer to the living room test is negative, there is a strong likelihood that the inclination to touch involves unhealthy motives and impulses on the part of the counselor or the client. Simon and Williams (1999) remind us that hugs are rarely free of an erotic element. Nonsexual touch that does not meet the living room test should be reconsidered and further examined in order to discover what hidden factors may be at play. Such inappropriate touching disrespects a client's dignity and violates the ethical principle of fidelity. Imposing the counselor's personal needs and drives onto the therapeutic relationship by touching the client in an unwelcome manner is an abuse of the power differential inherent in the counselor–client roles. That kind of boundary violation is clearly unethical.

What About Gifting and Bartering?

The subject of receiving gifts from clients brings to mind a colleague's case from a few years ago. A Japanese American family sought grief counseling, in part because of the acting-out behavior of one of their teenage children following an episode of loss. After a lengthy period of intense therapeutic work, the family had occasion to visit their homeland. Upon returning, the family brought the counselor an elaborately carved decorative tea service. The unwrapping of the tea set itself was done in a deliberate, almost ceremonial manner, so that even the presentation conveyed a message of gratitude and inclusion of the counselor as an honorary family member. Could this gift have been refused as too expensive or luxurious without shaming the family and denigrating their cultural values? Absolutely not! Instead, this vignette highlights the importance of counselor sensitivity to the motive, expectations, and cultural mores of clients bearing gifts. Context is crucial.

The traditional psychoanalytic position is that gifts should be interpreted rather than accepted. In a thoughtful reconsideration of whether the mental health professions have gone too far by misapplying the concept of boundaries in an overly rigid manner, Gutheil and Gabbard (1998) suggest that whether an event is *discussible* in the context of the counseling relationship is a pivotal indicator of whether crossing a boundary can be constructive. What about in the case of clients gifting?

It is our observation that gifting by clients varies, not just culturally but also regionally. Although the tea service was a dramatic example, in some parts of the country it is common for clients to give baskets of fruit or baked goods at holidays in a spirit of seasonal generosity. When consistent with regional customs, they can be accepted with a reciprocal attitude of cheerful thanks. In rural areas, gifts of largesse will appear when backyard vegetable gardens come into season, and such offerings are understood as being neighborly. We recommend sharing such consumables with office staff who contribute to the mission of caring for clients. Such token gifts, provided they are not obligatory or habitual, rarely involve an agenda beyond human kindness.

On the other hand, gifts of expensive theatre or sports tickets, invitations to use vacation condos or hunting leases, and proffers of fine cigars, perfumes, or spirits are more likely laden with complications. Perhaps the client seeks special status or treatment, wants a favor, or is attempting to influence the counselor's perception, judgment, or opinion. This type of gift should always be discussed and only rarely accepted. Clearly, it would make a difference if the skybox seats came from the team owner expressing gratitude for grief counseling received, rather than from a bereaved parent embarrassed that an extramarital affair had occurred during a period of acute grieving for a deceased child. In cases where clients want to bestow expensive gifts on the counselor, Welfel (2006) adroitly suggests that such gifts be redirected to charitable causes in order to avoid compromising the counselor's objectivity.

It may be difficult to discriminate a token gift from an expensive one. What about the client who pulls out $50 or $100, hands it to the grief counselor, and says, "I appreciate all you have done for me and my family. Use this and take your spouse [or partner] to dinner"? When money or gift cards are offered, a gentle explanation by the counselor is needed to clarify that paying the professional fee is fair compensation for services rendered, and no additional gratuity is necessary.

Some gifts have symbolic value and are judiciously acknowledged and handled accordingly. Once a client gifted the grief counselor with a fist-sized piece of flint discovered on a hiking trip because, to the client, it represented the counselor's strength on which the client had relied during bereavement. Or there was a client who gave the counselor a small, handblown glass bowl as indicative of how fragile and vulnerable the bereft client felt. Generally, our policy is to keep such symbolic gifts in the office as testimonials of how grief counseling impacts some clients.

The practice of bartering is a derivative of economic and cultural imperatives. Again, the traditional viewpoint is that professional fees should be paid in money as the acceptable "coin of the realm" (Simon & Williams, 1999). The argument favoring a fee-for-service plan is that a stable fee structure set by the counselor makes for the cleanest financial arrangement with minimal room for exploitation or confusion. Yet bartering may avert potential transference problems arising when clients cannot pay the fee, such as incurring feelings of shame or low self-esteem or, alternately, engendering feelings of special status or entitlement if the client is treated pro bono. In addition, equitable bartering can prevent potentially damaging countertransference on the part of the counselor who may feel compromised or resentful if reasonable remuneration is not forthcoming.

Bartering of goods, services, or other nonmonetary considerations, when necessary for economic reasons, needs to be undertaken carefully. An objective appraisal of the fair market value of any goods or services provided in exchange for counseling is key to an equitable barter. Even in the best of circumstances, either counselor or client may have reservations or misgivings about the exchange. Problems arise when either party feels an inequitable deal has been struck. In those instances, an additional relationship has inched into the picture; that is, besides the counselor–client relationship, the dimension of trade partners exists concurrently. Negative feelings originating with the party who believes the barter was unfair can contaminate the atmosphere surrounding the professional relationship. Consider the case of the artist who bartered a painting for grief counseling services. Later, as the value of the painting appreciated with the artist's growing reputation, the artist had second thoughts about the barter, which undermined motivation and investment in the grief counseling.

In some cultures, barter is a very accepted method in the marketplace, and so bartering to pay for professional services such as grief counseling may not be unusual. Welfel (2006) has suggested that refusing to barter in such instances runs counter to cultural norms and would be inadvisable. Again, respecting the client's cultural context is key to deciding if and when to barter, always keeping in mind that the client's welfare is the foremost consideration.

Akin to the living room test for determining whether physical touch during grief counseling is appropriate, we suggest the "newspaper test" for instances of gifting and bartering. Quite simply ask oneself, "If a report of this gift or an account of this barter appeared in tomorrow morning's newspaper, would my behavior meet the test of public scrutiny?" An affirmative answer indicates that ethical integrity has more than likely been maintained. A negative answer is cause for alarm because, should the grief counselor ever be sued over the matter, it is very possible that an account of the whole affair could appear in the local newspaper! Of course, applying the newspaper test, or any other, is only as good as the accuracy of the grief counselor's self-awareness.

One final note is in order about bartering in the United States. Goods or services received in exchange for professional grief counseling are required to be reported to the Internal Revenue Service as professional income. Then federal income tax is applicable to the fair market value of the goods or services received as barter. Not reporting such income is fraud.

HAZARDS OF MULTIPLE RELATIONSHIPS IN SEVEN DIFFERENT VENUES

The preceding sections concerned with power differentials, the grief counselor as friend, nonsexual touch, and gifting and bartering focus primarily on the first two elements in the Five P Model—client as *person,* including cultural context, developmental history, and current life situation as well as the *problem* or ethical dilemma. Yet, deciding how multiple relationships are navigated requires special consideration of the third element in the Five P Model—the *place* or setting in which the grief counseling is conducted. It is characteristic of grief counseling that many different professionals operating in many different work settings may provide this service. Thus, when the expectations associated with multiple roles collide, understanding the counseling venue yields valuable clues about how to manage multiple relationship dilemmas. In the following sections, we address potential ethical hazards found in seven unique practice sites: clinics and offices, hospitals, clients' residences, funeral homes, places of worship, educational environments, and legal arenas. Key constructs from this discussion are encapsulated in Table 7.1 for easy reference.

Clinics and Offices

The private consultation room in a clinic or office suite is conventional "home turf" to the grief counselor. This setting is probably most familiar to readers who can easily visualize many of the scenarios described in this book occurring in clinics or offices. The grief counselor is master of this domain. The consultation room is the counselor's professional home, and clients are visitors who are treated as important guests.

Nowhere is the power differential between counselor and client more sharply defined than in a clinic or office. Both the room itself and its contents—furniture, telephone, clocks, computer, books, client records—speak to the grief counselor's status and expertise. Therefore, even though this setting may be the one most comfortable for the counselor, it is also the one in which abuses of power in multiple relationships can occur most easily. Constant vigilance is required on the part of the grief counselor to use power respectfully and to adhere to professional responsibility as stated in the ADEC Code of Ethics.

> The primary obligations of members are to respect the integrity of and to promote the welfare of clients and students. (ADEC Code of Ethics, III. Responsibilities to Those Served, A)

Because the consultation room is the grief counselor's natural habitat, there is a temptation to believe that whatever is done in this venue

Table 7.1

HOW PLACE AFFECTS MULTIPLE RELATIONSHIPS IN GRIEF COUNSELING

PLACE	RELATIONSHIP DYNAMIC: COUNSELOR	RELATIONSHIP DYNAMIC: CLIENT	POTENTIAL ROLE CONFLICTS	KEY ETHICAL STRATEGY
Clinics and offices	Host/expert	Guest	Exploiting power differential	Use power respectfully
Hospitals	Landlord's (e.g., hospital's) associate	Tenant	Counseling in the client's "bedroom"	Avoid aloofness or undue familiarity
Clients' residences	Esteemed guest	Host	Entering client's liminal period of dying	Honor client's "here and now" experience
Funeral homes	Proprietor's (e.g., director's) employee	Customer	Marketing present or future services	Separate aftercare from preneed sales
Places of worship	Faith leader and authority figure	Congregant	Blending ministerial role with counseling or social roles	Compart-mentalize roles, not relationships
Educational environ-ments	Content expert and evaluator	Trainee	Exploiting power differential	Maintain supremacy of educational mission
Legal arenas	Expert witness	Claimant or litigant	Blurring allegiance to client vs. court	Preserve professional integrity

is the counselor's professional prerogative. Yet it is in clinics and offices that friendly behavior may be misconstrued, nonsexual touch misinterpreted, or inequitable bartering transacted. Simon and Williams (1999) cogently identify the segment of the treatment session "between the chair and the door" (p. 1445) as rife with opportunity for boundary crossings and boundary violations. It is in that space and time that the counselors and clients may prematurely cast off their respective roles in favor of launching into social exchanges or engage in questionable physical contact (e.g., hugs and pats), rationalized as part of the session's conclusion yet never discussed in therapy. The point is that the grief counselor's comfort level and power advantage in a clinic or office does not obviate the necessity for upholding professional decorum at all times.

Hospitals

In hospitals, the grief counselor must be an official staff member or have clinical privileges to practice there in order to conduct a paid consultation. Otherwise, only a social visit is permitted. Compared to clinics and offices, the sociology of a hospital room is a curious thing. Obviously, the space itself, with its technical equipment and trained personnel, *belongs* to the hospital. But the room is *occupied* by the patient who commands certain reign over the space as temporary domicile. It is much like a landlord–tenant arrangement, with each party retaining certain rights. However, any grief counselor who has visited a patient in the hospital cannot help but notice signs of the patient's ownership as occupant. Very often, boxes of food and bags of clothing are visible. Family members are present. The morning's shaving items or makeup kit may be nearby. The patient may be only partially clad or have undergarments showing. The hospital room is a bedroom that doubles as a consultation area.

When conducting a grief counseling session in a hospital room, place dictates a change in the rules. This is the patient's temporary residence, and the grief counselor is part host and part guest. Honoring the patient's physical as well as psychological privacy needs in a hospital environment is a cardinal rule. It is well-known that sitting down to talk with a hospital patient creates a subjective perception that the provider was in the room longer than if standing. But what if the only available space to sit is on the edge of the patient's bed? This necessitates juggling personal space, therapeutic effectiveness, and respect for body privacy all in the space of a six-foot twin bed!

There are other considerations as well when counseling a hospital patient. Control of time by the grief counselor is partial rather than absolute. Hospital routines, test schedules, arranged "shifts" of accompanying family members, and patient fatigue all define how time is spent. Also, preserving confidentiality, particularly information previously disclosed in an office setting, can be challenging with a hospital patient. Despite HIPAA (1996) guidelines, in a hospital there can be ambient expectations that the patient's information is openly shared with family and friends in attendance. Taking care to arrange a few minutes alone with the patient, or first ascertaining the patient's consent before including family members in the discussion, is required for sound ethical practice. If the family is included in the discussion, then this information should be documented in the patient's medical record.

In our experience, boundary crossings in hospitals sometimes take the form of going the extra mile in delivering compassionate care. For example, when is it appropriate to give the patient without transportation a ride home, or let the patient without resources use the counselor's cell phone to call home, or give money for cab fare and a meal to an indigent patient about to be discharged? Usually, these laudable efforts constitute good deeds done out of kindness that comport with Karl Menninger's dictum, "When in doubt, be human" (cited in Gutheil & Gabbard, 1998). However, in all things, even deeds of kindness, it is incumbent on the ethically poised grief counselor always to act in the patient's best interest rather than in self-interest. Because of medical illness, hospital patients are more vulnerable and less able to discriminate compassionate caring by a professional from what appear to be acts of personal friendship that may be confusing or ambiguous.

Clients' Residences

Hospice care is often delivered in the client's home and with it the grief counseling component of the program. Accordingly, the grief counselor making home visits discovers that the role reversal from host to guest that was partially applicable in the hospital setting is now complete. The grief counselor is a guest in the client's space. This new role creates an immediate duality in which the counselor is both expert consultant and esteemed (or suspect) visitor. How does the ethically conscious grief counselor manage this duality and maintain a professional stance while avoiding boundary violations when making home visits?

Readers may recollect that physicians have a long history of making house calls, as do other helping professionals such as midwives, home health workers, and massage therapists. Interestingly, the Hippocratic oath addresses protocol during home visits at the same time that it enjoins physicians from revealing what is learned about the lives of others in the course of caring for a patient, something particularly applicable when making a home visit.

> Into whatever houses I enter, I will go into them for the benefit of the sick, and will abstain from every voluntary act of mischief and corruption; and, further from the seduction of females or males, of freemen or slaves.

> Whatever, in connection with my professional practice or not in connection with it, I see or hear in the life of men, which ought not to be spoken of abroad, I will not divulge, as reckoning that all such should be kept secret. (Adams, 2005)

One way to avoid even the appearance of impropriety is to ensure that home visits are chaperoned. Typically, a family member or neighbor may be present in the home, albeit in a separate room, during the grief counselor's visit. Alternately, hospice staff may work in pairs. This strategy is especially advisable when a heterosexual client and the counselor are opposite sex, or when a gay or lesbian client and the counselor are the same sex. Generally, following the social etiquette of a polite guest is a safe strategy when visiting a client at home to conduct a grief counseling session.

There is another layer of meaning to consider when the grief counselor makes a home visit to a client on hospice. Being in the client's space means not only that the counselor is a guest in the client's home, but also that the counselor has entered into the client's experience of dying *as it is lived* rather than as it may be described in an office visit. Experiential theorists call this reality the "here and now" compared to the enterprise of "there and then" counseling discussions of a retrospective nature (Dayton, 1994; Yalom & Leszcz, 2005). The dying process is a transitional place in time sometimes referred to as a liminal period, that is, on the threshold between life and death. It is an existential moment—profoundly mysterious and intimate (Yalom, 1980). For many, it is an intensely spiritual moment as well. Grief counselors who make home visits to dying clients enter into that existential moment and participate in it in real time.

By participating in the liminal period of a client's dying, the grief counselor is given a great trust and honor. It can be very humbling to be included in a client's life at the time of death. At that moment, the grief counselor may be called upon to help in a variety of ways: listening, advice-giving or wisdom-imparting, simple companioning such as just sitting silently with the client, offering prayer or spiritual supplication, or extending reassuring physical contact such as holding a hand or even giving a hug. Guided by principles of respect and professional responsibility, the ethical grief counselor actively processes how to participate therapeutically with the client dying at home, ensuring that any boundary crossed is considered with the greatest of care and weighed always in favor of the best interests of the client.

Funeral Homes

In the last three decades, many funeral homes have begun to offer what is commonly referred to in the industry as *aftercare* (Johnson & Weeks, 2001). Aftercare means attending to the social, emotional, and psychological aspects of grieving experienced by the bereaved that extend beyond the time frame of customary funeral rituals. Although the two traditional functions of funeral homes have been the disposition of the body (or remains of the deceased) and the orchestration of social rituals of honor and farewell, aftercare attempts to address the ongoing grief of the bereaved.

Currently, we live in an era when funeral costs have been sharply criticized, cremation is increasingly common, and caskets can be purchased from major retailers or over the Internet. Thus, implementation of an aftercare program may be seen as a way that funeral homes can increase the perceived value of the services they offer. Some funeral homes provide aftercare not only to their own clients but also to the community as a public service. This service may be provided both because it is good for business and because it casts the funeral director more in the light of a helping professional rather than as simply someone running a business (Bendiksen, 2001).

When grief counseling is practiced in the funeral home setting via aftercare programs, a number of potential ethical conflicts can arise. Multiple-relationship dilemmas as a result of role incompatibility are the most likely problem. Because a typical aftercare program does not generate its own revenue stream, there may be a temptation to utilize aftercare providers in other activities within the funeral home that, consequently, present a conflict of interest. For example, if the grief counselor leading an aftercare program is also involved in preneed sales, the motives and integrity of the counselor can be called into question (Miletich, 2001). In that case, it is unclear whether the counselor is in the role of a helping professional dedicated to the human needs of grieving clients or in a public relations role promoting future sales among an emotionally vulnerable clientele. Using professional relationships to further the business interests of the grief counselor is inherently unethical as stated in the ADEC Code of Ethics.

This example is but one instance illustrating an overriding ethical question about grief counseling provided in a funeral home setting—is the individual or family being served a client in the sense of recipient of mental health services, or a customer in the sense of a business prospect or profit source? A genuine answer to this question may be *both*. Thus, clear delineation of how these dual statuses are served respectfully and ethically is a continuing challenge. From the perspective of the grief counselor working in or employed by a funeral home, careful attention to how this dichotomy impacts the counseling relationship is required.

There are several important ethical questions to ask about grief counseling in the aftercare program of a funeral home. Is access to aftercare programs contingent on the level of services the person purchased at the time of the loved one's death? Are there any limits to how aftercare programs or grief counseling may be used by clients? Is counselor–client confidentiality protected regarding what is conveyed in grief counseling, including grief support groups or memorial services, or is client information shared with other members of the funeral home staff, especially the funeral director who employs the grief counselor? When aftercare is accomplished in a facility separate from the funeral home, or with off-site providers contracted by the funeral home, who is ethically responsible for the quality of care received? How does the grief counselor affiliated with a funeral home address perceptions by clients that the funeral home first profited from the death of their loved ones and now profits from the survivors' grief?

From a marketing viewpoint, aftercare programs may be compared with the public education initiatives of many hospitals and surgery centers that offer no-cost educational seminars to the public about certain types of health problems and the range of treatments available. Such seminars are not a direct solicitation of business but carry an implied marketing message: "Should you ever need these types of services, we hope you will consider us." Similarly, grief counselors employed by funeral homes for aftercare are unspoken personal representatives of the business side of the firm and should be constantly mindful to clarify the boundaries of their professional role as grief counselors. It is their obligation to act in the best interest of the clients without being compromised by the fact that their clients are also customers, or potential customers, of the funeral home.

Places of Worship

Another outgrowth of the diversification beyond traditional mental health and medical settings is the provision of grief counseling in worship-related venues—churches, synagogues, temples, and mosques. Some larger or more affluent religious congregations have designated bereavement or family life ministers whose job descriptions entail providing services such as grief counseling to bereaved members of the congregation and their immediate families. Other congregations rely on specifically trained lay volunteers, such as the Stephen Ministers (Stephen Ministries, 2000), to help those hurting from loss and bereavement. In these cases, the same potential ethical challenges (e.g., confidentiality) exist as enumerated regarding aftercare in funeral homes. However, because places of worship do not have the same commercial interests as do funeral homes, those receiving grief counseling from a bereavement minister at church generally need not worry about financial encumbrances.

In places of worship, a potential multiple-relationship quandary is that of the minister concurrently wearing two hats: "counselor" and "evangelizer." Grief counseling provided by a minister based in a place of worship likely includes encouragement of faith-based perspectives as a source of understanding and comfort. As long as such evangelization efforts are not unwelcome and are not carried to the point of becoming onerous or compulsory, the client is not harmed or exploited for the sake of a proselytizing agenda because the client is free to employ or bypass such perspectives as seen fit. This influence is all the more important because many bereaved individuals find themselves questioning long-held beliefs about God or a deity, particularly when they sustain complicated or traumatic losses (Lord, 2006).

Probably only a minority of religious congregations in North America employ professionally trained grief counselors. More often, the presiding minister or an associate is seen as an individual to whom one turns at a time of loss. Thus a situation of multiple relationships, with the minister serving both as spiritual leader and as grief counselor, can result. Minister and longtime hospice chaplain Rodney Bolejack (personal communication, August 21, 2007) has warned that this can lead to tension within the minister (e.g., difficulty challenging a congregational leader within the counseling context without fearing a strain in the relationship surfacing later, as during a finance committee meeting), within the congregant (e.g., wondering if the minister can ever see the person at worship services without simply seeing the problems that arose in counseling), or within the congregation (e.g., should the larger group become aware of the counseling and place images upon the congregant as one having problems).

Yet experienced clergy often see little, if any, contradiction between the two roles of spiritual leader and grief counselor. The fact is, ministers have lived with the reality of multiple relationships for centuries by befriending the families in their congregations and sharing in the family milestones: birth, marriage, and death. Many ministers, especially those in smaller congregations or those who are unmarried like Roman Catholic priests, make it their objective to form a personal relationship with their congregants, even to the point of assuming the status of an honorary family member, and to minister from that context. In addition, clergy often view ministering in times of dying and death as one of their major pastoral functions.

So how do mature ministers avoid conflicts in their concurrent multiple relationships—minister to congregant, counselor to client, friend to friend—at times of death, particularly given that the minister may be grieving as well? How does the minister honor the pastoral role of spiritual leader while not seeming aloof or unfeeling? How can the minister bring a grief counselor's expert knowledge about human mourning to a grieving family without abandoning the faith perspective? How can a minister empathically companion congregational friends who are hurting from loss and still effectively counsel as a grief professional? The key is compartmentalizing. However, as aptly described by Barnett and Yutrzenka (1994), *compartmentalizing roles, not relationships*, is required. That is, ministers strive to maintain a constant interpersonal style while clearly delineating the role behavior in which they engage at a given moment. Similarly, Geyer (1994) urges grief counselors affiliated with places of worship to maintain flexibility and integrity when facing unavoidable situations of overlapping responsibility where personal and professional roles coexist.

This apparently seamless execution of multiple roles by a minister, all the while maintaining a consistent pastoral persona of warmth and acceptance, is well illustrated by the following story. A couple who had been strong members of their worship community for years suffered terribly when their teenager completed suicide. The couple sought both spiritual consolation and a friend's sympathetic presence from their minister. Precisely because of their close relationship, they wanted their minister to eulogize the deceased child at the funeral. In accommodating this request, their minister not only fulfilled the role of spiritual leader by using scriptural and theological resources during the funeral service but also delivered a moving eulogy by taking advantage of the special familial relationship with the deceased child to impart unique insights and memories of the child that comforted those mourning (cf. Kunkel & Dennis, 2003).

Yet even though mature ministers may blend such multiple relationships effortlessly, the enormous trust placed in clergy by their congregants should never be taken for granted. Clergy scandals of the past few decades have left the public wary of potential abuses (Cozzens, 2004). Therefore, prudent ministers who undertake multiple roles with their congregants, including grief counseling, need to honor consistently their pastoral relationship at the same time that they continuously clarify and maintain the boundaries appropriate to each role.

Educational Environments

Much like grief counselors in clinics and offices, death educators operate with a substantial power differential over students, supervisees, and clients (Biaggio, Paget, & Chenoweth, 1997; Burian & O'Connor Slimp, 2000). This power differential has its basis in the educator's role as evaluator of trainees and in the educator's authority in the subject matter (Blevins-Knabe, 1992). This makes the terrain in educational environments difficult to traverse should the faculty trainer engage in multiple relationships. Most professors have some fairly benign forms of multiple relationships with trainees (e.g., instructor and colleague on research projects). However, death educators are well advised to proceed with caution in instances where multiple relationships with students may involve concurrent counseling, business, or social relationships.

When students or supervisees require counseling, the best practice is to refer them to someone with whom they have no other professional relationship (O'Connor Slimp & Burian, 1994). This enables both parties to avoid potentially awkward situations wherein the educator is both professor and grief counselor to the trainee, and the educator's knowledge of the trainee from one interaction may carry over to another. This certainly could happen in the example cited earlier in this chapter about the faculty investigator who agrees to provide grief counseling to his research assistant. Learning details of the research assistant's partner relationship prior to the suicide may alter the investigator's appraisal of the research assistant's work performance. Or concerns about deadlines associated with the research project may influence how the investigator handles confrontation of difficult material in the counseling sessions. In fact, there are many ways the grief counseling or the research program, or both, could be compromised in this multiple-relationship scenario. This illustrates how crossing a boundary can easily become a boundary violation resulting in harm to the educator's employee/client.

Many students and trainees, of their own volition, confide personal material to a professor in the course of instruction or supervision. Sometimes students seek wise counsel from their faculty educators about a wide range of life issues, even without the structure of a formal counselor–client arrangement. How does the faculty member deal with such personal information, which is very similar to material disclosed in counseling? Certainly, confidentiality is important. So is maintaining the integrity of the educator–student relationship without being unduly influenced, either to the positive (e.g., having sympathy for the student) or to the negative (e.g., assuming a character flaw in the student), by information trainees volunteer about themselves. One sage professor explained the strategy this way: "I don't 'counsel' students, I 'mentor' them." Indeed, for death professionals in educational settings, mentoring with noncoercive guidance may be a useful model to employ in parallel with the educator–student model when personal information is disclosed by trainees. To ensure that mentoring does not evolve into counseling, a cross-check with trusted fellow faculty can help death educators avoid a blind spot in this area.

Business relationships are sometimes superimposed on the professor–student relationship in educational environments. How often do educators hire their students to babysit, house-sit, do yard work, or make repairs? Seen as nothing more than an extension of a teaching assistant's role, such business relationships may appear innocent and advantageous for both parties. Professors find energetic, willing workers whom they know and can trust with their children or their possessions; students find a convenient opportunity to earn much-needed income.

However, below this surface harmony can lurk other motives that complicate such multiple relationships. Does the professor actually use the power of the educator position as a form of intangible collateral to ensure proper discharge of duties or ready availability by the student? Do students attempt to ingratiate themselves to professors by taking on noneducational roles in which they perform well or make themselves indispensable? Not unlike barter arrangements that are perceived as inequitable by one party, when multiple relationships of professor–student and employer–employee occur, they are fraught with potential problems such as disguised motives of manipulation or influence-seeking. That is why many educators employ only students or trainees from outside the department in which they work (Koocher & Keith-Spiegel, 2008).

Finally, a word about social relationships between faculty and students is in order. Some institutions intentionally foster team building through activities such as department picnics, holiday parties, brain bowls, intramural athletic squads, or organized trips in which faculty and students fraternize. It is also the case that educators actually may have more in common with students or trainees who share their specialized interest, such as thanatology, than with other faculty in an academic department (Burian & O'Connor Slimp, 2000; Koocher & Keith-Spiegel, 2008). This similarity may foster the inclination for faculty and students to socialize or spend personal time together. O'Connor Slimp and Burian (1994) contend that even seemingly benign social relationships with laudable intentions can have an adverse effect on the pedagogical process. Personal esteem and likeability generated by an amiable social relationship can distort objective evaluation of a trainee's progress or potential for future employment. Harm may also occur indirectly for the trainee if the appearance of favoritism creates "sibling rivalry" within a training cohort (Burian & O'Connor Slimp, 2000). Whenever a death educator engages a trainee in multiple relationships, such as concurrent roles of both trainer and friend, it is the responsibility of the educator, who holds greater power, to maintain clear boundaries and avoid exploitation or harm of the trainee. The educator's responsibility is underscored by research showing that students can be very uncertain about the appropriateness of therapeutic, business, or social relationships with their faculty trainers (Holmes, Rupert, Ross, & Shapera, 1999).

Legal Arenas

Extreme caution should be exercised when grief counselors step into legal arenas (Koocher & Keith-Spiegel, 2008). The role incompatibilities between sensitive grief counselor and effective expert witness are so pronounced that such multiple relationships should be studiously avoided whenever possible (see Chapter 12, "Grief Counselor as Expert Witness," for more extensive analysis of the ethical dilemmas in forensic work). Most importantly, those counseling the bereaved for purposes of achieving emotional healing and restoration should recuse themselves from any role as forensic evaluator for those same clients. Conversely, when a grief counselor performs forensic evaluations for the court, for which there are discipline-specific guidelines available (cf. Committee on the Revision of the Specialty Guidelines for Forensic Psychology, 2008), the individuals evaluated should not be accepted subsequently as clients in the evaluator's counseling practice.

Of course, it may be impossible to avoid situations where the grief counselor is compelled to provide testimony for the court as an expert witness. Such testimony could happen when a client suffers a traumatic loss of a loved one in a car crash before, or during, counseling and a lawsuit ensues. Or a client who is a bereaved parent may become party to a dispute over custody of a surviving child during a subsequent divorce. Even when boundary demarcations are clearly defined, and the responsibilities in both roles are discussed with the client before a grief counselor testifies, the potential for misunderstanding and harm to the counseling relationship is enormous.

One of the fundamental sources of conflict in multiple relationships involving legal arenas is the difference in how truth is defined. Good grief counseling starts with nonjudgmental acceptance of a client's *subjective reality* of perceptions, recollections, and attributions from which the counselor builds an understanding of the individual's worldview and story of loss. As Strasburger, Gutheil, and Brodsky (1997) explain, counseling is more a search for narrative truth than historical truth as the counselor attempts to see the world through the client's frame of reference. On the other hand, legal investigations and courts of law are concerned with fact finding, historical veracity, and *objective reality*. Clients' thoughts and feelings that figure so prominently in counseling have little place in forensic considerations of who did what to whom and when and how events transpired. Unfortunately, clients involved in litigation sometimes find that their "day in court" becomes a "day in Hell" wherein their subjective experiences are discounted or discredited and their internal vision of justice proves to be a vanishing mirage.

The relationship between grief counselor and client is essentially an empathic one. The counselor is charged with working to benefit the clients' mental health, promote healing, and assist the client in developing more accurate self-awareness, better self-efficacy, and greater independence. The process is one of *advocacy*. In judicial settings, the grief counselor turned expert witness is transformed into an agent for the law to resolve disputes between opposing parties, each vigorously making its case before a judge or jury of peers. The process is an *adversarial* one. The disparity between a counseling context, with its respect for subjective reality and its emphasis on advocacy, and a judicial context, with its quest for objective reality and its adversarial process, makes these very different *places* indeed. In the legal arena, the grief counselor who is also giving expert witness blurs the boundaries between these two contradictory endeavors and, in so doing, risks compromising allegiance to the client (Strasburger et al., 1997) and violating the ethical principle of fidelity.

When such problematic multiple roles are unavoidable (e.g., when the grief counselor is served with a subpoena to testify in court), the grief counselor's initial duty is to clarify in advance with all parties the respective role requirements involved. To the greatest extent possible, the ethically conscientious grief counselor maintains the advocacy role appropriate to counseling while acting with professional integrity and speaking the truth at all times—a difficult balancing act at best. A disclaimer that the grief counselor, by virtue of the therapeutic relationship, lacks the objectivity of an independent evaluator for rendering an expert opinion on legal questions may be employed, if necessary, to preclude offering objective certainty about subjective counseling data (Strasburger et al., 1997).

SUMMARY

It should be abundantly clear to the reader that the ethical challenges inherent in multiple relationships are enormous. Grief counselors need to exercise due discretion whenever they have an association, or potential association, with a client beyond the primary professional one of counselor–client. A general policy for practice is to avoid such situations whenever possible and, in the case of sexualized multiple relationships, to avoid them completely. Respect for the client demands a healthy acknowledgment of the enormous power differential between counselors and clients. Although there is no single formula for how to proceed in every instance, a useful heuristic is gauging the degree of incompatibility present in multiple roles as well as the presence of divergent or conflicting obligations in the multiple roles being considered.

Sound ethical practice of grief counseling means clients are neither harmed nor exploited when the counselor assumes more than one role with them. Subjecting oneself to the crucible of public scrutiny, as in the living room test or the newspaper test, or to the judgment of a trusted colleague can be an effective reality check on the counselor's choices or inclinations. Finally, place, the third element in the Five P Model for ethical decision making, is of critical importance in understanding the various contexts in which multiple relationship dilemmas arise. Ethical management of multiple relationships in grief counseling entails determining an appropriate course of action based on privileging the client's welfare above any competing interests.

8 Ethnic, Cultural, and Spiritual Considerations

Television and computers have brought diversity of cultures, religions, and lifestyles into the homes of many people for the first time in human history. No longer do people grow up in the sort of insular provincialism that once defined many communities. At a young age, children see cartoons with characters of different races. By school age, children may be enrolled with students from ethnic, cultural, or religious heritages different from their own. Many school curricula promote a multicultural perspective.

In the United States, non-White ethnic groups now account for approximately one-third of the population. In the 2000 census (U.S. Department of Commerce, Economics and Statistics Administration & U.S. Census Bureau, 2006), approximately 65% of the population identified themselves as White. The remainder identified themselves as African/Black (13%), Hispanic (13%), Asian/Pacific Islander (4.5%), American Indian/Alaskan Native (1.5%), and two or more races (2.5%). Truly, many societies around the world, including the United States and Canada (Statistics Canada, 2001), are becoming more pluralistic and multicultural. It is essential for ethical practice that grief counselors recognize this diversity and be skilled in counseling clients within the context of the client's own heritage and tradition.

DEFINITIONS

The terms *ethnicity, culture, religion,* and *spirituality* are sometimes used interchangeably to designate individual differences arising from many different sources (American Psychological Association, 2003; LaRoche & Maxie, 2003). Such unfortunate habits of speech disregard authentic aspects of a person's uniqueness, blur important behavioral characteristics that derive from diversity, and contribute to conceptual confusion. Table 8.1 lists definitions of important terms used throughout this chapter in order to clarify their meaning.

Table 8.1

IMPORTANT TERMS FOR UNDERSTANDING DIVERSITY

- *Race*—A biological descriptor, based on the person's family lineage or bloodline, designating membership according to physical characteristics such as skin color, hair type, or facial features. Clearly, a person may be of mixed ancestry. Race may or may not carry other ethnic, cultural, religious, or spiritual characteristics.
- *Ethnicity*—From one's *ethos,* generally understood as one's background with a particular people or nation. Large ethnic groups are often classified according to common racial, tribal, linguistic, national, religious, or cultural origins.
- *Culture*—A broad term that refers to the environment in which a person lives. Culture may include customs, attitudes, mores, and social structures based in geography, race, ethnicity, religion, or social group. The term *majority culture* may be used to describe the broadest common denominators among the dominant people in a specific area or country, in contrast to other subgroups.
- *Minority*—A term generally connoting a group that has suffered discrimination or oppression as a result of reduced power, compared to those in the cultural majority. *Minority* is used less frequently in the current literature on multiculturalism.
- *Religion*—An organized set of beliefs, rituals, practices, and morals pertaining to God, a supreme being, or the supernatural. An organized religion generally refers to some recognizable group with an established creed, codified doctrines and practices, a designated ministry, and some hierarchy of authority.
- *Spirituality*—A personal conviction about God's existence (or some form of higher power), or one's sense of connection with the divine or the transcendent. Intrinsic spirituality is an organizing principle in how a person lives. A person may be spiritual without being religious, that is, without identifying or affiliating with a particular religion. Or a person may be very active in practicing the external trappings of an organized religion without cultivating intrinsic spirituality. Or a person may be both religious and spiritual.

The *myth of sameness* is the belief that people from certain places or members of a particular race or religion are all the same (Hardy, 1989). This myth can lead to serious misunderstandings. For example, a White person from the United States and a Black person from the United States may have more in common than a White person from the United States and a White person from Russia. But someone who saw these three people standing on a street corner in a major U.S. city may assume, incorrectly, that the two White people have more in common with each other than with the Black person.

Jennings (2005) writes, "While it is important to appreciate the ways religious traditions shape [clients'] understandings of the end of life and expectations regarding care, it is equally important for caregivers to remember that no faith or cultural tradition is monolithic" (p. 96). In other words, no matter how much grief counselors study diverse groups and their varied ways of finding meaning in dying, death, and bereavement, the actual experience is still an individual one. Each person makes meaning in these circumstances according to his or her own experiences and background. Jennings cautions against "reverse stereotyping" or "losing sight of the individual [client] within well-meaning cultural generalizations" (p. 96). Werth, Blevins, Toussaint, and Durham (2002) concur: "in writing about cultural diversity, summarizing research on various groups, and using case examples, both authors and readers alike run the risk of stereotyping people" (p. 205).

The myth of sameness and reverse stereotyping can be very destructive to genuine understanding of the client seen for grief counseling. Such illusory thinking can be punctured easily by reading Braun and Nichols's (1997) account of their ambitious study of cultural variations in response to dying and grieving among four Asian American populations: Chinese, Japanese, Vietnamese, and Filipino. Even though all these groups would be lumped together by census-takers under the label of "Asian/Pacific Islander," Braun and Nichols provided a fine-grain analysis of each focus group's philosophies about death, approaches to funerals, attitudes toward advance directives and organ donation, and advice for health care workers. Both *between*-group and *within*-group differences were found. The authors acknowledged that other factors besides cultural heritage influenced their findings, such as length of time in the United States, number of generations since immigration, educational attainment, and socioeconomic standing. Nonetheless, their study is a testament to how much individual variability exists among members of the same group or class.

In another way, differences between immigrant groups and members of the majority culture may be muted somewhat by those who do not want to draw attention to themselves. However, in order to maintain their ethnic or religious identity, there may be limits to how far some immigrants will go in order to accommodate or acculturate. Regardless of how subtle the differences may be, they often emerge in the context of existential issues such as dying, death, and bereavement. For many people, care of the deceased body, funeral traditions, and grief rituals represent primal connections with their ethnic, cultural, and religious heritage.

OBLIGATIONS OF THE GRIEF COUNSELOR

The ADEC Code of Ethics addresses the ethical obligation of the grief counselor to respect individual differences and honor the fundamental human dignity of every person who is served.

> The member takes care to know the student or client. Good education and counseling are based upon an understanding of, and a respect for, the student's or client's cultural background, developmental status, perceptions, and other individual differences and needs. (ADEC Code of Ethics, Basic Tenets, 3)
>
> Members provide their professional services to anyone regardless of race, religion, gender, sexual orientation, socio-economic status, or choice of lifestyle. When the member cannot render service, the member makes an appropriate referral. (ADEC Code of Ethics, I. General Conduct, D)
>
> In providing professional services to clients or students, members neither violate nor diminish their legal or civil rights. (ADEC Code of Ethics, III. Responsibilities to Those Served, D)
>
> Members work to prevent and to eliminate discrimination against any person or group on the basis of age, color, race, gender, sexual orientation, lifestyle, religion, national origin, marital status, political belief, or mental or physical disability. (ADEC Code of Ethics, VII. Responsibility to Society, A)
>
> Members act to ensure that all persons whom they serve have access to the resources, services, and opportunities they require. (ADEC Code of Ethics, VII. Responsibility to Society, B)

The thrust of the multicultural provisions in the ADEC Code of Ethics parallels the ethics code of the ACA (2005a) in promoting what LaRoche and Maxie (2003) call the *transcendist* perspective—believing that people from diverse backgrounds can work together and, specifically, that psychotherapists can learn to effectively and competently treat clients with dissimilar ethnic, cultural, or religious backgrounds.

Although there are no absolute rules for how to work with clients who present diversity, some theoretical and practical models have been proposed (American Psychological Association 2002, 2003; Sue & Sue, 2003). Foremost is for the grief counselor to maintain sensitivity, openness, and respect—all derivatives of the ethical principle of fidelity. Autonomy demands that the counselor honor the client's prerogative for self-determination when it comes to adhering to specific cultural norms or religious practices in grief. When language barriers exist, it is important to verify informed consent and keep confidentiality by using an objective translator familiar with the process of grief counseling or experienced in medical translating, if at all possible. Sometimes there is no alternative to using a bilingual family member, such as an adult child of a first-generation immigrant, as a translator. However, this arrangement always presents the possibility that the client will filter information requested by the grief counselor for sake of not disclosing something to the family member who is translating or that family translators will modify questions or statements according to their own sensibilities (American Psychological Association, 1993; Flores, 2006).

So how does an ethically minded grief counselor maintain sensitivity and uphold autonomy when the counselor does not know what is important or meaningful to the client with ethnic, cultural, or religious differences? Historically, autonomy and protection of individual rights are highly valued in the United States, especially among Whites of European descent, whereas other cultures de-emphasize autonomy, perceiving it as isolating rather than empowering (Searight & Gafford, 2005; Werth, Blevins, et al., 2002). In some non-Western cultures, beneficence is valuing family and community decision making, especially in such significant decisions as end-of-life treatment. This thinking is similar to feminist ethics with its emphasis on connectedness and relationships. Nonmaleficence may operate in some cultural groups as protecting patients, especially the revered elderly, from direct discussions of death or end-of-life care, in contrast to the milieu of truth-telling promoted by the majority culture in the United States. Finally, non-Whites have consistently lower rates of completing advance directives, a finding that could have a variety of interpretations: distrust of the health care system, such as a suspicion that "not everything" would be done for the patient in a life-or-death situation; the preeminence of surviving, with a conviction that life always has some value; or a sense of obligation to care for the elderly, while the elderly feel a responsibility to continue living for their adult children.

Some mental health professionals adopt a fallback position when unfamiliar with, or ignorant about, the values and customs of a client who presents diversity. They cast themselves in the learner role by telling the client, "Teach me about your experience. I want to understand how you view this problem and what it means to you." This approach is an acceptable *starting* point, particularly if the situation is unforeseen, but it is not sufficient by itself. It is incumbent upon the ethically conscious grief counselor to seek out knowledge about the client's ethnicity, culture, religion, or spirituality independently of what is learned directly from the client. Otherwise, the practitioner is just winging it, improvising without doing the research needed to counsel the client effectively.

Depending solely on clients to educate the counselor about their ethnicity, culture, or religion places too great a burden on the clients, who are already distressed and vulnerable. In the process, the counselor risks overlooking something significant or inadvertently saying something insensitive or disrespectful. In working with clients of different backgrounds, it is important for the counselor to create an environment of trust and respect, so that clients will not feel pressured or threatened. A helpful comment may be something like, "I only want to be of help. If I say anything in our counseling that does not fit with your values, beliefs, or life experiences, please tell me. I would like you to challenge me on these differences because I think it will be useful in our working together. Please know I would never do anything intentionally to hurt you or offend you" (cf. LaRoche & Maxie, 2003). Admitting that one does not know everything may be a useful heuristic, as long as the grief counselor makes a concerted effort to learn more about the client's norm group.

When physicians encounter a syndrome or disease with which they are unfamiliar, they go to medical journals, textbooks, or Internet sources seeking additional information about the symptoms, underlying cause, prognosis, and treatment options for that illness until they know better how to treat their patient. Or they refer the patient to a trusted colleague or specialist who may know more about the disease than they do. To do anything less would be considered irresponsible practice and a disservice to the patient.

When confronted with a client whose ethnicity, culture, or religion is dissimilar, grief counselors can augment their knowledge in the following three main ways:

1. Reading scholarly literature on multicultural counseling or on the specific reference group in question
2. Seeking supervision or consulting someone reputably knowledgeable about the specific ethnicity, culture, or religion involved
3. Attending continuing education seminars

For reading, Bryant's (2003) *Handbook of Death and Dying* as well as Sue and Sue's (2003) *Counseling the Culturally Diverse: Theory and Practice* are both good sources. The objective is not to find out all the answers about an individual based on their class membership, but to learn what factors may be pertinent, what unique perspectives or sensibilities may exist, when nuance is needed, and what questions may draw out latent attitudes, beliefs, and practices. Pope and Vasquez (2007) say it eloquently:

> Knowledge of cultural and socioeconomic contexts becomes the basis for informed inquiry rather than the illusion of uniform group characteristics with which to stereotype the client. Neither variation between groups nor within groups can be discounted or ignored. (p. 227)

The only responsible alternative is to refer the client to a colleague who may be in a better position to work with that individual.

When working with clients of diverse backgrounds, it is important to be aware of how one's own ethnicity, cultural context, and religious training may influence one's perception of the client and the communication process. In effect, the counselor is constantly asking his- or herself, "If I am different from you, then how can I be sure that the difference does not interfere with our communication and the tasks we are trying to accomplish?" Grief counselors may hold ethnocentric attitudes that are not politically correct or they may have conditioned responses to individuals different from themselves that are not emotionally correct (Pope, Sonne, & Greene, 2006). The mandate from the ADEC Code of Ethics for grief counselors to work toward preventing and eliminating discrimination requires counselors to be aware of prejudicial attitudes and practices within themselves and in others.

Welfel (2006) outlined a five-step procedure for counselors to avoid insensitive behavior and ethical missteps when dealing with ethnic, cultural, and religious diversity. First, adopt an attitude of openness toward other cultural views of the world. Second, operate with knowledge of the specific culture, consistent with our earlier recommendation. Third, consult with other support people from the client's cultural group, such as elders, community leaders, or clergy, to become better informed. Of course, given that many subgroups are tightly knit, due discretion is necessary to uphold confidentiality. Fourth, modify interventions to make them applicable within the client's cultural context. Fifth, develop tolerance for ambiguity and divergent views of appropriate behavior.

What happens when the counselor belongs to a diverse ethnic, cultural, or religious group and is working with a client of the majority culture who discloses prejudicial or bigoted attitudes? Does the counselor challenge the client or let it go? We believe that a grief counselor's obligation as a mental health professional is to confront misperceptions and misrepresentations of a particular group or class of people in the interest of educating the client and helping that person to grow. As always, this must be done tactfully and earnestly but not punitively. Statements such as "I'm not sure you realize how hurtful that term can be" or "You may not be aware that many people find comments like that offensive" can open a useful dialogue about the client's behavior and clearly communicate the message that prejudice is not condoned.

Calling attention constructively to a client's discriminatory comment without shaming or demeaning the client is a delicate balancing act. Hinrichsen (2006) described an encounter between a young African American counselor and an older White client. Obviously uncomfortable with the counselor to whom he was assigned, the client proceeded to reminisce about "Negro fellas" with whom he had served in the military. It appeared to be an ingratiating effort on the client's part designed to allay his own discomfort. Without rancor or defensiveness, the counselor observed, "I guess you noticed I'm Black." This disarmingly simple comment identified the proverbial elephant in the living room and led to a constructive discussion about the client's fears and concerns about the interviewer's ethnicity. This vignette is an excellent example of how good counseling practice is sound ethical practice.

ETHNICITY

A favorite teaching story of ours is the case of Angus McDougall (a pseudonym). After inviting students to ponder how they begin to form an impressionistic understanding of who the client is based on initial demographic information, such as age, gender, and surname, we describe our surprise at the person who answered to the name "Mr. McDougall." We encountered an older man with obvious Hispanic features and skin color. He spoke English very properly, yet was bilingual in Spanish. Having a sense of humor, he took some delight in the game of confusing those meeting him for the first time with his unique mix of racial, cultural, and linguistic traits.

Mr. McDougall indulged us with a brief biography of how his great-great grandfather had immigrated to Texas through the port of Galveston in the 1800s and had married a local woman of Mexican lineage. He was a direct descendent from the paternal branch of the family tree and thus had retained the original Scottish surname. However, because his great-grandfather, grandfather, and father had also married Hispanic women, Mr. McDougall's racial ancestry was increasingly Hispanic with each succeeding generation. Spanish was spoken in the home when he was growing up. He recalled with dismay and anger how he was mistreated by elementary school teachers who responded only to his skin color and disbelieved that "McDougall" was his real name. The family attended a Presbyterian church, even though sometimes within their own congregation they were seen as an anomaly. Through perseverance and higher education, Mr. McDougall perfected his English skills, all the while maintaining his native Spanish tongue.

In the United States, stories such as Mr. McDougall's are commonplace. A deeply held American ideal is "the land of opportunity." Here, all who work hard can become equal members in the great melting pot of society. However, that melting pot metaphor may be less applicable as new immigrants continue to bring the uniqueness of their own ethnicity and culture to the United States. Clinebell (1981) suggested that a better term would be *stew pot,* where each part flavors the whole without losing its own distinct characteristics.

The obvious moral to the story is that racial and ethnic characteristics are only part of the client's story. Although a counselor makes an initial notation of variables such as gender, age, physique, race, and language fluency, none of these factors tells the whole story. As Mr. McDougall's case illustrates so well, the element of ethnicity is necessary but not sufficient for understanding a person's background. By the time the initial interview of Mr. McDougall was complete, a richly textured picture had emerged of a man who was a product of his genetic endowment and ethnic heritage with its unique blend of Scottish and Hispanic elements, together with bilingualism. However, he was not defined entirely by these characteristics. His education level, socioeconomic attainment, work history, and matriculation within the broader society showed considerable acculturation. Names, like appearances, can be deceiving.

The myth of sameness can obliterate ethnic identity that may be very important to an individual. The vast continent of Asia hosts many different countries and nationalities. Referring to all people from Asia as "Chinese" is not only inaccurate but also very insulting to someone from Korea, Japan, Vietnam, the Philippines, or other countries. Likewise, Hispanics come from a variety of backgrounds in Europe, Mexico, and Central and South America. Someone from Spain speaks Spanish, but identifies as a Spaniard, not as a Mexican, who is someone from Mexico. A Puerto Rican from New York City may be totally different from a native living in Puerto Rico. Some Hispanics have a mixed heritage. Many were originally Native Americans who were mixed with the Europeans who conquered them, such as the Spanish and the Portuguese mixing with the Inca and Aztec native population. Some in the Caribbean Islands mixed with the African slaves who were brought there to do plantation work. Ethnic variations are endless.

Additionally, immigrant status can overlap with ethnicity and bring its own set of stressors. Many immigrants face an uphill struggle, often with few or no resources. Their ability to navigate in a new environment may be limited by being able to communicate with only a limited number of people. Even if highly educated in their native land, immigrants may not be able to secure employment in their chosen field and must take low-paying jobs instead. Immigrants may have very limited access to health care or social services. Mental health practitioners who are aware of multicultural factors realize that immigrants may experience culture-bound syndromes or disorders that have no Western equivalent. Korean women may experience *hwa-byung*, a suppressed anger syndrome characterized by diffuse symptoms of insomnia, fatigue, fear, indigestion, palpitations, and aches (American Psychiatric Association, 2000). The Korean language has no word for depression, but a Korean may speak of being "a little bit irritable" or having a "down heart." In addition, a Korean may tap a fist against the chest while speaking to indicate this disorder of suppressed anger.

Particularly pertinent for grief counselors is a body of research showing that ethnicity can be an important variable in how health care is provided, particularly pain management at the end of life (Werth, Blevin, et al., 2002). Members of non-White ethnic groups experiencing severe medical pain or cancer-related pain tend to receive fewer analgesics than European Americans and are at risk of being under-medicated by health care workers. Clearly, such inequity violates the ethical principle of justice. Grief counselors involved with end-of-life care, especially in hospitals, need to be vigilant toward such subtle biases. Ersek, Kagawa-Singer, Barnes, Blackhall, and Koenig (1998) summarized and extended a number of helpful suggestions originally proposed by Koenig and Gates-Williams (1995) for making end-of-life care more sensitive to ethnically and culturally diverse populations:

- Determine the degree of openness in discussing diagnosis, prognosis, and death
- Establish the locus of decision making (e.g., the individual patient or the family/social group)
- Solicit the patient's and family's view about location and timing of death, including the preferred role of health care providers
- Attend to the level of fatalism or activism regarding end-of-life decisions
- Consider gender issues and power relationships within the decision-making unit
- Assess religious beliefs about the meaning of death, the existence of an afterlife, and the possibility of miracles
- Honor how hope is maintained
- Account for historical and sociopolitical factors, such as past discrimination, poverty, or refugee status, that may influence attitudes toward end-of-life care
- Seek information from community elders, religious leaders, and language interpreters

CULTURE

Within any ethnic group there may be numerous cultures or subcultures. Each subculture may have its own language or religious identities. For example, on the Indian subcontinent of south Asia alone, including India, Bangladesh, Pakistan, and Sri Lanka, conservative estimates put the number of spoken languages at more than 300 (Khulpateea, 1998). India itself has 28 different states, each with its own character and identity. Clearly, these regional divisions and the multiplicity of languages make any one culture there difficult to define. Yet, there may be overarching similarities resulting from religion as a unifying factor. More than 80% of the inhabitants of India are Hindu according to the 2001 census, with the remainder of the population affiliating as follows: Muslim (13.4%), Christian (2.3%), Sikh (1.9%), Buddhist (1.5%), and other (<1%; The World Factbook, 2008). Thus, the Hindu practice of cremating the dead can be seen as a cultural norm, based in religious tradition.

Generally, when a Hindu dies, the body is washed, anointed, and covered with flowers. The body is then disposed of as quickly as possible to hasten the time it takes for the soul to reach the heavens. Hindus cremate the body of the deceased, either on a funeral pyre or in a modern crematorium. The chief mourner, usually the eldest son, lights the pyre. The family watches the fire burn the body, particularly concerned that the skull will open up during the burning, in order for the spirit to escape the body. If the skull does not open, then a mallet or bamboo pole may be used to break it open, although this aspect of the ritual is becoming less common (Kamat, 2005; Rambachan, 2003).

The relevance of these data for grief counselors is to provide a context for understanding the sensibilities of clients from an Asian Indian heritage who retain these cultural norms surrounding the cremation ritual when a loved one dies. Even more acculturated, Westernized Asian Indians who are Hindu are likely to retain those cremation practices consistent with their heritage. Agarwal (1991) wrote a fascinating account of how cultural values and practices among post-1965 Asian Indian immigrants in the United States have shifted based on generational succession and about the confusion sometimes resulting from the homogenization of two disparate cultures.

The point of this discussion about individuals of Asian Indian ancestry is to illustrate the overlapping influences of race, ethnicity, and religion onto what is understood as *culture.* A similar analysis could be applied to any country or peoples across the globe in an effort to comprehend what may be normal for that group. For example, in the Middle East, many people speak Arabic. Arabic is a language, not a nationality or religion. To presume that all Arabic speakers have the same country of origin or that all practice Islam is inaccurate. In Iraq, there is a large Christian population known as Chaldean Christians. Although they share many of the customs of the predominant Islamic-based culture where they live, they are not Muslims. In Israel, there are many non-Jews who are Palestinians. The Palestinians speak Arabic, yet some are Muslim, and some are Christian. Besides attending to these potentially significant differences in cultural norms between groups, the culturally sensitive grief counselor also keeps in mind that within-group differences and individual differences can modify further even those working assumptions (cf. Sue & Sue, 2003).

SEXUAL AND GENDER DIVERSITY AS A SPECIAL POPULATION

Under the rubric of cultural considerations, there are many special populations that could be deemed minorities deserving attention in a chapter on ethical practice, such as individuals with disabilities, the deaf community, older adults, or the economically oppressed. Also, even though women are the majority of the population, historically they have been treated as holding minority status because of power arrangements favoring men. Exploring each of these minority groups with respect to ethical practice of grief counseling is beyond the scope of this text. Instead, we discuss only individuals presenting sexual and gender diversity, as an example of one of these special populations, to illustrate how unique subgroup dynamics may present additional challenges regarding health care, end-of-life issues, and grief counseling.

The acronym LGBT stands for lesbian, gay, bisexual, and transgender. The terms *homosexual* and *gay* may refer to males or females but often are used only for males. LGBT generally refers to (L) lesbian women, (G) gay men, and (B) bisexuals of either gender who are attracted both to their same sex as well as to the opposite sex. The (T) transgender person is someone born with male or female sexual anatomy but who identifies with the opposite gender, feels like a person of the other gender, and is uncomfortable with his or her anatomically assigned gender. Often there is a subjective sense of having been born in the wrong body. Some transgender people choose to have a sex-change operation that surgically remakes them into the gender that they believe themselves to be. Additionally, some individuals may be questioning or exploring their emerging sexual identity and experimenting with bisexual or homosexual relationships. This questioning of one's sexual identity was exemplified by a trainee's report during a supervisory session of how the client had said, "I am 'bi-curious.'"

LGBT individuals continually struggle with discrimination, misunderstanding, and marginalization (Gilbert, 2003). Often acceptance comes only from others like themselves. Many know friends who are

HIV-positive or have lost friends to AIDS, particularly gay men. An AIDS death may invoke guilt, anger, or fear in the partner. How did the AIDS patient contract the HIV virus? Did the partner/lover transmit it to the one who is dying? Did the virus come from an outside liaison? Might the partner now be infected as well? These kinds of questions and concerns are very common within the LGBT community in times of grief and loss. Goldblum and Erickson (2000) make many helpful suggestions for grief counselors working with AIDS-related bereavement. They emphasize validating the loss (e.g., of a partner/lover) that often is not recognized by society; using problem-solving techniques to neutralize risk factors specific to AIDS bereavement, such as caregiver burdens and lack of social support; and using intensive grief counseling when personal impediments or psychodynamic blocks to grief resolution warrant it.

A very real ethical dilemma emerges when a homosexual person is dying in the hospital, but the natural family has never accepted the sexual orientation of the person, either for personal or religious reasons. This attitude disenfranchises the patient's "family of choice" that may include a partner and homosexual friends (Doka,1989; Piazza, 2005). As loved ones gather at the hospital for visitation and support, the partner and friends of the homosexual patient may be excluded or discounted by the natural family or by hospital policy (Jelinek, 2002). Likewise, if the homosexual patient does not have a durable power of attorney for health care or a designation of a proxy for health care decisions, those closest to the patient emotionally, such as a life partner or dear friend, may be unable to speak for the patient's wishes. If the hospital interprets the customary hierarchy of surrogate decision makers literally, then the parents of an "unmarried" and "childless" homosexual patient may be designated as the ones to make end-of-life treatment decisions.

If the natural family of the dying homosexual patient denies access to the partner and close friends, then a critical element of interpersonal and emotional support for the patient is missing. The end of life may present a major crisis for a family who has never acknowledged that the family member is homosexual or never recognized the status of the partner/lover. Usually, the partner is well aware of how the family feels from years of being excluded and ignored. This exclusion may carry over to funeral and memorial services. Lack of access to compassionate, understanding clergy may result in denial of required ritual or spiritual practices associated with dying and death (Corless, 2001). Conflicting agendas, competing allegiances, and control struggles can characterize these situations at their worst. Culturally attuned grief counselors, particularly those with pastoral training, may be called on to mediate such conflicts. Sensitivity must be shown to people from all different sides who want to honor the deceased and have the opportunity to receive care and solace. The emphasis should be on inclusion, tolerance, and mutual respect (Piazza, 2005). Such long-term family conflicts cannot be resolved by changing one's sexual identity for the purpose of pleasing the family or by unwelcome parties just going away.

RELIGION

Traditionally, the world's major organized religions have been designated as Judaism, Islam, Christianity, Buddhism, and Hinduism (Smart, 1996). There are many subdivisions and sects within each of these major world religions. In addition, there are numerous other religions in the world that are practiced by millions of people, such as animism, Shinto, Rastafarianism, Universalist Unitarian, Bahai, Native American religions, and many others. For members of the U.S. armed forces requesting military burial, there are at least 39 different emblems of belief available to designate a veteran's religion on headstones or grave markers (U.S. Department of Veterans Affairs, 2008).

Within any of these major or secondary religions, there may be strict fundamentalists who interpret doctrine literally and practice the rituals meticulously (i.e., follow the letter of the law). By contrast, there may be more moderate or liberal adherents who also embrace the beliefs and follow the practices, albeit with less rigidity (i.e., follow the spirit of the law). For example, within Judaism, there are Orthodox, Conservative, and Reformed groups. Orthodox Jews follow a more strict adherence to the principles of Judaism, living scrupulously according to Hebrew law. Conservatives accept much of the law but are not as strict as the Orthodox. Reformed Jews are more open and accommodating to modern culture, while still maintaining their Jewish identity. An open-ended query by the grief counselor—"How do you practice your faith?"—will usually elicit descriptions that enlighten the counselor about the prominence of religion in clients' lives and whether clients are more conservative or liberal in their practices.

Interestingly, some distinguish "religious Jews" (e.g., those who are more careful about keeping the Law and the Sabbath) from "nonreligious" or "secular Jews" (e.g., those who are Jewish only by parentage). In fact, one of the continuing conversations within Judaism pertains to *who is* a Jew. Is a Jew a person who has a certain racial and ethnic pedigree or someone who practices Judaism as a religion? It is an unresolved issue. However, it illustrates very well how race, ethnicity, culture, and religion can all become intertwined in defining a person's identity and outlook. This fluid interplay of factors only reinforces the importance of grief counselors getting to know the role of religion in the client's life, rather than making assumptions based on group assignment.

Broadly speaking, in addition to the conservative–liberal dimension, the world's major religions are sometimes divided according to Eastern and Western traditions. Among the Eastern religions are Buddhism, Hinduism, Confucianism, Taoism, and Shinto. Generally, in the Eastern traditions, there are multiple deities, and there is considerable emphasis on developing one's individual religious life through private meditation, devotion, and prayer. The Western religions are Judaism, Islam, and Christianity, which all trace their origins back to the Hebrew patriarch Abraham. Jews and Muslims, who often are publicly presented as being at odds with one another, actually share a common ancestry through Abraham as well as a common prohibition against eating pork. The three major Western religions are sometimes called *monotheistic* traditions because they believe in one God. The Western traditions tend to have more corporate worship rituals. Beliefs about cremation are another example of East–West contrasts: for Hindus and Buddhists, cremation is normal; for Muslims and Orthodox Jews, cremation is largely rejected (Davies, 2003).

SPIRITUALITY

Defining spirituality in terms of an individual's personal conviction about the existence of a higher power, or an internalized sense of connectedness to the divine, is stepping onto shaky conceptual ground. Zinnbauer et al. (1997) criticized *spirituality* as a fuzzy concept with diverse meanings and connotations, depending on the perceiver's vantage point. Gamino, Easterling, and Sewell (2003) spoke for many grief counselors when they summarized how religion and spirituality seem to be two distinct phenomena:

> Pastoral caregivers have long suspected that those persons who simply perform religious rituals or routinely attend worship services do not necessarily cope better with bereavement or other personal crises. Rather, those

> individuals who are able to *actualize* their spiritual experience in times of crisis and *apply* their belief system to life difficulties such as bereavement seem to cope more adaptively. (p. 13)

Spirituality is subjective and reflects a constellation of *inner* beliefs, attitudes, motivations, and experiences. In that way, spirituality can be differentiated from external religious practices, such as attendance at worship services. The latter are easier to measure but may be less meaningful. In other words, a person may attend worship services for many external reasons: habit, social status, belonging, or perceiving it as being good for business. Because of its subjective nature, intrinsic spirituality can be difficult to identify and appreciate in another person without exploring it in some detail. Easterling, Gamino, Sewell, and Stirman (2000) recommend that practitioners *listen* for how closely the client has found God (or a higher power) to be present in life or how likely the client is to think about God (or a higher power) at times of trauma or loss. Some sensitively posed inquiries along these lines can draw out the discussion without forcing the issue. For example, "Is faith or spirituality a resource for you in making decisions such as these (i.e., end-of-life), or in how you think about death and what it means?"

For the grief counselor, the salience of a client's spirituality is twofold. First, intrinsic spirituality is associated with positive health benefits, both psychologically and medically (Koenig, George, & Peterson, 1998). Among bereaved people in particular, these benefits appear to go beyond any that may accrue simply from attendance at worship services alone (Easterling et al., 2000). Second, intrinsic spirituality may be a key to unlocking adaptive strategies for grievers at a time of loss and poignant pain. Gamino et al. (2003) refer to this as a "reachable moment":

> For the survivor, death often brings to the surface existential concerns about mortality, the meaning of life, ultimate purpose, the possibility of an afterlife, and so forth. In this process of confronting life's greatest mysteries, the mourner may be "primed" to consider (or reconsider) the role of his/her spiritual experiences in how death is understood and how grieving is construed. Thus, a unique "reachable moment" exists when, with the assistance of a well-trained clinical or pastoral caregiver, a mourner may be able to access relatively *dormant* intrinsic spirituality and utilize it to cope with one of life's ubiquitous challenges, the death of a close loved one. (p. 24)

How people derive personal meaning at a time of dying and death often involves their spirituality, regardless of religious affiliation. For example, some people will construct elaborate explanations of how this or that happened "according to God's will" (Anderson, 1989). All major world religions have devotees who fervently believe that all things happen according to God's will or according to some divine plan or destiny and that making sense of what has happened is an important part of their faith life. Others may view their human faculties as gifts from God, believing that this endowment was given for the purpose of figuring out for oneself the meaning and significance of life events, including death and loss. Or, the individual may view death as a type of metamorphosis from a temporal existence to some kind of ethereal, cosmic unity with a higher power or supernatural force (cf. Yalom, 1980), in effect, a transformed state with which one can maintain communication and a continuing bond (Richards, 2001).

Death can shake a person's spirituality to its core. Yet, no one can construct a meaningful attribution about death based on spirituality for another person. Suggestions can be made, thoughts can be provoked, or questions can be posed, but the answer must come from within the client. Trying to force a spiritual meaning for death is both insensitive ethically and ineffective therapeutically. For example, some may attempt to explain the tragic death of a child using spiritual constructs, as evidenced by comments often made to grieving parents: "God needed your son/daughter more than you did," or "You have given God a great gift, just as God gave his son for you," or "God is testing your faith to see how strong it is, like Abraham." Most bereaved parents find such comments to be cruel, not comforting. Usually, the sympathizers are engaging in a kind of psychological projection—in trying to explain the loss of the child to the parents, they are really trying to explain it to themselves.

We recall the case of a bereaved mother who lost one of her two children in an accident, even though she had prayed many times for her children's safety. Her child's death prompted a crisis of faith where she felt betrayed by God for not answering her prayers. Enraged and powerless, she protested to her grief counselor, "All I can say is God is mean. Just plain mean. God *killed* my child." Formulaic promises of God's divine comfort offered by denominational clergy seemed hollow and pointless to her.

The grief counseling sessions provided a forum in which the bereaved mother could verbalize whatever she was thinking or feeling. She finally determined not "to grow old and bitter" and acknowledged begrudgingly some fulfillment in parenting her living child: "I hate to admit it, but people are right. I still have another child who needs me."

The counselor respected the client's process of reconsidering and reformulating her long-held religious beliefs that were called into question by the death of her child. Gradually, the client recast her worldview and found some consolation in identifying love as the ultimate priority. Even though her child's lifetime was short, the mother drew comfort from having loved her child fully and lavishly. She felt connected to her deceased child whenever she gave love or experienced love richly again, and this became her spiritual meaning.

DIVERSITY AND THE FIVE P MODEL

When encountering ethical challenges presented by a client's diversity, application of the Five P Model can help grief counselors demonstrate appropriate professional sensitivity while providing effective counseling services.

Case Example

A Chinese American woman in her early 40s consulted a grief counselor following the death of her elderly father. The client had an advanced degree and a successful career in the information technology field. Although unmarried and without children, she did have a supportive partner relationship. As the eldest daughter, she lived at home and helped her elderly parents, neither of whom spoke much English. They emigrated from China when the client was a child and made their living with a small retail business that her brother still operated. Having spent most of her life in the United States, the client thought of herself as "80% American, 20% Asian." Neither she nor her family attended church or temple regularly. When asked about religious affiliation, she responded, "Confucianism, I guess," although she was not even sure what that designation implied.

When her father became ill, no one really knew what was wrong with him. He developed breathing problems. After finally consulting physicians, it was discovered that he had lung cancer. The client and her siblings were devastated. Aggressively, the doctors outlined a treatment course to include chemotherapy and radiation. The client thought her father would live a few more years with treatment.

When he declined rapidly, she took him to the emergency department one night. Because her father spoke almost no English, the client served as translator. The doctors were trying to talk to him about how ill he was and to determine his wishes regarding treatment options. Even so, she thought they were being somewhat circumspect in their questions and descriptions. Grief-stricken herself at what was happening and not sure if her father would live through the night, she did not know whether to simply translate precisely what the doctor said or to engage her father in a more extended discussion about end-of-life decisions. She elected just to translate literally, but she was never sure whether her father really understood what was happening.

Ultimately, he was placed on a ventilator and sent to the intensive care unit. She recalled tearfully asking an experienced nurse in the emergency department whether patients in her father's condition ever survived. The nurse was kind but direct in explaining to the client that with "end-stage disease" like her father's, it was "rare" to survive.

When the client's mother arrived at the hospital, she was accompanied not only by the client's siblings but also by certain elders of a Buddhist-affiliated cultural group of which her father was a member. In the client's estimation, the elders proceeded to take over by advising her mother about what was proper and "auspicious" with regard to his care. As the patient's spouse, the medical staff looked to the client's mother as the decision maker, and the mother looked to the elders for guidance. The client's role was reduced only to translator.

The client's father spent a week in intensive care but only deteriorated. The doctor suggested withdrawing life support, and the family concurred because "there were so many needles and tubes going in and out and he was not getting better." The Buddhist elders determined that her father should be "let go" in the morning to facilitate the "spirit journey." The same pattern of advice-giving continued throughout the next few days, with members of the Buddhist group directing decisions about the funeral arrangements and the cremation. They insisted on certain ceremonial aspects such as incense, candles, and chanting, and the client's mother passively acquiesced. In her own state of acute grief, the client was too paralyzed to protest or even ask for explanations. The whole experience was kind of a "blur" to her. She mainly remembered crying a lot.

The father's death was the first major loss the client had sustained in her life. She felt there was really no way she could have prepared herself for it, and she recognized she was having trouble coping. Her mother seemed lost in her own world of mourning, did not ask much of her daughter, and could offer little comfort to her children. The client's siblings all had spouses and children with whom they were busy. The client's partner was very understanding and provided solace.

Much of the therapy discussion consisted of revisiting the time of the father's death and addressing the client's doubts about whether more could have been done medically for her father. Also, the subject of the Buddhist elders was reviewed. The elders' involvement was a confusing and disconcerting aspect of the events. The client was not sure whether she felt grateful or angry about their participation. Mostly, she did not understand what their rituals meant. The whole sad experience led her to question the meaning of life and death, what happens after a person's death, and whether Confucianism offered any insight for her. Simply put, she was not sure what she believed, or why. Largely acculturated into American society, the client did not feel she had either a religious grounding or a cultural tradition on which to rely at this difficult time.

The grief counselor faced several ethical dilemmas. First, the counselor had limited experience with Asian clients and had worked before with only one Chinese family. A potential resource for the counselor was a faculty colleague who was Chinese and quite open to discussion of cross-cultural issues. Second, the grief counselor had no working familiarity to speak of regarding Confucianism or Buddhism. Related to that, the counselor had no clear indication of whether the client maintained any intrinsic spirituality. Third, as a practicing Christian with strong convictions about the afterlife, the counselor could readily see how meaning consistent with that framework could be found in the client's experience. The question concerned how to probe for or guide the client toward finding her own understanding of her father's death and what the experience meant to her, without pushing or suggesting ideas from a Christian perspective.

Analysis With the Five P Model

Person

Who is the client as a person? She is a bilingual woman in her early 40s whose ethnicity is Chinese but whose citizenship is American. Having lived in the United States since childhood, she considers herself fairly acculturated. Her graduate education and successful career likely contribute to that identification as American. She lives with her elderly mother but does not appear to have much support from her mother or her siblings. She has a supportive partner but mentions no other friends.

Her religious affiliation is Confucianism, although she does not practice or even seem to know the tenets of her faith tradition. The death of her father is the first significant loss she has sustained in her life.

Problem

In terms of the grief counseling, the client's problem is a familiar one—how to cope with the loss of her elderly father. The client is self-aware enough to realize that she is struggling and so seeks professional help. Beyond having a supportive partner relationship, she has few social resources to draw on in attempting to adjust. Her main assets are her intelligence, education, and drive. She has no experience with a major loss.

The ethical problem really rests with the grief counselor. Fortunately, there is no language barrier, but does the counselor have the specific competencies necessary to work with a Chinese American client? Does the counselor grasp the cross-cultural issues presented by this case? What about the element of religion? How does the counselor deal with the factors of Confucianism and Buddhism that are part of the client's story? Does the counselor's Christian perspective enter the picture? How does the counselor try to guide the client's quest for understanding and meaning without imposing on the client the counselor's own religious beliefs or spiritual values?

Place

At a micro level, the counseling takes place in an office setting. The necessary parameters of consent, confidentiality, privacy, and a professional atmosphere are assured. There are no multiple relationship issues associated with place. At a macro level, the counseling takes place within a broader social world that constantly provides messages about ethnic and cultural differences (LaRoche & Maxie, 2003). The grief counselor must be constantly aware of how such influences can shape the perception of the client.

Principles

Two main ethical principles apply to this case scenario. Beneficence is the first consideration. In the interest of accomplishing something helpful or beneficial for the client, does the counselor have the knowledge and expertise needed in light of the ethnic, cultural, and religious diversity presented? Would it be in the client's best interest to refer her to another professional with greater familiarity with Chinese Americans or with Confucianism and Buddhism?

The second consideration is one of autonomy, but not in the classic sense of the client's right to self-determination and the right to choose treatment. In this case, respecting autonomy concerns more subtle factors. Specifically, the counselor needs to respect the client's right to develop her own unique formulation and understanding in regard to her father's death and what it means to her. This requires respecting her freedom to incorporate or reject the traditions of Confucianism or Buddhism as potential avenues to meaning making. The subject of the counselor's Christian perspective may or may not have a place in the therapeutic dialogue, depending on whether the client introduces it or whether it seems beneficial to advance the discussion. Respecting the client's autonomy regarding religious beliefs precludes any unilateral moves by the counselor to promote a Christian viewpoint (i.e., proselytizing).

Process

Possessing basic demographic information prior to the initial appointment, including the client's name, age, marital status, education level, occupation, and language fluency, the counselor knew the client was Chinese. However, until meeting and talking with her, the counselor did not know the client's degree of acculturation or how well they would be able to relate. The counselor did not want to prejudge the client or make attributions based on the myth of sameness.

In this case, rapport developed rather rapidly, and the counselor was aware of the client's efforts to connect with the counselor and her earnestness in laying out her therapy agenda. The counselor was aware of a feeling of likeability between them from early on in the discussion. Later in the session, when the counselor inquired about the client's comfort level with the interaction, they shared a chuckle about the client's response, "Oh, I checked you out before I came. They said you were 'very good,' and I can see that you are." Based on all these factors, the counselor decided that this was a case that could be competently handled, provided that the counselor took some initiative to get better educated about Chinese culture as well as Confucianism and Buddhism.

To that end, the counselor took several steps. The faculty colleague who was Chinese American allayed many of the counselor's concerns and emphasized that for highly acculturated Chinese, treating the person in any fashion *other than* that of a fellow American would be seen as demeaning or disrespectful. When the counselor told the colleague about the client's sense of humor, the colleague suggested employing a reciprocal device if the subject of her Chinese ethnicity came up (e.g., telling the client with a smile that the counselor had "checked out" what it meant to be Chinese American!).

As further steps, the counselor sought out and read book chapters on cultural experiences of Asian Americans in the United States and on Confucianism and Buddhism. The counselor telephoned a colleague knowledgeable in Buddhist beliefs and practices, trying to understand better the Buddhist cultural group that the client mentioned and Buddhist death rituals. Having exercised due diligence in gaining additional knowledge about the various cultural and religious factors pertaining to the client's case, the counselor was more confident in asking questions and discussing those subjects. Instead of instructing the client that she would have to teach the counselor about her ethnic background and religion, or saying nothing at all, the counselor was able to respond, "My reading and sources tell me [thus and so]; how does that correspond with your experience?" This educational aspect of the counselor's process of resolving the ethical dilemma was especially important because the client herself was not very knowledgeable about Confucianism or Buddhism.

Finally, the subject of Christianity never came up directly in the counseling sessions. The counselor realized latently that the initial thought of introducing a Christian perspective came from two sources: the counselor's uneasiness about lack of knowledge of the client's religion and a brief moment of death anxiety linked to the fact that the counselor's elderly father was about the same age as the client's deceased father (i.e., countertransference feelings). Later, the counselor did draw on Christian beliefs *indirectly* by raising the notion of afterlife as "a feature of many religions" and initiating a dialogue regarding the client's viewpoint on that concept.

There is a postscript to this case. Months later at the next ADEC annual conference, the counselor made a point of attending sessions on East–West differences in grief and bereavement. Not only were these enlightening, but also the counselor contributed to the development of other professionals by sharing the case example and what had been learned. Thus, the counselor provided excellent service to the client, managed the ethical dilemmas involved, enhanced the counselor's own knowledge, and helped other grief counselors learn from the experience.

SUMMARY

The ethical principles of autonomy and beneficence are particularly salient when grief counselors work with clients and families from diverse backgrounds. Whether it is diversity of race, ethnicity, language, culture, religion, spirituality, or some other element, each person must be respected and honored as having value and a right to self-determination. As challenging as counseling may be when one does not understand another person's context, ethically conscious professionals approach such situations with the welfare of the client as the foremost consideration in deciding whether to treat or refer. It is constructive to view work with clients from diverse backgrounds as an opportunity for learning and furthering professional development. Such an attitude can be transformative in augmenting the grief counselor's skills, advancing the field of thanatology, and enhancing tolerance throughout our society and global community.

9 Grief Counseling on the Internet

Picture the following scene: a client enters a coffee shop on the entry level of a large office building in a major U.S. city on the eastern seaboard and selects a comfortable, overstuffed chair in a secluded corner. With the technological assistance of a very smart phone and local wireless access to the Internet, the client participates in a real-time, videoconference grief-counseling session with an expert provider located on the West Coast, who was recommended as the best counselor available for the client's particular loss. The client wears a wireless headset to hear the counselor's comments and responds into a sensitive microphone that transmits clearly what the client says when speaking no louder than a library voice. On the telephone screen, the client can see the grief counselor, who is seated at a desktop computer with Webcam in an office at the counselor's home 3,000 miles away. When the client's cup of coffee is finished, and the 50-minute therapy "hour" is over, both parties sign off, and the bill is paid over the Internet by credit card. Does this sound futuristic?

In a brave new world of grief counseling on the Internet, this scene could become commonplace. In some parts of the United States, and around the world, it already is a frequent occurrence. Given that online mental health service delivery is underway and likely to expand in the future (Rochlen, Zack, & Speyer, 2004), contemporary grief counselors need to be apprised of the ethical challenges associated with providing professional services via the Internet. First, we consider how the Five P Model applies to the unique practice demands of Internet counseling. Then we describe the various forms of online counseling, explore the advantages and disadvantages of Internet counseling, identify potential ethical problems linked to Internet modalities, and review available standards and guidelines for providers offering Internet counseling.

INTERNET COUNSELING AND THE FIVE P MODEL

Internet counseling is a new and emerging field of practice. Therefore, grief counselors should exercise appropriate caution and seek special training and preparation before attempting to include Internet counseling in their repertoire of professional services. Following the organization of this book, professionals who want to offer Internet counseling need to consolidate the ethical steps of establishing competence, obtaining informed consent, and maintaining confidentiality. As Maheu (2001) warns, "it is imprudent to use e-mail and chat rooms to establish or maintain psychotherapeutic relationships with unscreened, undiagnosed, unseen, unheard, and unknown consumers through the Internet" (p. 7). Instead, grief counselors interested in Internet modalities will have to modify their administrative procedures and adjust their practice styles to meet the specific demands of the Internet as a medium. How does one authenticate the identity of prospective clients and conduct the process of informed consent both before grief counseling begins and during sessions?

The hypothetical case of grief counseling via transcontinental videoconferencing described at the beginning of this chapter illustrates how the element of place in the Five P Model is particularly important to consider in meeting the specific ethical challenges presented by Internet counseling. Internet counseling happens over an electronic network instead of in a geographic location. So how does one ensure confidentiality and keep others from eavesdropping on the teleconference? Furthermore, cyberspace is a virtual place not governed by licensing boards and jurisdictional statutes. It has been said that Internet counselors practice "with one foot in the jurisdiction where they work and one foot in the jurisdiction where the client resides." The Internet as the place of service delivery requires grief counselors to make special arrangements for intervening in the event of a crisis and to take special precautions for meeting state or jurisdictional rules in order to conduct themselves in an ethically sound manner.

However, the same basic ethical principles that govern grief counseling in traditional practice settings apply also to Internet counseling: respecting a client's autonomy to choose counseling and negotiate the terms of a working agreement for online services; making the client's welfare a priority and striving to obtain a good outcome for the client (beneficence); avoiding any harm to the client through misuse or mishandling of the Internet as a medium (nonmaleficence); treating the client fairly within the parameters of available resources, especially utilizing online sources of mental health information (justice); keeping trust and good faith by honoring the professional integrity of the counselor–client relationship (fidelity).

TYPES OF INTERNET COUNSELING

Teletherapy. E-therapy. Online counseling. Internet-mediated psychological services. Telehealth. WebCounseling. Cyber-therapy. E-mail counseling. Internet therapy. Web-based counseling. A variety of names are found in the scholarly literature to describe mental health services delivered on the Internet (Heinlen, Welfel, Richmond, & Rak, 2003). For purposes of this chapter, we use the term *Internet counseling* as a convenient description. Borrowing from Rochlen et al. (2004), we define Internet counseling broadly as any professional interaction that makes use of the Internet to connect qualified mental health providers and their clients. Potentially, Internet counseling is available to any client with a computer and Internet access that can connect with a grief counselor. Similar options would be cell phone texting or "telemedicine" delivered through closed-circuit television or satellite. However, we will not address the topic of computer-administered mental health treatments where the computer effectively replaces the human therapist (Cavanagh & Shapiro, 2004; Cavanaugh, Zack, Shapiro, & Wright, 2003).

Some have argued that Internet communication, or "e-therapy," between a provider and a client is not really counseling or psychotherapy because it does not consist of diagnosing and treating mental disorders (Grohol, 1999; Manhal-Baugus, 2001). For us, making a distinction between e-therapy and formal grief counseling or psychotherapy is superfluous hair-splitting. Barnett and Scheetz (2003) cite how courts tend to see the existence of a professional relationship when an individual pays a fee to a professional for advice given, especially when multiple communications occur. Thus, we encourage grief counselors to acknowledge that offering help and advice online to clients for a professional fee constitutes grief counseling and requires them to adhere to all applicable rules of professional conduct and ethics in providing such service.

Internet counseling can be either *asynchronous* or *synchronous*. Asynchronous means the parties respond to one another on a time-delayed basis, such as exchanging e-mail or posting entries to a Web-based message board. Synchronous means the interchange occurs in real time with both parties online simultaneously, such as chat modes like instant messaging, live voice streaming, or videoconferencing, as in the hypothetical scenario portrayed at the beginning of this chapter (Recupero & Rainey, 2005; Rochlen et al., 2004; Stofle, 2002). As a function of technology, the majority of Internet counseling provided at the time of this writing is through asynchronous e-mail (Heinlen et al., 2003; Rochlen et al., 2004). As technology advances, live videoconference could well become the preferred modality.

Providing some form of Internet counseling can be an adjunct to traditional, face-to-face sessions. For example, some counselors give out their e-mail address for brief communication between sessions. As with telephone calls, the counselor then must set clear boundaries about what kind of information will be acknowledged between sessions and what will be carried over to the next session (see Appendix D, "Sample Client Information Brochure for Informed Consent for Grief Counseling"). Should a client whom the counselor knows well move to another locale, they may agree to continue via Internet counseling (see Chapter 13, "Moving or Closing a Practice"), with e-mail or instant messenger. Or some grief counselors may encourage clients, especially adolescents, to stay connected electronically through e-mail, Web logs known as "blogs," or designated chat rooms in order to build rapport and give clients the opportunity to communicate on their terms.

Some practitioners may offer Internet counseling as an independent, stand-alone service without ever having any in-person contact with the client. Interestingly, survey data shows that Internet counseling for grief and bereavement is much less common than online treatment for depression, anxiety, family problems, and relationship difficulties (Cook & Doyle, 2002; Maheu & Gordon, 2000). On the other hand, Vanderwerker and Prigerson (2004) studied a community-based sample of bereaved persons and found that 59% reported using the Internet, and 50% used e-mail, although their data did not indicate whether this usage included health information seeking or Internet counseling. Perhaps because of the intensely personal nature of grief counseling, an Internet modality may be less preferred than traditional face-to-face sessions (J. Bissler, personal communication, September 29, 2008).

IS INTERNET COUNSELING ADVISABLE?

Like it or not, Internet counseling appears to be here to stay and will likely only increase in the future (Maheu, 2001; Nickelson, 1998; Rochlen et al., 2004). Skinner and Zack (2004) trace the history of indirect treatment back to Freud's practice of providing psychoanalysis by letter when necessary because of geographic distance. In other words, communicating through writing with clients is not really a new idea. Still, many scholars continue to debate the potential advantages and disadvantages of Internet counseling (Fenichel et al., 2002; International Society for Mental Health Online [ISMHO], 2000; Leibert, Archer, Munson, & York, 2006; Maheu, 2001; Manhal-Baugus, 2001; Ragusea & Vande-Creek, 2003; Robson & Robson, 2000; Rochlen et al., 2004; Shaw & Shaw, 2006). For discussion purposes, we summarize in the following sections the principal issues involved in the debate over the advisability of Internet counseling.

Advantages of Internet Counseling

Convenience and ease of use are often mentioned as prime advantages to Internet counseling. In short, clients can reach out to their counselors when the moment of need occurs, regardless of whether it is the middle of the night or they are traveling away from home (cf. Ainsworth, 2002). There is no telephone tag, there are no obstacles to getting an appointment, and conceivably, the client can choose from a more extensive panel of providers. Additionally, Internet counseling increases access to mental health treatment by dissolving geographic boundaries and empowering clients in remote locations with few providers or in areas where there is a language barrier. Internet counseling may provide an avenue for mental health treatment for the homebound, those disabled with mobility problems, the deaf, and those reluctant to seek treatment face-to-face because of shame or embarrassment.

Suler (2004) wrote an oft-cited paper describing the "online disinhibition effect" as one of the potential advantages of Internet counseling.

Without the perceived necessity of negotiating social personas and expectations, clients may feel less restrained and engage more quickly in a high degree of intimate self-disclosure. Clients may reveal personal material to an online counselor that they would never admit in person. Suler believes that the anonymity of Internet counseling and the fact that clients are invisible physically to their counselor give them the courage to speak out more, an assertion supported by early empirical data (Cook & Doyle, 2002). However, Suler also describes how the disinhibition effect can enable acting-out behavior, making it a disadvantage at times.

Another advantage to Internet counseling is that both the client and the counselor have the capability of downloading the conversation and printing out a transcript of the counseling session(s). Clients can reread and ponder the words of the counselor any time after their exchange. Rereading can help promote a reflective stance, extend the therapeutic value of the counselor's input, and enhance the client's internalized sense of the counselor's ongoing presence (Fenichel et al., 2002). The time delay involved in asynchronous forms of Internet counseling affords freedom from having to respond immediately to the other party, thus allowing both counselors and clients an opportunity to contemplate the therapy dialogue and formulate their thoughts by writing.

Related to this, the fact that clients must write out their responses in e-mail or message board–style Internet counseling may be a salutary process in and of itself (cf. Pennebaker, 1997; Smyth & Pennebaker, 2008; White & Epston, 1990), especially for bereaved clients (Neimeyer, van Dyke, & Pennebaker, 2008). For the client who enjoys journaling, e-mail exchanges with an Internet counselor may be a natural way to think through various concerns and identify potential strategies for coping. Writing helps the client find connections and patterns in responses and relationships, both internally and with others. (See Chapter 10 on journaling and letter-writing as therapy techniques with bereaved clients.)

Two other advantages to Internet counseling concern finances and educational resources. As a general rule, professional fees for Internet counseling, particularly text-based options like e-mail and message-posting, may be less than fees customarily charged for face-to-face counseling (Heinlen et al., 2003; Manhal-Baugus, 2001). Presumably, this is because overhead costs such as office space, staff salaries, supplies, and so forth are significantly less, particularly for those practitioners who offer Internet counseling as a stand-alone service or who work from home. Finally, because clients often ask for educational materials pertaining to their specific problems, such as books or Web sites, Internet counseling has the advantage of enabling the counselor to create hyperlinks easily when typing a response to direct clients to Web locations with helpful information or resources.

Disadvantages of Internet Counseling

The most frequently mentioned disadvantage to Internet counseling with text-based modalities is the absence of nonverbal cues. Most therapists trained in traditional, face-to-face counseling pay close attention to numerous nonverbal signals, including facial expression, body language, and voice stylistics, in making an assessment of a client and conducting therapeutic interventions. The totality of data accrued from visual, aural, olfactory, tactile, and intuitive channels contribute to an accurate anamnesis of the client. Ekman and Friesen (2003), citing decades of research, assert that facial signals are the primary system for expression of emotion. Mehrabian (2007) hypothesizes that, in any conversation, 93% of the meaning is communicated through nonverbal cues such as facial expression, behavior, and voice quality, with only 7% of the actual message communicated by the words themselves.

Consider the following examples. An acutely grieving client who states, "I'm doing pretty well with the loss," while leaking tears throughout the session presents an incongruity that a counselor will explore. A client with terminal lung disease who smells of tobacco and has a pack of cigarettes in a shirt pocket will have a difficult time convincing the counselor that very little smoking is occurring. A bereaved parent whose voice conveys angry overtones while describing forgiveness for the driver at fault for the fatal car crash that killed the child may be in a state of denial that needs to be addressed. The client who responds with a fearful deer-in-the-headlights expression when asked why the opportunity was not taken to say goodbye to the loved one dying in the hospital is telling the counselor something that would never be conveyed through asynchronous e-mail. Many practitioners admit readily that they would not be comfortable forgoing these important nonverbal aspects of grief counseling and consider such information vital to a complete understanding of the client.

Proponents of Internet counseling counter by arguing that novelists and poets throughout human history have succeeded in capturing the richness of the human experience in the written word alone (Fenichel et al., 2002). Supporters of Internet counseling believe that enterprising clients can use a variety of compensatory techniques to enliven and imbue their writing with an emotive, conversational quality. Examples include use of emoticons (either symbols formed from aggregated keystrokes, such as frowny faces, or cartoon-like icons representing a wide array of moods and affects); parenthetical expressions that convey subvocal nuance, such as (sigh); CAPS for emphasis; bracketed labels of [emotion]; use of similes and metaphors; and trailers (. . .) for transitions, to name a few (Fenichel et al., 2002; Manhal-Baugus, 2001).

These arguments on the adequacy of the written word to convey truth about the human heart and spirit have not persuaded everyone. Shaw and Shaw (2006) worry that developing adequate rapport can be a problem with a client never seen face-to-face, a worry founded on data indicating that as much as one-fourth of the therapeutic effect of counseling is based on establishing a working alliance (Hubble, Duncan, & Miller, 1999). Barnett and Scheetz (2003) warn that cultural differences, such as those addressed in Chapter 8, may be even more difficult to detect and account for in a text-only interchange. Others have charged that relying on text-only communication modes in Internet counseling results in a subtle form of socio-intellectual elitism by selecting only those clients most adept at a written medium, thus neutralizing arguments of increased access and availability (Manhal-Baugus, 2001; Ragusea & VandeCreek, 2003).

There are other potential disadvantages such as the time delays that occur with asynchronous Internet counseling. The immediacy of the client's ability to talk to the counselor any time of the day or night can create an unrealistic wish or expectation for an expedited response. Clearly, e-mail or message-posting modalities require some mutual understanding between clients and counselors about the time frame in which the client can reasonably expect a response, typically within 24–72 hours (Manhal-Baugus, 2001). Just as traditional therapists have office hours during which appointments are taken, Internet counselors are not online all the time, and clients need to be prepared for inevitable time delays.

Internet counseling depends on technology in a manner that face-to-face counseling does not. Anyone with a computer is aware of the many exasperating ways that technology can break down as a result of hardware failure, software malfunction, transmission problems with one's Internet provider, power outages, bugs and viruses, and many other potential problems. Obviously, when technical problems occur, interruptions in the anticipated schedule of Internet counseling will follow, and this is a major disadvantage. Counselors who plan to offer services over the

Internet need to become skilled at troubleshooting and solving technical problems that interrupt service provision, both as a business practice and as a model for clients who rely increasingly on the Internet for vital life activities, including their counseling (Ragusea & VandeCreek, 2003; Skinner & Zack, 2004).

Many scholars suggest that certain types of emotional disorders are not amenable to Internet counseling. Usually, this list includes unstable bipolar disorder, borderline and other personality disorders, eating disorders, substance misuse, dissociative disorders, psychotic disorders with a perceptual distortion of reality, sexual abuse, and violent relationships. A client in an abusive or violent relationship who accesses Internet counseling from home may risk the perpetrator finding out that family secrets are being revealed and incur additional risk as a result (Robson & Robson, 2000). Although everyone may not agree on what kind of problems should be excluded from consideration, there appears to be broad consensus that depression, anxiety, and relationship or interpersonal problems lend themselves most readily to Internet counseling. To the extent that there are limits to which problems can be addressed suitably through Internet modalities, this can be considered a disadvantage.

RESEARCH DATA ON INTERNET COUNSELING

As an emerging treatment modality, Internet counseling does not yet have a substantial body of research validating its efficacy. Yet, early tests of its effectiveness compared to face-to-face counseling or wait-list controls are promising (Rochlen et al., 2004). One early test of the therapeutic effectiveness of Internet counseling came from Cook and Doyle (2002), who compared the relative strength of the perceived therapeutic alliance by clients in both Internet and face-to-face counseling. In their small, mostly white female sample of volunteers, empirical ratings of the counselor–client working alliance were higher in the group of online clients than in the norm group of clients in face-to-face counseling on whom the empirical scale was validated.

In a similar study, Leibert et al. (2006) investigated client perceptions of Internet counseling and the therapeutic alliance. They noted that previous research showed individuals who were lonely, socially anxious, and struggling with forming relationships in person were more likely to develop relationships online. Online clients in their study were predominantly female, White, unmarried, young adults (average age was 29 years old) who had some college, were already regular Internet users, and enjoyed the convenience and anonymity of the service. Almost one-third of the sample mentioned cost considerations as a factor. Regarding modality of Internet counseling, 59% reported e-mail contact, and 33% had used instant messaging. Only 2% used videoconferencing. Interestingly, nearly 80% of the sample had *previously* attended face-to-face counseling.

In a cross-sectional comparison, Leibert et al. (2006) found that online counseling clients were generally satisfied with their counseling, but their satisfaction ratings were not as high as a comparative group of clients who received only face-to-face counseling. Clients who received face-to-face counseling reported a stronger therapeutic alliance with the counselor than those clients who received counseling online. The researchers concluded that some people are clearly at ease with Internet counseling. Their sample of young adult women may represent a generation that has grown up using the Internet on a daily basis, so they embrace the anonymity and convenience of Internet counseling and generally feel safe online.

A randomized controlled trial of Internet counseling for complicated grief was reported by Wagner, Knaevelsrud, and Maercker (2006). German-speaking clients in Europe and elsewhere who responded to Internet notices of the study were carefully screened online and eliminated from consideration if they met any of the following exclusion criteria: younger than age 18, receiving mental health treatment elsewhere, time since death less than 14 months, abusing substances, reporting severe depression or suicidal intentions, and indicating dissociative or psychotic tendencies. It is noteworthy that this screening process began with 213 requests for the questionnaires, of which 143 were returned. After screening, only 55 persons entered the random treatment allocation. The authors' efforts to ensure an appropriate sample for their study illustrates how important it is to screen Internet applicants for research or counseling.

Wagner et al.'s (2006) study sample was predominantly younger females (average age was 37), of whom 61% were bereaved parents. This suggests they closely resemble the population of troubled grievers who seek mental health treatment because of problems coping (see Chapter 10, "Ethical Controversies in Grief Counseling," specifically on whether grief counseling is effective). Clients were randomly assigned either to 5 weeks of cognitive-behavioral treatment delivered entirely through e-mail communication or to a 5-week waiting list control group (who then received the treatment sequence). Based on Stroebe and Schut's (1999) dual-process model of grief, the treatment focused on deliberate exposure to bereavement cues such as thinking about the most distressing aspect of their loss, cognitive restructuring to begin thinking of the deceased in a more comforting way that incorporated new perspectives, integrating the death by reflecting on how the loss had changed them, and envisioning the future. Clients receiving the cognitive-behavioral treatment showed significant symptom reduction after 5 weeks compared to the waiting list group. They maintained those gains at follow-up 3 months later. Most clients felt that the contact between the therapist and them was personal and expressed satisfaction with the Internet counseling. Only 20% of the clients reported missing face-to-face contact with the therapist. Wagner et al. concluded that Internet counseling for complicated grief can be as effective as, if not more effective than, traditional therapy.

ETHICAL CHALLENGES WITH INTERNET COUNSELING

Five major areas of ethical challenges emerge from the scholarly literature available on Internet counseling. These include authenticating identity, obtaining informed consent, securing confidentiality, intervening in a crisis, and establishing jurisdictional and administrative governance.

Authenticating Identity

Most readers of this text will probably have heard at least one news story, personal account, or client disclosure of an individual impersonating someone else on the Internet for purposes of voyeurism, exploitation, criminal activity, or other mischief. An example was the case of Missouri teenager Megan Meier (Scott & Huffstutter, 2008). The mother of one of Megan's neighborhood girlfriends enlisted the help of some other teenage girls to fabricate an identity as a male admirer and begin chatting with Megan on her MySpace page. The hoax was intended as an effort to learn what Megan was saying about the neighbor's daughter. Later, the fictitious boy broke off contact with Megan in messages that turned vindictive and mean—"The world would be a better place without you." Megan subsequently hanged herself. The ringleader mother was indicted by the State of California for violating the rules of MySpace, creating a false identity, and using it to solicit personal information from a minor. In a controversial verdict based on a federal statute designed to combat computer crimes, the mother was convicted of misdemeanor charges of computer fraud in creating the phony account (Steinhauer,

2008). The point of this vignette is that anyone can impersonate someone else on the Internet, and this can happen in the course of Internet counseling as well.

Authentication of identity is critical, and the process starts with the counselor. Counselors who plan to practice Internet counseling should be willing to provide their real name and their educational credentials, training experiences, state license, and pertinent certifications. A Web page listing this information should include hyperlinks to licensing boards or professional associations enabling potential clients to verify independently a counselor's identity and licensure status. Legitimate counselors with appropriate training and credentials should have no hesitation providing this basic information.

An example of how large, online clinics handle authentication is http://www.letstalkcounseling.com. The site lists numerous counselors from various locations around the United States and Canada. There is also a thorough list of topics addressed, including Grief/Loss. Each counselor for the site has a page that includes a picture, an address, and the counselor's training, license and certification, and fees for service. Fees vary for e-mail, telephone counseling, chatting online, videoconferencing, and face-to-face counseling in the office. The Web site lists the professional organizations that certify the various counselors. Potential clients can select a topic, such as grief counseling, and enter their state of residence, and the site will list counselors who are geographically close.

Authenticating the identity of potential clients is trickier. Specifically, an individual must be at least 18 years old to give consent for counseling. Because Internet counseling is paid for by credit card, one cross-check is to match the client's reported demographic information with credit card information. It is always possible for minors to masquerade as their parents for purposes of engaging a counselor online and to use the parents' credit card to pay for it. That is why it is sometimes helpful to ask for a second form of identification, such as a photocopy of a driver's license, to verify identity. Of course, in order for clients to feel safe providing this kind of personal information about themselves, they must first be convinced of the counselor's authenticity.

Obtaining Informed Consent

Moving from traditional office practice to Internet counseling is not a reason to abandon the dynamic model of informed consent as a continuous consensual process (see Chapter 4, "Consent"). The same information contained in the sample client information brochure in Appendix D needs to be conveyed to potential online clients, together with modifications appropriate to Internet modalities, such as the time window in which a response can be expected, the nature of emergency backup, confidentiality safeguards (and the client's responsibilities in that regard), fee schedules for different types of service, and so forth. The challenge is ensuring that the client not only understands the parameters of grief counseling but also freely agrees to the proposed course of action.

In lieu of face-to-face discussion between counselor and client about informed consent, some interchange verifying the client's understanding and noncoerced agreement is necessary. When initial consultations are conducted in person, by telephone, or through videoconference, this interchange resembles customary discussions of informed consent prior to the initiation of counseling. When e-mail is the intended format, some exchange between prospective client and counselor is necessary to confirm consent. What is *not sufficient* is using "click-wrap agreements" in which the client reads a consent form or information page and indicates consent for counseling simply by clicking on a button saying, "I accept" or "I agree." Such shortcuts do not constitute discussion informing consent for grief counseling (Recupero & Rainey, 2005).

Securing Confidentiality

Conducting Internet counseling through e-mail or real-time chat via "open air" transmission with a commercial Internet service provider is open to eavesdropping and does not at all secure confidentiality. The only way to have the kind of privacy that clients enjoy in traditional face-to-face counseling behind a closed office door is to use encryption technology to protect the communications over the Internet. No system is completely foolproof, but there are some alternatives available that meet HIPAA (1996) standards for securing protected health information in transit.

Most readers will have at least some familiarity with encryption technology from making purchases over the Internet or banking from home. Financial transactions over the Internet commonly employ an encryption process called Secure Sockets Layer (www.verisign.com). Applied to the situation of Internet counseling, Secure Sockets Layer (SSL) would originate with the counselor's Web site. Conceptually, it creates an encrypted tunnel between the client's computer and the counselor's Web site destination that protects the information as it travels online. The primary advantage of SSL is that it can be activated by most common Internet browsers such as Internet Explorer, AOL, and Netscape Navigator and usually does not require the client to add or install hardware.

Another alternative is to use an encryption program such as Pretty Good Privacy (www.pgp.com), which encrypts files prior to sending them over the Internet. It requires the recipient to enter a password to decrypt the file and thereby access it. Thus, the password or key must be shared between the sender and the recipient. Also, the software program has to be installed on both computers in order for encryption and decryption to take place. For Internet counseling, the client would have to have the same encryption program as the counselor in order for a system such as Pretty Good Privacy to operate. Without encryption technology, it is possible for clients to install a Trojan horse program on the practitioner's computer and download all the contents of the practitioner's computer onto a remote computer (Maheu, 2001).

It is important to acknowledge to clients that e-mail and text-based messages are stored on local servers and that agency or institutional supervisors and information technology (IT) personnel have the right to read e-mail records of counselor-employees (Manhal-Baugus, 2001). Another security consideration with Internet counseling is the fact that texts that are deleted do not really disappear. Whatever has been typed into the system is discoverable by legal process. All the documents that have been a part of the counseling can be ordered legally from the online service provider. Under subpoena, these documents are discoverable for use in a court of law. Further, some countries outside of the United States regularly intercept e-mails and messages. Any international Internet counseling may be subject to these intercepts.

As described in Chapter 5, "Confidentiality," electronic data downloaded to discs or remote storage devices, or printed on paper, require the same secure storage as conventional counseling records. Lax procedures by practitioners who work from home computers that are either shared by family members or located in common living areas of the house can breach confidentiality, even if elegant encryption programs are in place. With wireless Internet access becoming more commonplace, Internet counseling could be conducted from almost anywhere via laptop computers, which are particularly vulnerable to security breaches resulting from human error or theft (Zur & Barnett, 2008). Practitioners intent on providing Internet counseling can refer to Fisher and Fried (2003) for an excellent summary of how to protect confidential counseling information online.

Intervening in a Crisis

In Chapter 5, we detailed counselors' responsibilities in instances of clients posing danger to themselves or others. Those same responsibilities apply in Internet counseling. However, the geographic distance that may be insignificant for an Internet connection between a counselor in one locale and a client in another can become, in turn, a formidable barrier to intervening effectively in a crisis if advance arrangements have not been made. This is another reason, in addition to authenticating a client's identity, for knowing where clients live.

Even if potential clients do not see the reason or need, certain basic information about the client's locale is needed in order to activate a crisis intervention plan in the heat of the moment. At a *minimum,* this includes telephone numbers for the local police department and a local hospital emergency department. Also helpful are telephone numbers for community crisis lines or hotlines where distraught individuals can call at any hour of the day or night, as well as telephone numbers for local support groups. Ideally, a practitioner providing Internet counseling to a client in a remote location would also have the name and telephone number of a nearby mental health or medical provider in order to link the client to a local resource should a crisis develop. Of course, lack of qualified local providers may be the very reason that the client is seeking Internet counseling in the first place, so this recommendation may be difficult to carry out in some instances.

Establishing Jurisdictional and Administrative Governance

Cyberspace is not a specific geographic location, so it is not immediately clear what entity has jurisdictional governance of Internet counseling activity. Does it take place in the state or jurisdiction where the counselor works and holds a license? Do the laws of the client's home state or jurisdiction apply? Is it a case of interstate, or international, commerce where federal regulations prevail? Given these unanswered questions, to whom can one complain if the counseling process goes awry, or if clients believe they have been harmed or mistreated? Koocher and

Keith-Spiegel (2008) offer a humble, straightforward admission regarding these vexing questions about Internet counseling: "We simply do not know the answers at this time" (p. 144). (See Chapter 13, "Moving or Closing a Practice," for a specific discussion of telephonic or electronic communication between counselors and clients following an out-of-state relocation by one of the parties.) However, Barnett and Scheetz (2003) believe unequivocally that a professional license is needed in the jurisdiction where the client resides.

Grief counselors legitimately interested in offering Internet counseling as part of their service line must address this jurisdictional dilemma. The most conservative approach would be restricting one's online practice only to clients who reside in the state(s) where the counselor is licensed. A cavalier approach would be interpreting the lack of regulatory guidelines as a carte blanche to offer Internet counseling to any willing, paying client from anywhere. Unfortunately, unlicensed individuals may exploit lack of regulations to pass themselves off as counselors to unsuspecting or naive clients, as evidenced by survey studies of Web sites that advertise Internet counseling (cf. Heinlen et al., 2003; Shaw & Shaw, 2006).

Koocher and Morray (2000) polled U.S. state attorneys general about regulations governing the practice of Internet counseling. At that time, only 3 of 42 responding jurisdictions had statutes in place that specifically addressed provision of psychotherapy by telephone, Internet, or other electronic means. However, almost half of the responding attorneys general claimed regulatory authority over mental health practitioners residing outside the state who offer Internet therapy to residents of that state. Thus, these states consider Internet counseling to be an instance of crossing state lines. Koocher and Morray urge practitioners who provide Internet counseling to consult in advance with their professional liability carrier to make sure that coverage is in force (cf. Heinlen et al., 2003). Given this variability in how Internet counseling is viewed in different jurisdictions, prudent grief counselors will contact attorneys general and state licensing boards in jurisdictions where clients reside to determine the status of the counselor's ability to offer Internet counseling and whether any special statutory or credentialing obligations exist.

A related administrative issue concerns charging third-party payers for Internet counseling. Conscientious grief counselors must make it clear to third-party payers if they are providing services via the Internet, rather than face-to-face, in order to avoid any fraudulent representation in charges. Medicare authorizes reimbursement for some telehealth services, including psychotherapy, rendered to individuals residing in geographic areas with provider shortages, but such coverage is by no means automatic or universal (Nickelson, 1998). Again, the best policy is clarifying in advance the client's eligibility for insurance coverage of Internet counseling.

ETHICAL STANDARDS AND GUIDELINES

Several provisions in the ADEC Code of Ethics address the ethical challenges presented by the prospect of Internet counseling. Most important, the professional standards embodied in the ADEC Code of Ethics are in force regardless of the modality used to deliver counseling services. Therefore, the same principles and aspirations that apply to face-to-face service delivery also apply to Internet counseling services.

> The Ethics Code applies across a variety of contexts, whether in person or by postal service, telephone, internet, and/or other electronic transmissions. (ADEC Code of Ethics, Introduction)

In addition, given the specific confidentiality concerns raised by the mechanics of Internet counseling, special emphasis is given to protecting clients' confidentiality when depending on the Internet or any other type of electronic medium.

> Members who offer services, products or information via electronic transmission inform their clients and students of the risks to privacy and the limits of confidentiality. (ADEC Code of Ethics, III. Responsibilities to Those Served, E)
>
> Members safeguard written and recorded information about clients and are alert to potential threats to confidentiality in duplications processes, in use of computer equipment, and in electronic mail and facsimile transmission. (ADEC Code of Ethics, VIII. Confidentiality and Privacy, F)

American Counseling Association

The Code of Ethics of the ACA (2005a) contains detailed provisions pertaining to technology applications in counseling. Because of the importance of these admonitions in addressing ethical challenges presented by Internet counseling, we list these provisions in their entirety in Table 9.1. The ACA provisions include general directives concerning use of computer technology and distance counseling services as well as specific directives regarding informed consent and the use of the World Wide Web in Internet counseling.

These exhaustive standards embodied in the 2005 ACA Code of Ethics were preceded by a series of guidelines provided in a 1999 document published by ACA titled *Ethical Standards for Internet Online Counseling.* Though no longer available, its provisions were incorporated in the 2005 revision of the ethics code that superseded it. However, the 1999 document was the basis for an impressive study by Shaw and Shaw (2006) that assessed compliance with these initial standards by 88 online counseling Web sites that were surveyed. The authors performed a total of 16 specific checks:

1. Is the full name of the counselor given?
2. Does the site clearly identify the state from which they are operating?
3. Are degrees listed?
4. Are areas of study and university given for degrees?
5. Is the address or the phone number of the counselor given for backup purposes?
6. When requesting client information, does the site require client's full name and address?
7. Does the site clearly state that clients must be 18 years or older or have consent of a legal guardian?
8. When requesting client information, does the site require client's age or birth date?
9. Does the site have an intake that clients must fill out before counseling can begin?
10. Does the site have a statement stating that online counseling is not the same as face-to-face counseling?
11. Does the site have a statement stating that not all problems are appropriate for online counseling?
12. Does the site refer clients to traditional forms of counseling, or provide other suggestions (crisis lines, etc.) for clients who are not deemed appropriate for online counseling?
13. Does the site have a statement indicating that ensuring complete confidentiality over the Internet is not possible?

Table 9.1

AMERICAN COUNSELING ASSOCIATION (2005A) CODE OF ETHICS, SECTION A—THE COUNSELING RELATIONSHIP, A.12. TECHNOLOGY APPLICATIONS

A.12.a. Benefits and Limitations

Counselors inform clients of the benefits and limitations of using information technology applications in the counseling process and in business/billing procedures. Such technologies include but are not limited to computer hardware and software, telephones, the World Wide Web, the Internet, online assessment instruments, and other communication devices.

A.12.b. Technology-Assisted Services

When providing technology-assisted distance counseling services, counselors determine that clients are intellectually, emotionally, and physically capable of using the application and that the application is appropriate for the needs of clients.

A.12.c. Inappropriate Services

When technology-assisted distance counseling services are deemed inappropriate by the counselor or client, counselors consider delivering services face to face.

A.12.d. Access

Counselors provide reasonable access to computer applications when providing technology-assisted distance counseling services.

A.12.e. Laws and Statutes

Counselors ensure that the use of technology does not violate the laws of any local, state, national or international entity and observe all relevant statutes.

A.12.f. Assistance

Counselors seek business, legal, and technical assistance when using technology applications, particularly when the use of such applications crosses state or national boundaries.

A.12.g. Technology and Informed Consent

As part of the process of establishing informed consent, counselors do the following:

1. Address issues related to the difficulty of maintaining the confidentiality of electronically transmitted communications.
2. Inform clients of all colleagues, supervisors, and employees, such as Informational Technology (IT) administrators, who might have authorized or unauthorized access to electronic transmissions.
3. Urge clients to be aware of all authorized or unauthorized users including family members and fellow employees who have access to any technology clients may use in the counseling process.

(continued)

Table 9.1

AMERICAN COUNSELING ASSOCIATION (2005A) CODE OF ETHICS, SECTION A—THE COUNSELING RELATIONSHIP, A.12. TECHNOLOGY APPLICATIONS *(continued)*

4. Inform clients of pertinent legal rights and limitations governing the practice of a profession over state lines or international boundaries.
5. Use encrypted Web sites and e-mail communications to help ensure confidentiality when possible.
6. When the use of encryption is not possible, counselors notify clients of this fact and limit electronic transmissions to general communications that are not client specific.
7. Inform clients if and how long archival storage of transaction records are maintained.
8. Discuss the possibility of technology failure and alternate methods of service delivery.
9. Inform clients of emergency procedure, such as calling 911 or a local crisis hotline, when the counselor is not available.
10. Discuss time zone differences, local customs, and cultural or language differences that might impact service delivery.
11. Inform clients when technology-assisted distance counseling services are not covered by insurance.

A.12.h. Sites on the World Wide Web

Counselors maintaining sites on the World Wide Web (the Internet) do the following:

1. Regularly check that electronic links are working and professionally appropriate.
2. Establish ways clients can contact the counselor in case of technology failure.
3. Provide electronic links to relevant state licensure and professional certification boards to protect consumer rights and facilitate addressing ethical concerns.
4. Establish a method for verifying client identity.
5. Obtain the written consent of the legal guardian or other authorized legal representative prior to rendering services in the event the client is a minor child, an adult who is legally incompetent, or an adult incapable of giving informed consent.
6. Strive to provide a site that is accessible to persons with disabilities.
7. Strive to provide translation capabilities for clients who have a different primary language while also addressing the imperfect nature of such translations.
8. Assist clients in determining the validity and reliability of information found on the World Wide Web and other technology applications.

14. Is e-mail secure via an SSL or via encryption software?
15. Does the site have a statement about conditions under which confidentiality must be breached for legal reasons?
16. Does the site have a waiver that clients must electronically sign or mail in before beginning counseling that specifically states the limits of ensuring confidentiality over the Internet?

Shaw and Shaw (2006) found that counselors who identified themselves as licensed or affiliated with a professional association and who clearly identified the state in which they were practicing had significantly higher compliance ratings on these indices. Fewer than half of the Web sites surveyed included even 8 of the 16 required items. Only two sites met all criteria! The authors noted soberly that informed consent procedures and disclosure of limits on confidentiality were woefully lacking in almost two-thirds of the Web sites surveyed. This is unacceptable professionally and ethically. In the case of Web sites offering Internet counseling, as in all other aspects of ethical practice, it is clear that "a lack of awareness or a misunderstanding of an ethical standard is not itself a defense to a charge of unethical conduct" (ADEC Code of Ethics, Introduction), a standard mirrored by the ACA Code of Ethics (2005a).

Part of the problem identified by Shaw and Shaw (2006) was the fact that there are many unlicensed, unaffiliated individuals holding themselves out as counselors and not conforming to professional and ethical standards. Also disturbing was the fly-by-night nature of many Web sites offering counseling. Within a 2-month period, fully 20% of the Web sites surveyed had disappeared, were for sale, or were no longer offering Internet counseling. Clearly, the adage *caveat emptor*, Latin for "let the buyer beware," applies to Internet counseling. Withdrawing unilaterally or disappearing altogether from a counseling relationship constitutes abandonment of clients and is clearly unethical (cf. ADEC Code of Ethics, GC-I., Responsibility to Those Served, J).

National Board for Certified Counselors

Another professional society that has published specific guidelines governing the practice of Internet counseling is the National Board for Certified Counselors (NBCC). NBCC has provided standards for Internet counseling since 1997, and the most current revision of its document, *The Practice of Internet Counseling*, contains 14 key provisions (NBCC,

2007). These NBCC guidelines are summarized in Table 9.2. (Readers should consult the original document to view the standards in their entirety.)

Similar to Shaw and Shaw (2006), Heinlen et al. (2003) surveyed 136 Web sites to assess compliance with NBCC standards for ethical practice of Internet counseling. The criteria were based on an earlier version of the NBCC standards; nonetheless, the results were disappointing. No

Table 9.2

SUMMARY OF NATIONAL BOARD FOR CERTIFIED COUNSELORS (2007) STANDARDS FOR THE PRACTICE OF INTERNET COUNSELING

1. Address imposter concerns by verifying identity and using code words or numbers.
2. Obtain parental/guardian consent for minors and verify identity of consenting person.
3. Explain procedures for contacting the counselor when the counselor is offline and indicate how often e-mail messages will be checked by the counselor.
4. Discuss and make provision for technology failure.
5. Explain how to deal with potential misunderstanding in absence of visual cues.
6. Identify resources local to the client for crisis or emergency situations.
7. Make client aware of free-access Internet resources for information or guidance.
8. Make Web sites barrier-free to clients with disabilities.
9. Remain aware of language, time zone, cultural, and local factors impacting clients.
10. Use encryption methods whenever possible and inform potential clients of those methods. When encryption is not used, warn clients of the hazards of unsecured transmission on the Internet.
11. Inform clients whether session data is stored and for how long.
12. Follow appropriate procedures for release of confidential counseling information to other electronic sources.
13. Review pertinent legal and ethical codes regarding the practice of Internet counseling, both in the counselor's home jurisdiction and in that of the client.
14. Provide links to Web sites of all entities by which the counselor is licensed or certified.

Adapted from *The Practice of Internet Counseling,* © 2007 National Board of Certified Counselors, Inc.™ & Affiliates; 3 Terrace Way, Greensboro, NC 27403-3660. Reprinted with permission.

Web site met all the measured criteria, although licensed counselors showed a significantly higher level of compliance. Heinlen et al. found five major shortcomings in Web sites surveyed. First, providers showed inattention to safety matters such as seeking permission from parents or guardians before counseling minors, ensuring emergency backup, and making provision for when the counselor is offline. Second, there was inadequate explanation of the limits of confidentiality. Third, Internet counselors were more concerned with protecting credit card information used to pay for services than protecting personal information disclosed in counseling. Fourth, Web-based counselors were unreliable providers—37% of the surveyed sites were no longer operating 8 months later (cf. Shaw & Shaw, 2006). Fifth, unqualified endorsement by Web sites of the efficacy of Internet counseling exceeded scientific evidence of its merits.

International Society for Mental Health Online

ISMHO (2000) has endorsed principles for the online provision of mental health service. Their guidelines cover three basic areas: informed consent, standard operating procedure, and emergencies.

Under the umbrella of informed consent, ISMHO (2000) recommends that clients be fully informed about the process of Internet counseling, including the limitations of text-based modalities, expected turnaround time for the counselor's response, and the counselor's right to privacy. ISMHO insists that clients should know the name and qualifications of their counselor as well as contact information for relevant institutions that can verify their counselor's credentials. Clients should be informed of the advantages and disadvantages of Internet counseling. Risks to confidentiality as well as safeguards in place to enhance confidentiality (e.g., encryption) should be disclosed. Alternatives to Internet counseling should be described, including acknowledgment that there are many information sources on the Internet that may be helpful for coping with grief, such as the Web site maintained by the Dougy Center for grieving children and families (www.dougy.org).

ISMHO (2000) encourages counselors to follow the same operating procedures with clients when practicing Internet counseling as when providing face-to-face counseling. Such procedures include the following: practicing within one's areas of competence; obtaining appropriate training; determining with clients the frequency, cost, and modality of sessions; evaluating clients' needs; ensuring confidentiality; and maintaining accurate records. Also, following discipline-specific and domain-specific ethical guidelines is important.

Finally, ISMHO (2000) directs Internet counselors to discuss with clients what procedures to follow in the event of an emergency, recognizing that the counselor might not immediately receive an online communication of distress. This may involve identifying a local backup who could be contacted by the client, if necessary, or by the counselor if there is reason to believe the client presents a danger to self or others.

SUMMARY

Because Internet counseling is a new and emerging practice option for grief counseling, providers bear an additional burden of mastering the techniques of online communication needed for Internet counseling—demonstrating competence, meeting the specific ethical challenges posed by authenticating the identity of the parties involved, ensuring that the informed consent process is adequate, securing confidentiality, intervening in a crisis, and establishing jurisdictional and administrative governance. Many of these challenges are a function of the Internet as a unique place of service delivery, the third dimension of the Five P Model.

Fortunately, the detailed guidelines provided by the ACA (2005a), the NBCC (2007), and the ISMHO (2000) give clear directions to professionals contemplating Internet counseling. Also, Barnett and Scheetz (2003) provide practitioners with detailed recommendations for ethical practice of Internet counseling. By acquiring the specific knowledge needed and addressing adequately the ethical issues raised, grief counselors can offer Internet counseling as an option to clients who have a legitimate reason for choosing this treatment modality.

10 Ethical Controversies in Grief Counseling

Ever since publication of George Engel's (1961) paper asking the question "Is grief a disease?" debate has ensued between those who view the grief process through a medical or psychopathological lens and those who view grieving as a natural human function. Derivatives of this debate appear in current controversies about whether grief counseling is necessary at all, whether it is effective when applied, and how to formally diagnose grief-related problems that are the reason for consultation. These controversies have become more heated in recent years with the publication of several studies questioning the efficacy of grief counseling interventions. In an era of evidence-based practices where there is a push to provide empirical substantiation for claims of treatment efficacy, many hard-working grief counselors are scratching their heads over how to *prove* what seems obvious—clients report getting better and genuinely appreciate help received.

Controversies about the efficacy of grief counseling raise important ethical questions. Who should be treated with grief counseling after a significant loss? How do grief counselors know for sure that the services they provide are effective? How do grief counselors avoid inflicting harm while intending to accomplish good when counseling the dying and the bereaved? How does one diagnose a bereavement-related condition that is the reason for seeking grief counseling? Is it ethical to charge a professional fee for services if efficacy is undocumented or doubtful? This chapter is intended to guide practitioners toward ethical practice of grief counseling in the face of these scientific and administrative controversies.

DO GRIEVERS NEED COUNSELING?

In the past two decades, several scholars have challenged some time-honored assumptions in the field of grief counseling. Wortman and Silver (1989, 2001) questioned whether grievers need to display socially expected symptoms of sadness and mourning. Often, a dearth of such signs is thought to indicate delayed or absent grief, ostensibly because grievers' inevitable negative affect has been suppressed. In short, an assumption of "grieve now or grieve later" has been prevalent in the field. In part, this assumption was based on earlier scholarly work (Parkes & Weiss, 1983; Raphael, 1983) that appeared quite influential on professionals' attitudes, as documented by survey data (Middleton, Moylan, Raphael, Burnett, & Martinek, 1993) and promulgated by popular counseling textbooks (Rando, 1993; Worden, 2009). Wortman and Silver argued that not everyone shows intense grief distress, and there are some grievers who show few signs of sadness. Therefore, if a normal variation in bereavement patterns is minimal distress, where is the need for grief counseling? After all, Stroebe, Hansson, Stroebe, and Schut (2001) assert that the majority of bereaved people have no pathological indicators and do not usually require the help of professional counselors or therapists.

George Bonanno and colleagues (Bonanno, 2004; Bonanno et al., 2002; Bonanno, Wortman, & Nesse, 2004) introduced the concept of resilience to explain how many grievers weather the loss of an important loved one. Drawing on data from a large prospective study of aging adults, investigators had the advantage of both preloss and postloss measures (at 6 and 18 months afterward) of participants' functioning on a variety of psychometric indices. They found 46% of participants reported low levels of depression before and after the deaths of their spouses, as well as relatively few grief symptoms during bereavement. They classified this pattern as *resilience.* Resilient participants were not unmoved by their loss; instead, their emotional perturbations were transient and did not interfere with their ability to function in other life areas, including the capacity for positive affect. Significantly, resilient grievers reported that positive memories of their deceased spouse were comforting, a finding that contradicted any suggestion that they were not strongly attached to their partner.

On the other hand, only 4% of bereaved participants showed a delayed grief pattern—that is, low preloss depression, no change at 6 months, and a grief reaction at 18 months (Bonanno et al., 2002; Bonanno et al., 2004). However, 16% of participants with low preloss depression levels developed *chronic grief* reactions characterized by higher postloss depression and grief symptoms at both measurement periods. In this group, the distress was due primarily to the cognitive and emotional upheaval surrounding the loss of a spouse. Bonanno et al. (2002) also found that 11% of their sample displayed higher postloss distress at 6 months yet returned to baseline levels of lower distress at 18 months, a pattern they called *common grief.* Additionally, 8% of the sample displayed *chronic depression* before and after their loss, together with markedly higher grief symptoms. This group's distress was more likely due to enduring emotional difficulties exacerbated by spousal loss. When those displaying the delayed grief pattern are combined with the chronic grief, common grief, and chronic depression groups, *distressed individuals account for 39% of Bonanno's sample.* We believe experienced counselors will recognize readily these four distress groups as representative of individuals who may seek grief counseling after their loved one's death. The very fact that they are nonresilient in their adaptation following loss is a strong indicator that professional help may be warranted.

IS GRIEF COUNSELING EFFECTIVE?

Although previously cited studies seem to challenge whether most grievers even need professional assistance to cope, the results of several meta-analytic studies and literature reviews of bereavement interventions lead to questions about the effectiveness of grief counseling when it is applied. Allumbaugh and Hoyt's (1999) review found a moderately small but positive treatment effect for individuals receiving grief counseling compared with nontreatment controls, although the expertise of the practitioner and treatment modality made a difference (i.e., professionals were better than trainees or nonprofessionals, and individual counseling was better than group therapy). Quite telling was the fact that self-selected clients who actively sought treatment for bereavement showed a much more pronounced positive effect than study participants recruited merely on the basis of their bereaved status.

In an overview of psychological interventions for the bereaved, Kato and Mann (1999) examined treatment effects on somatic ailments as well as depression and other psychological symptoms from a smaller, more restricted set of bereavement intervention studies. They found a small positive treatment effect on self-report of physical symptoms but not on more objective measures of illnesses, such as doctor visits or medication use. With depression and other psychological symptoms, they found a positive treatment effect so small as to be considered negligible, a finding from which they concluded that psychological interventions for bereavement are just not effective.

Schut, Stroebe, van den Bout, and Terheggen (2001) surveyed studies of bereavement interventions to determine who really benefits from them. Intervention programs open to all bereaved people, such as support groups for widowed persons, yielded few enduring positive effects for participants. The results were only slightly better when participants were screened as being "at risk" for developing complications in grieving. Those individuals showed modest improvement at best, and sometimes that was only temporary. However, their findings from studies of participants who either sought help on their own or were referred for treatment are encouraging for providers of grief counseling. In these cases, treatment effects were still modest yet produced positive and lasting results. Clearly, these latter samples resemble more closely the cohort of grievers that most professional counselors encounter in practice.

Probably the most pessimistic view on the efficacy of grief counseling came from a review article by Neimeyer (2000) in which he reported unpublished dissertation data compiled by Barry Fortner. In the meta-analytic review, the treatment effect was positive but small, comparable to the negligible effect found by Kato and Mann (1999). More disturbing was the assertion, based on an inferential statistical method, "that nearly 38% of recipients of grief counseling theoretically would have fared better if assigned to the no-treatment condition" (Neimeyer, 2000, p. 545). He referred to this iatrogenic worsening of problems as "treatment-induced deterioration." Secondary analyses found normal grievers realized no measurable effect from grief interventions, whereas more distressed grievers showed a reliable positive effect similar in magnitude to that found by Allumbaugh and Hoyt (1999). Neimeyer (2000) concluded,

> Grief therapy is appropriately offered to mourners experiencing protracted, traumatic or complicated grief reactions. Conversely, existing evidence

> from scientifically credible controlled outcome trials suggests that grief therapy for normal bereavement is difficult to justify. (p. 546)

The controversy does not end there. Larson and Hoyt (2007) published a scathing critique of Neimeyer's (2000) assertions about treatment-induced deterioration and decried the number of other scholars who uncritically accepted his results and gave them undue credence by citing them. Larson and Hoyt demanded a published retraction on the basis that the inferential statistical method used to generate the claim of 38% of treated participants doing worse by virtue of receiving grief counseling was flawed, and therefore the results were spurious. They concluded there is no compelling evidence that bereaved clients are harmed by grief counseling or that grief counseling, as typically practiced, is less efficacious than other forms of counseling and psychotherapy.

In response, Neimeyer and colleagues (Currier, Neimeyer, & Berman, 2008) undertook an impressive, methodologically meticulous meta-analytic review of 61 controlled-outcome studies in order to provide the best scientific assessment currently possible of the effectiveness of psychotherapeutic intervention for bereaved persons. Each of the surveyed studies compared those receiving grief counseling to bereaved persons who did not receive any active type of intervention (e.g., wait-list control groups). Most of the interventions used a group modality (63%), although individual (25%) and family (12%) approaches were used as well. Overall, bereavement interventions showed a small positive effect, outperforming no-intervention control conditions immediately following treatment, even though no measurable benefit could be found at follow-up. On average, follow-up measures were taken at 36 weeks posttreatment, but there was wide variability ranging from 2 weeks to 72 weeks.

Most pertinent to the debate over the efficacy of grief counseling was Currier et al.'s (2008) results after studies were coded as to whether researchers' interventions were *universal* (i.e., intended for any bereaved person), *selective* (i.e., focused on bereaved individuals thought to be at higher risk of distress based on nuclear family relationship to the deceased or on grieving a violent death), or *indicated* (i.e., targeted for participants manifesting bereavement-related difficulties before intervention began). In Currier et al.'s coding scheme, which parallels the classification employed by Schut et al. (2001), the indicated group most closely approximates individuals typically seen in grief counseling practices. Outcomes of interventions with grievers showing poor bereavement adaptation *before* treatment—generally individuals who were either self-referred or referred by another health care professional—showed moderate positive effect sizes both at posttreatment and at follow-up. The authors attest that these results compare favorably with outcome studies of psychotherapies for other difficulties. Currier et al. concluded,

> The present comprehensive review documents the relevance of attending to the targeted population and reinforces the growing consensus that psychotherapeutic interventions for bereaved persons can be effective in instances when researchers and clinicians focus on persons who are genuinely in need of help. (p. 656)

Most impressive was Currier et al.'s (2008) finding that there were no signs of deterioration for the typical intervention recipient. Instead, all of the positive intervention effects resulted from greater reductions in distress in intervention recipients relative to those who went without formalized help. This suggests that the earlier warning sounded by Neimeyer (2000) about treatment-induced deterioration effects was premature. Based on the most current data, it is reasonable to conclude that grief counselors can make a positive difference in the lives of suffering grievers and that concerns about grief counseling making clients worse are unfounded.

LACK OF DIAGNOSTIC CATEGORY

While the scientific controversy over the efficacy of grief counseling continues to evolve, there are other administrative issues that pose a challenge to ethical and effective practice of grief counseling. In clinics, offices, and hospitals where professional counseling is rendered fee-for-service and where governmental or commercial insurers pay at least part of the bill, administrative difficulties can arise when bereaved clients seek grief counseling. The only grief-related diagnostic code in the latest edition of the *Diagnostic and Statistical Manual of Mental Disorders* (*DSM-IV-TR*; American Psychiatric Association, 2000) is a category designated "bereavement." Bereavement is not listed as an actual disorder, and therefore services addressing it are generally not reimbursed. The rationale for this was based on a good-faith attempt to preserve the notion that normal bereavement is not a psychiatric condition, although it may be a focus of clinical attention. Only when a griever's clinical course manifests more enduring interference in social or occupational functioning, defined as longer than 2 months from the time of death, does it constitute a disorder. Although a time interval of 2 months to make such a distinction may seem arbitrary, it is based, in part, on psychiatric lore originating with Lindemann's (1944) investigation of survivors of Boston's infamous Cocoanut Grove nightclub disaster, in which over 400 people perished in a flash fire. Lindemann found that most acute grieving among survivors ran its course over about a 6-week period thereafter.

So when distressed grievers seek professional consultation or are referred for grief counseling in mental health settings, the available (and reimbursed) diagnostic codes pertain primarily to depression, anxiety, adjustment, or other symptom-based disorders. This situation forces grief counselors to conceptualize cases and plan interventions based on alternate diagnoses. To paraphrase Engel (1961), if grief *is* a disease, it must be a hidden one, for nowhere it is found in contemporary diagnostic nosology.

This situation angers supporters on both sides of the debate about human grief. Practitioners viewing grief through the medical model are upset that troubled grievers are not recognized in the current diagnostic code and that legitimate grief counseling provided to such persons must be carried out under a disguised rubric. They believe designating grief as a distinct diagnosis would enfranchise those grievers who need help and may not be able to obtain it under the present classification system. But their efforts to have complicated grief included as a diagnostic category in the next edition of the *DSM* upset those in the thanatology community who seek to de-pathologize human grief. Opponents of an official diagnosis object to imposing a psychiatric label, with its stigmatizing connotation, on individuals already reeling from the pain of loss. They reason that if grief is a normal response to the loss of an important figure in a person's life, it is a violation of the griever's basic human dignity to call it a disorder that requires psychiatric treatment.

A major impetus in the movement for revision of the *DSM* comes from the work of Selby Jacobs and Holly Prigerson, who initially proposed a diagnostic category called *traumatic grief* (Jacobs, 1999; Jacobs, Mazure, & Prigerson, 2000; Jacobs & Prigerson, 2000; Prigerson & Jacobs, 2001). They argued that there is evidence for traumatic grief as a unified syndrome, with symptoms distinct from those of bereavement-related depression and anxiety, and that traumatic grief creates significant distress and debility in those who suffer it. They conceptualized the reaction to be a stress response syndrome similar to posttraumatic stress disorder (PTSD) but based on separation trauma. Together with Stanislav Kasl, they developed a scale to assess symptoms of the disorder, the Inventory of Traumatic Grief (ITG; Prigerson & Jacobs, 2001).

In a later review making the case for incorporating a grief-related disorder in *DSM-V* (Lichtenthal, Cruess, & Prigerson, 2004), the authors acknowledged first using the term *complicated grief* to describe their proposed diagnostic entity and then changing the designation to *traumatic grief* based largely on the contributions of a consensus panel of experts they convened. According to their explanation, they reverted to the term complicated grief after the terrorist attacks of September 11, 2001, to avoid confusion and to differentiate their concept more clearly from PTSD.

The initiative for development of a grief-related diagnostic category that is distinct from other mental disorders has involved a lengthy process of scholarly refinement (Lichtenthal, Cruess, & Prigerson, 2004). At times, the process has met with opposition (Hogan, Worden, & Schmidt, 2003–2004, 2005–2006). However, when Prigerson and Maciejewski (2005–2006) presented a subsequent iteration of criteria for a proposed complicated grief diagnosis, they focused mainly on separation distress and de-emphasized the traumatizing aspects of the griever's distress. Also, to qualify as a disorder, they proposed that symptom disturbance must persist for at least 6 months, in contradistinction to normal grieving that is thought to be self-limiting. Experienced practitioners recognize that imposition of hard and fast time limits following a loss before a griever could qualify for mental health services is a potential problem, given the individual differences observed in bereavement trajectories. From our perspective, the muddy waters engulfing a diagnostic category for grief were not clarified when Prigerson and colleagues again renamed the proposed diagnosis *prolonged grief disorder* (Boelen & Prigerson, 2007; Goldsmith, Morrison, Vanderwerker, & Prigerson, 2008).

At present, the movement continues for including in *DSM-V* a diagnosis befitting troubled grievers who need professional grief counseling. Unfortunately, as in most human endeavors decided by committee, the scholarly research that informs this process is considered in concert with medical, economic, and political agendas. Therefore, the final decision may reflect all four influences, not just the scientific one. In our view, the construct of *complicated bereavement* is one that most readily fits contemporary practice paradigms in grief counseling (cf. Rando, 1993; Worden, 2009). We know many practitioners would welcome the introduction of complicated grief as a diagnostic category in order to simplify dilemmas about diagnosis and reimbursement and to empower them to legitimately care for those in need because of grief-related distress (Horowitz, 2005–2006).

CHARGES TO GRIEF COUNSELORS

In light of these ethical controversies in grief counseling, we have compiled a series of seven charges or mandates for practitioners who are committed to ethical practice of grief counseling. Reprising a principal theme of this book, ethical practice means more than the omission of ethical errors or lapses. Grief counselors have an ethical obligation to screen clients appropriately, provide sound counseling interventions, and evaluate the results of their professional work in an ongoing effort to tailor services to the specific individual, family, or group receiving them. In doing so, the chances of inadvertently harming a client through professional misjudgment or misapplication of technique are minimized.

These procedural rules of thumb are intended to serve as a broad practice guide when counseling the dying or the bereaved. They can help conscientious grief counselors remain alert to some of the potential problems posed by scientific challenges to the necessity for and efficacy of grief counseling, as well as by administrative challenges regarding diagnosis and reimbursement. These mandates are not a substitute for professional training or credentials. They do not preclude a thorough working familiarity with both discipline-specific codes of ethics and ADEC's domain-specific code of ethics. And they are not a shortcut obviating the requisite death competence discussed in Chapter 3.

Heeding these seven charges can enhance the likelihood that grief counseling is rendered only when necessary and executed in a manner that promises to be most effective. Our mandates include screening clients carefully, employing risk-factor algorithms, monitoring potential growth factors, assessing quality of attachments, using proven methods, exercising caution in group work, and educating the public. Grief counselors are advised to measure their practice patterns against these general guidelines as part of a systematic review designed to enhance the efficacy of their counseling services and ensure that the highest ethical standards are maintained at all times.

Screen Clients Carefully

The findings of Allumbaugh and Hoyt (1999), Schut et al. (2001), Currier et al. (2008), and even Neimeyer (2000) show that mourners seeking help for self-identified bereavement-related distress or those referred by another professional, such as a physician, were most likely to profit from grief counseling. This contrasts with those recruited for grief counseling programs simply because they were bereaved. Zisook and Lyons (1988–1989) devised a very basic screening question that effectively discriminated individuals with unresolved grief from individuals managing to fare on their own. They asked, "Are you having trouble dealing with the death?" Those who answered affirmatively also reported more difficulty coming to terms with the death of their loved one. Thus, a simple yes or no answer may go a long way toward narrowing the field of those who may need grief counseling.

Data from the Scott and White Grief Study (Gamino, Sewell, & Easterling, 1998) replicated the clinical utility of Zisook and Lyon's screening question. In our study, we found that grievers who endorsed having trouble dealing with the death consistently scored higher on psychometric measures of grief distress. This self-identification of problems with grieving is exactly what meta-analytic reviews (Allumbaugh & Hoyt, 1999; Currier et al. 2008; Neimeyer, 2000; Schut et al., 2001) promote as a subjective indicator of who is most likely to benefit from counseling.

When screening clients as potential candidates for grief counseling, we suggest starting with the Zisook and Lyons' (1988–1989) question, "Are you having trouble dealing with the death?" For those who answer affirmatively, we propose a follow-up probe: "Are you interested in seeing a grief counselor to help with that?" Those who acknowledge grief distress but who may be disinclined to seek counseling as the solution, such as those with avoidant (Bonanno, 1999) or instrumental (Martin & Doka, 1999; Martin & Wang, 2006) coping styles, will less likely accept referral or return for a subsequent visit. Also, individuals who experience their grief primarily through somatic symptoms or who lack psychological-mindedness regarding their emotional makeup (cf. Bauer & Kobos, 1987) may answer negatively to both of these screening questions. From an objective standpoint, these individuals may seem like they could benefit from grief counseling, but they are not yet amenable to taking that step. Persons who answer both questions affirmatively (i.e., those who identify their own grief distress and are motivated for professional help) are clear candidates for grief counseling. Referencing the findings of Bonanno et al. (2002), individuals who answer both screening questions affirmatively may well be among the 39% who display distress over their bereavement (e.g., chronic, common, or delayed grief, or chronic depression).

Employ Risk-Factor Algorithms

Most readers will have at least some familiarity with the risk-factor profile used by physicians when evaluating an individual's potential vulnerability to heart disease. This includes factors that may be controlled or influenced by health habits and medical treatment, such as diet, exercise, smoking, and blood pressure, as well as factors that cannot be controlled, such as age, male gender, and family history. This approach enables the clinician to gauge the relative risk for heart disease facing a particular individual by considering the entire panel of known risk factors. Assessment of an individual's degree of risk for complicated or problematic grief can be conducted in a similar manner. Parkes (1990) recommended using bereavement risk factors for two reasons: to identify people likely to have difficulties so as to focus grief counselors' care where it is most needed and to provide clues as to the causes of good and bad outcomes after loss.

There are several risk-factor models available in the bereavement literature. In Rando's (1993) landmark text on complicated mourning, she identified seven high-risk factors associated with poorer outcomes. These include *death circumstances,* such as sudden, unexpected, or traumatic death, death following an overly lengthy illness, death of a child, and preventable death. They also include *mourner characteristics,* such as presence of a problematic relationship (defined as conflicted, ambivalent, or overly dependent) between mourner and decedent; a history of unaccommodated losses, stress, or mental health problems; and a perceived lack of social support. Worden (2009) uses the term *mediator variables* to compile a comparable risk-factor profile: relationship (i.e., both kinship and functional) between mourner and decedent, nature of the attachment, mode of death, mourner's mental health history, personality and coping style, social support, and concurrent stresses. Jordan and Neimeyer (2007) incorporate factors with greater emphasis on evaluating the mourner's narrative understanding of the death experience and its aftermath.

Although the applicability of these risk factor algorithms will vary according to one's practice setting and theoretical frame of reference, an algorithm helps ensure not only thorough assessment of a client but also recognition of the level of complication a given client may encounter when coping with loss. This is particularly germane to our discussion of the efficacy of grief counseling because, like Currier et al. (2008), Schut et al.'s (2001) comprehensive review of intervention studies concluded that "the more complicated the grief process appears to be or to become, the better the chances of intervention leading to positive results" (p. 731).

A final word is needed about employing risk-factor algorithms to assess complications. Although one sometimes hears the terms *high-risk griever* or *complicated bereavement,* we conceptualize complicated grief as a continuous rather than a categorical variable. It is not a simple matter of a high-risk versus low-risk griever or of complicated versus noncomplicated bereavement. Instead, the greater number of risk factors operating in a given loss situation increases multiplicatively the challenges facing a client who is dying or bereaved, particularly as many of these factors interplay with one another (Gamino et al., 1998). Again, the most distressed grievers are the ones most likely to benefit from grief counseling.

Monitor Potential Growth Factors

At the same time that one assesses risk factors for complications in grieving, monitoring for indications of personal transformation or growth following bereavement is important too. For many, loss brings not only grief but also gain. Jordan and Neimeyer (2003) urge consideration of *salutogenic outcomes* of bereavement as landmarks of clients' progress, instead of relying exclusively on desired changes in pathogenic outcomes as treatment goals. In other words, helping a client find meaning in and unanticipated benefit from a loss experience are valid aims in grief counseling, just as achieving relief or diminution of a client's suffering are legitimate objectives. In fact, research has shown an inverse relationship between self-report of personal growth following bereavement and subjective grief misery (Gamino et al., 2000; Hogan, Greenfield, & Schmidt, 2001). Thus, personal growth may be an antidote to the anguish of grief and loss.

Understanding that personal transformation and growth can be a pathway to adaptation following a major loss or trauma (Hogan & Schmidt,

2002), the astute grief counselor will listen for descriptions conveying such positive outcomes or themes suggesting that possibility. Findings from the scholarly literature in thanatology (Frantz, Farrell, & Trolley, 2001; Gamino, Hogan, & Sewell, 2002; Gamino & Sewell, 2004; Gamino et al., 2000; Nadeau, 1998) and traumatology (Calhoun & Tedeschi, 2001, 2006; Tedeschi & Calhoun, 1995) converge regarding the types of positive outcomes discovered. Generally, these fall into three categories: changes in self, changes in relationships, and changes in life philosophy. Changes in self may include developing greater compassion for others or realizing one's latent personal strengths and capacities. Changes in relationships may include drawing closer to loved ones or coming to value connections with people over acquisition of material possessions. Changes in life philosophy may include greater existential awareness of the preciousness and brevity of life or resolving to live more authentically in the moment (e.g., smelling the roses along the way).

Davis, Wohl, and Verberg (2007) studied 52 adults, all of whom had lost a loved one in a tragic mine explosion. These investigators were in the unique position to study different bereavement trajectories of grievers whose losses all stemmed from the same event. The nature of the mine explosion carried with it circumstantial risk factors—sudden, unexpected, violent death that was widely considered preventable, yet no party was ever held accountable. A cluster analysis found participants congregated into three principal subgroups: rebuilt self, minimal threat/minimal growth, and no meaning/no growth. The *rebuilt self* group showed definite signs of posttraumatic growth. Even though the loss struck to the core of their lives and their beliefs, they were able to make some sense of their loss, gain inner strength, learn something about themselves, and take heart from the fact that laws and regulations had changed for the better as a result of their tragedy. By contrast, individuals in the other two groups did not necessarily search for meaning (i.e., minimal threat/minimal growth), thought the deaths were senseless and shattered their beliefs in a just world (i.e., no meaning/no growth), and concluded that nothing good had come of the tragedy. Posttraumatic growth was not evident in these latter groups.

Additional data on the role of growth factors in bereavement recovery comes from Phase 3 of the Scott & White Grief Study (Gamino et al., 2008). The likelihood that bereft participants involved themselves in grief counseling was a function of both distress (i.e., pathogenic) and growth (i.e., salutogenic) indicators. Individuals characterized by higher levels of grief distress, as well as those demonstrating higher personal growth, utilized grief counseling much more frequently than grievers who appeared less impacted emotionally by the loss of their loved one (cf. Bonanno et al., 2002). Ostensibly, high-distress grievers self-select into counseling primarily to find relief, whereas high-growth grievers matriculate into counseling both to find ways to cope and to find ways to grow from their bereavement experience. This suggests that grief counseling is potentially efficacious not only as a treatment to salve the suffering and anguish of highly distressed grievers but also as a vehicle to facilitate salutary personal growth and transformation following loss.

Assess Quality of Attachments

One of the exciting, cutting-edge developments in thanatology is a renewed interest in the role attachment plays in complicated grief. Bowlby's (1969, 1980, 1988) pioneering work postulated that attachment behavior in humans persists throughout the life cycle and is strongly influenced by developmental experiences. According to Bowlby, responsive and consistent caregiving early in life helps a young child form secure attachments, which are the basis of healthy adult relationships. Lack of dependability or disruptions in the caregiver–child relationship breed insecure attachment. Children are thought to develop internal working models of the self and of attachment figures that function as basic schemas for viewing the world and that guide formation and maintenance of future relationships. Additionally, attachment style has enormous implications for how a bereaved person grieves.

Subsequent empirical research delineated four fundamental styles of attachment (Ainsworth, Blehar, Waters, & Wall, 1978; Main & Hesse, 1990). Although the majority of individuals are capable of forming secure attachments, a sizeable minority displays some variation of insecure attachment: anxious/ambivalent, dismissive/avoidant, or disorganized/disoriented. These insecure attachment styles put grievers at risk for complicated bereavement reactions when the problematic attachment figure dies. Anxious attachments, evident in clingy or overly dependent relationships, can lead to prolonged or chronic grief, whereas an avoidant attachment style is thought to correlate with delayed or inhibited grief when the loved one dies (Parkes, 2001; Stroebe, 2002). A disorganized attachment style may be related to unresolved grief in the sense that these individuals have limited capacity to negotiate changes or disruptions in relationships with any coherency of thought or action (Shaver & Tancredy, 2001). Even though theoretically consistent, some researchers have questioned these inferential relationships between attachment style and grief reactions (Bonanno et al., 2002; Fraley & Bonanno, 2004).

For the grief counselor seeking to assess the quality of a client's attachments, a thorough developmental and social history is crucial. This begins with a comprehensive review of the individual's relationships with primary caregivers and nurturers from childhood and adolescence. How secure did the client feel with these formative relationships? Was there abandonment, disruption, neglect, abuse, trauma, or any other untoward occurrences contributing to insecure attachment? In the adult years, the quality of the client's attachments to partners, siblings, close friends, relatives, and coworkers is instructive. How well has the client achieved intimacy (Erikson, 1963) in these relationships? Finally, the grief counselor endeavors to understand the nature of the client's attachment to the deceased person. A history of insecure attachments, especially when replicated in the mourner–decedent relationship, may be a harbinger of problems in grieving that could become the focus of grief counseling.

Another reason for grief counselors to assess the quality of a client's attachments is to clarify whether to promote or encourage bereaved clients to maintain continuing bonds (Klass, Silverman, & Nickman, 1996; Klass & Walter, 2001) with the deceased loved one. Evidence now suggests that this may be constructive for individuals with secure attachment styles who enjoyed a generally positive relationship with the decedent (cf. Bonanno et al., 2004). Many benefits, such as retaining access to comforting memories, talking with the deceased, or using the deceased as a sort of moral guide, can accrue from such a postdeath, metaphysical affiliation. Generally, prototypically secure individuals can experience and express their grief in the context of continuing bonds without feeling overwhelmed (Shaver & Tancredy, 2001).

Conversely, those with insecure attachment styles associated with complicated grieving may not be helped, and may even be harmed, by fostering continuing bonds with the decedent. Seeking continuing bonds under conditions of insecure attachment—relationships characterized by extreme dependency, unpredictability, or love–hate dynamics—could be detrimental during bereavement because of lingering preoccupation, dependence, ruminative grieving, or problems moving on with life (Stroebe, Schut, & Stroebe, 2005). In part, this is why Rando (1993) and Worden (2009) emphasize quality of attachment to the deceased when considering risk factors for complicated grieving. Understanding clients' attachment histories, as well as the nature of their specific bonds with the decedent, can provide valuable clues about how to proceed in grief counseling in a manner most likely to help and least likely to hurt.

Use Proven Methods

Once we have identified clients who are having trouble dealing with the deaths of their loved ones, who pose the highest risk for complications in mourning, or who evidence insecure attachment patterns, the search turns to which intervention methods are most demonstrably effective when counseling them. This question is reminiscent of the decades-old psychotherapy quandary—*when* to use *which* treatment for *what* problem experienced by *this* particular client seen by *which* counselor? In addition to the trusted triad of empathic listening, normalizing, and psycho-education, ethically conscientious grief counselors rely on sound empirical findings of best practices when crafting counseling interventions. Although a comprehensive review of grief counseling methods is beyond the scope of this text, we mention briefly here some illustrative examples of both the best-researched therapies and some tried-and-true techniques that have passed the test of time.

A randomized controlled trial by Shear, Frank, Houck, and Reynolds (2005) compared the effectiveness of interpersonal therapy designed for treatment of depression-spectrum disorders (Weissman, Markowitz, & Klerman, 2000) with complicated grief treatment customized to address bereavement. Their complicated grief treatment was based on Stroebe and Schut's (1999) dual process model of coping with bereavement and was designed to focus on both loss-oriented problems (i.e., grief work) and restoration-oriented processes (i.e., going on with life). For grief work, they used techniques such as having clients retell the story of the death, actively confront their distress, and connect with the deceased through memory triggers and simulated conversations. For restoration work, clients defined personal life goals and were encouraged to consider what they would like for themselves if their grief were not so intense. Although both treatment groups improved, participants in the complicated grief treatment fared better by logging a higher rate of improvement, scoring significantly lower on measures of depression and grief distress, and reporting better work and social adjustment. Although preliminary in nature, the work of Shear et al. points to the benefit of applying well-grounded methods in grief counseling.

A recent study by Boelen, de Keijser, van den Hout, and van den Bout (2007) compared simple supportive counseling with cognitive-behavioral therapy for complicated grief, based on the work of Aaron Beck (Beck, Rush, Shaw, & Emery, 1979). The cognitive-behavioral therapy featured *exposure* strategies that forced participants to confront loss reminders as well as *cognitive restructuring* approaches that challenged negative thought patterns. The cognitive-behavioral therapy produced more improvement in grief symptoms and general psychopathology than did simple supportive counseling. Like Shear et al. (2005), these results suggest that treatment interventions tailored specifically for individuals with complicated grief have a higher probability of success.

Two popular time-honored techniques in grief counseling are journaling and letter writing. Journaling is prescribed as a way for clients to have a ready outlet for documenting their thoughts, feelings, and reactions about their loss (cf. Neimeyer et al., 2008; White & Epston, 1990). Sometimes, these writings are read or referred to in counseling sessions, but more often they form a private record in which clients endeavor to assign meaning and coherence to their bereavement experience (cf. Jordan & Neimeyer, 2007). Research has shown that having people write regularly about emotional upheavals can improve their physical and psychological health, especially when "working through" is evident in changed perspectives (Neimeyer et al., 2008; Pennebaker, 1997; Pennebaker, Zech, & Rime, 2001; Smyth & Pennebaker, 2008). In this case, empirical research has substantiated the efficacy of what has been a common counseling technique.

Writing a letter to the decedent is a variation on journaling. Obviously, the letter cannot be delivered in a physical sense. However, like journaling, the process of self-expression in writing the letter may itself be salutary. Typically, this technique is employed when clients have unfinished business with their deceased loved one, such as things left unsaid or incomplete leave-taking (Worden, 2009). The letter serves as a vehicle for communicating symbolically with the deceased. The effect can be heightened by having the client read the letter aloud in a counseling session, read it at the cemetery, or share it with a confidante.

Grief counselors trained in experiential methods have amplified these forms of communication with the decedent through the Gestalt empty-chair technique (Jordan & Neimeyer, 2007; Klass & Walter, 2001; Worden, 2009). In a simulation exercise, the griever is instructed to talk directly to the deceased using the present tense, just as if the decedent were occupying the empty chair. There is an option for the client to take the seat, and role, of the deceased and talk back to the client as the decedent might. Both the empty chair and psychodrama-style conversations (Dayton, 1994) can be particularly helpful when there has been unresolved conflict. However, we join Jordan and Neimeyer in cautioning that such methods are best reserved for those with the clinical experience and training necessary to capably handle the intense affect that can be generated.

We recall a particularly dramatic case where, after months of intense work with a bereaved mother grieving the death of her youngest son in an ambiguous truck–pedestrian collision, the empty-chair technique allowed the client to "converse" with her deceased son about how his death happened and whether it was an accident or suicide (as asserted by the truck driver). When assuming the role of the son, the client was able to articulate that the son misjudged traffic as he tried to cross the highway on foot at night, that he did not intend to die, and that he was sorry for hurting her so much by his fatal mistake. Of course, these attributions came from within the client herself, based on a mother's knowledge of her own child. Nonetheless, "hearing" this explanation brought enormous relief to her restless spirit and enabled her to assimilate his loss in a new way.

We intend the above examples to illustrate that there are both research-based and time-tested techniques in grief counseling that should form the bulk of a grief counselor's armamentarium. Using proven methods helps ensure effective counseling work and sound ethical practice. All the while, we advocate retaining the freedom to explore and creatively devise new approaches in grief counseling, which remains a blend of science and art.

A timely example of a new approach that may become a classic is Byock's (2004) concept of "the four things that matter most" for individuals and their loved ones facing developmental tasks at the end of life. From his experience in emergency medicine and palliative care, Byock advocates "Please forgive me," "I forgive you," "Thank you," and "I love you" as part of saying goodbye. These four basic phrases help people reach completion in their relationships in a manner that can afford much healing and eliminate or minimize regrets later. Although no single technique is a panacea, Byock's prescription for dying well has the potential for becoming a standard intervention when counseling those who are terminally ill and their loved ones.

Exercise Caution in Group Work

A great deal of grief counseling takes place in groups, especially in hospital-based or hospice bereavement programs, funeral home aftercare programs, and places of worship. There are many varieties of bereavement groups: professionally facilitated groups; peer support groups such as the Compassionate Friends for bereaved parents or Survivors of Suicide; volunteer-led bereavement groups; and groups formed primarily for educational or social purposes. Yalom and Leszcz (2005) summarize several therapeutic factors that operate in group therapy. Most applicable to grief counseling groups are instillation of hope, universality (e.g., finding out others share similar experiences and reactions), imparting information, altruism (among group members), group cohesiveness, catharsis, and existential factors such as recognizing that life can be unfair and unjust, or realizing there is no escape from some of life's pain or death itself. Clearly, much good can be accomplished in group counseling with the bereaved.

Several cautions are needed when a grief counselor contemplates using a group format. First, learning to counsel individual clients does not necessarily prepare one for grief counseling in a group. Different skills are required to facilitate a group effectively, and specialized training is needed. Second, sometimes administrative pressures prompt use of group formats. Staff reductions or limiting benefits to group therapies may thrust grief counselors into group leadership roles for which they are unprepared. Just because it is more economically efficient to counsel people in groups does not guarantee that counseling groups will be therapeutically efficacious. Third, sometimes mental health professionals accustomed to overseeing employees or supervising work groups believe erroneously that running a counseling group is a similar proposition. Having experience running departments, work teams, or office groups does not automatically endow one with the skills to run a grief counseling group. Fourth, depending exclusively on psycho-educational materials, workbooks, or religious tracts to structure a grief counseling group is an insufficient basis for handling the challenges that can arise in this work, such as display of intense emotions of anger, sadness, and guilt or transference-type reactions toward the facilitator. Fifth, one of the cardinal rules in therapy groups is a pledge of confidentiality on the part of every member in order to ensure safety in self-disclosure. In our own group work, we recite unfailingly a mantra from our own medical records department as the group's norm: "What you see here and what you hear here needs to stay here when you leave here." Sixth, simply assembling a group of individuals with similar losses and thinking that spontaneous caring and sharing will make the group process effective is naive. Although homogeneity indeed fosters universality and group cohesiveness, it does not ensure a constructive outcome without capable leadership.

Jordan and Neimeyer (2003) address problems related to membership composition in grief counseling groups. Because homogeneity is helpful, particularly in early stages of group formation, they caution that clients who do not identify with the other group members gravitate into an outsider position within the group and are less likely to have a positive experience. Fundamental demographic differences—such as gender differences, class or culture differences, marked differences in levels of distress, or striking differences in types of loss (e.g., suicide deaths versus natural deaths) or relationship to the decedent (e.g., mixing widows/widowers with bereaved parents)—can leave some members feeling marginalized or alienated. Jordan and Neimeyer suggest careful prescreening of clients, much as we have mandated, to minimize such detractions from a healthy group process.

At the extreme, there is always a risk of "casualties" from therapy groups. Early in the encounter group movement of the 1960s and 1970s, Yalom and Lieberman (1971) studied such group casualties and found 7%–10% of participants could have an enduring, significant, negative outcome to their participation in group. Even though the encounter groups they studied are not really representative of the way most bereavement groups are conducted, it is worth reviewing the reasons they found for casualties: attack or rejection by the leader or by the group; failure to attain unrealistic goals; group pressure to experience and express emotion (which may be off-putting to instrumental grievers; cf. Martin & Doka, 1999; Martin & Wang, 2006); and input overload or too much stimulation. An illustration of the latter occurred at a rather large support group for bereaved parents wherein, by the time introductory accounts of the causes of death of their children were complete, some attendees felt numbed and overwhelmed at the tragic sadness of so many anguished stories.

One suggestion by Yalom and Lieberman (1971) was to follow the example of a leader with a low-risk style who very explicitly asked members to make the choice of what they wanted to work on and how far to proceed in any particular meeting. Such nonjudgmental empowerment gives potentially vulnerable group members sufficient freedom to self-determine the extent of their participation and the depth of their self-disclosure.

A basic counseling axiom is that group treatments are not for everyone. Extrapolating from Yalom and Leszcz (2005), potentially vulnerable clients who are poor candidates for group intervention include those with low motivation, pronounced personality disorders, extreme mood disorders (especially mania), social phobia, active psychosis or paranoia, alcohol or drug addictions, brain impairments, or any other impediment that precludes the person from meaningful participation in the group task. These same individuals have the greatest chance of being identified, sociologically speaking, as outsiders or deviants and pushed to the periphery of the group process. Again, screening is the key to detection of these exclusion factors when considering formation of a grief counseling group.

Educate the Public

Controversy over the efficacy of grief counseling has found its way into the popular press. Begley's (2007) *Newsweek* article "Get Shrunk at Your Own Risk" carries the following subheading: "A study found that 4 in ten people who entered grief therapy after losing a loved one would have been better off without treatment" (p. 49), an uncited reference to Neimeyer's (2000) assertions about treatment-induced deterioration. Brody's (2004) article in the *New York Times* concluded, "Often, time beats therapy for treating grief," based on Bonanno et al. (2002) and Neimeyer (2000). These articles call into question the working assumption that a "talking cure" (i.e., grief counseling) helps. Instead, they deem newsworthy any research suggesting that grief counseling is not always helpful and may even be harmful for some bereaved persons. Hopefully, the results of Currier et al. (2008) will begin to assuage those fears, but media reports such as these show how hard it is to influence public opinion once an unfavorable view is promulgated.

The ethical obligation of grief counselors is to stay abreast of developments and scholarly literature in the field and to be willing to engage quizzical members of the public about the controversy. Accordingly, one must be cognizant of arguments on both sides of the issue and able to explain *when* and *for whom* grief counseling is most appropriate. In order to accomplish this, grief counselors have an obligation to teach each other and, ultimately, to share knowledge of dying, death, and bereavement with the general public. The ADEC Code of Ethics spells out this general obligation to educate the public.

> Based on quality research and theory, the Association provides information, support and resources to its multi-cultural, multidisciplinary membership and, through it, to the public. (ADEC Code of Ethics, Preface)

> The member works to promote greater understanding among lay persons and professionals of dying and death so that each member of society can achieve a more satisfying life and personal acceptance of death. (ADEC Code of Ethics, Basic Tenets, 9)

In parallel, some mental health professionals are called on repeatedly to answer the question, "What's the difference between a psychologist and a psychiatrist?" For grief counselors, the never-ending question may well be some variation of, "Does grief counseling really help, or not?" The preceding sections of this chapter are intended to provide a summary answer to this question. *Grief counseling practiced by competent professionals can help those individuals struggling to accommodate to their loss and is especially helpful for those who self-identify their need or whose personal history and circumstances make it even more difficult than usual to cope with their loss.*

A final caveat is in order about educating the public. When answering questions about the efficacy of grief counseling, one wears two hats simultaneously—the hat of educator and the hat of counselor. Giving a brief, well-reasoned, knowledgeable answer to such a question, delivered in a down-to-earth, understandable manner, discharges the professional obligation of educator. Should one's answer inspire confidence in the questioner, the exchange may also advertise the counselor's practice. If an inquiry is made about grief counseling, one can legitimately inform the inquirer whether one is accepting new clients and, alternately, about the presence of other competent grief counselors in the community. In these instances, educating becomes advertising even though that is not the original intent of the interaction, and there is no ethical breach involved.

In Chapter 7, "Multiple Relationships in Thanatology," we addressed how intentional advertising is sometimes camouflaged as educating. Unethical self-promotion occurs if the grief counselor's answer to a sincere question by a member of the public follows the theme, "Make an appointment to see me and I'll explain it to you." Nor is such a question grounds for an ill-advised exploration into the inquirer's personal circumstances of loss when such inquiry is clearly not welcomed or occurs in a noncontrolled setting where confidentiality and a professional relationship have not been established. One's ethical obligation as grief counselor is to educate the public without shameless or opportunistic self-promotion (see Chapter 11, "Potential Pitfalls of Public Service") and without launching impromptu counseling in a public venue.

SUMMARY

In closing, despite the ethical controversies surrounding grief counseling, there remains considerable optimism for the future of professional efforts to assist the dying and the bereaved. Following the mandates enumerated in this chapter can help grief counselors operate in a manner that conforms closely to established best practices in counseling and ensures that the services they provide are professionally defensible and ethically sound.

11 Potential Pitfalls of Public Service

- Pan Am 103, Lockerbie, Scotland—1988
- Murrah Federal Building, Oklahoma City—1995
- Columbine High School, Littleton, Colorado—1999
- World Trade Centers, New York City—2001
- Nightclub fire, Warwick, Rhode Island—2003
- Earthquake and tsunami, Indonesia and India—2004
- Hurricane Katrina, New Orleans, Louisiana—2005
- Shooting massacre, Virginia Tech University—2007

These familiar names and places bring to mind large-scale disasters and scenes of mass casualties caused by terrorists, weather, human error, negligence, or mechanical failures. Often, grief counselors and mental health workers are present in large numbers to help with the emotional aftermath of these major calamities. On a smaller scale, grief counselors may be called in their home communities following fires, car wrecks, murders, suicides, tornados, or floods to assist with the perceived mental health needs of bereft survivors. Although grief counselors may respond to such tragedies with a reflexive altruism, there are several ways that well-intended efforts to help can become ethical problems. The subject of this chapter is how to faithfully discharge a professional obligation to use one's expertise in thanatology for public service, including disaster work, support groups, educational roles, and media contacts, without compromising one's ethical principles in the process. *Any form of public service is, by definition, the practice of grief counseling and requires adherence to ethical principles and standards of conduct.*

LARGE-SCALE DISASTERS

Massive tragedies such as those listed at the beginning of this chapter send out shock waves in all directions. Those immediately affected by the events may be traumatized by their losses or injuries. Families may be frantic to find out if loved ones are safe or harmed, and they often seek expeditious reunion as their highest priority. First responders and emergency personnel may be profoundly affected by the horrendous sights, sounds, and smells of destruction and death. Community members and the general public, possibly a national or even global audience, remain riveted to news programs or the Internet, seeking information and visual reports. Media representatives swarm to cover the emerging saga, often with graphic images or wrenching human interest angles.

Grief counselors are not immune from sensationalism and morbid curiosity. We, too, watched video replays of the twin towers falling and the tidal waves of the tsunami crashing ashore. We, too, listened to the harrowing tales of peril and escape and the awful stories of those who lost everything except their very lives. The sense of dread and horror that seized other onlookers penetrated us as well. Our position as grief counselors prepares us to respond empathically to those in pain from trauma and loss, and our training as helpers may mobilize us to seek an active role in serving disaster survivors. However, freelance volunteering just showing up to provide supportive mental health care—is unlikely to result in making a meaningful contribution; rather, it may create additional confusion. Unless one understands what needs to be done after large-scale disasters and knows how to help during such catastrophes, one may do more harm than good. Noble intentions are not enough.

A few years ago, we attended a professional meeting that featured some speakers sharing their experiences following a major disaster in which they were asked to help, despite lacking any formal training or preparation. These counselors, who were accustomed to a predictable clinic practice, were thrust onto a disaster scene with the expectation of aiding victims suffering emotional trauma and grief. Most of the counselors' experience consisted of coming to grips with the fact that they were "not in Kansas anymore" and trying to grasp how to talk purposefully to people in those crisis conditions. Raphael (2007) described the uncertainties that arise for practitioners who are used to structured office settings when they arrive at the site of a disaster: "Response to such emergencies requires a whole new set of scientific understandings and interpersonal skills" (p. 330). Despite their honorable intentions, these practitioners displayed questionable professional judgment by attempting to provide counseling services in an emergency—a task for which they were utterly unprepared.

In the following discussion, we employ the Five P Model of ethical decision making to help grief counselors navigate the vagaries and chaos inherent in mass disasters. Applying the model with flexibility (e.g., considering the component dimensions in a different sequence) can enable grief counselors who volunteer during large-scale disasters to practice ethically and avoid potential pitfalls associated with such fieldwork.

Principles

We start with the ethical principles that inform the decision making of grief counselors involved in large-scale disasters. Beneficence, the wish to do something helpful, is the motivating force behind public service. An ennobling aspect of all the health professions, grief counseling included, is the ideal that one's specialized skill and training may be applied on an emergency basis when circumstances warrant it. Indeed, the ADEC Code of Ethics specifies this calling as a societal duty.

> Members provide their appropriate professional services in public emergencies. (ADEC Code of Ethics, VII. Responsibility to Society, D)

The complementary consideration to beneficence-based strivings is the principle of nonmaleficence—avoiding harm. If one does not know the difference between counseling actions that can help during large-scale disasters and interventions that could harm, the specific competencies needed for good counseling practice and sound ethical practice may be missing. When competing ethical values are involved in a dilemma, one makes a reasonable effort to reconcile the opposing arguments and ferret out the greater good. In this case, priority is assigned to the notion that grief counselors confine professional activities to those positions or assignments for which they are adequately trained (cf. ADEC Code of Ethics, II. Competence, B). Thus, the immediate impulse to volunteer for disaster fieldwork may be tempered by a simple question: "Do I really know how to help in an emergency?" Any affirmative response must be grounded in appropriate training and preparation, not a naive assumption that what works in the office will work in the field.

A third ethical principle particularly applicable to emergencies and large-scale disasters is autonomy. Victims and survivors are not clients in the conventional sense, yet they certainly retain all the prerogatives of self-determination. In fieldwork, obtaining informed consent does not involve a sheaf of papers on a clipboard that the individual is asked to sign. Rather, consent is established during a brief introductory encounter in which providers introduce themselves by name and describe their role in the disaster response efforts. They then ask for permission to talk with the survivor, always respecting that some may not need or want such contact (Rosser, 2008; Ruzek et al., 2007). As defined in Chapter 4, consent is reassessed continuously during the exchange between the counselor and the survivor and can be electively retracted at any point should the survivor decide to discontinue.

Place

Grief counselors responding to large-scale disasters leave their own turf and enter someone else's domain. Understanding the importance of place is paramount for sound ethical decision making during disasters. It is important to respect the sociocultural makeup of the locale in which the disaster occurs and work collaboratively to utilize the community's strengths. Mendenhall (2006) terms this *co-owning* relief-oriented initiatives and calls for members of mental health teams who come into a disaster area to help community members who are already there. Failing to exercise cultural sensitivity when entering a disaster area may result in being seen as intrusive or irrelevant. Intrusiveness not only violates ethical standards but also defeats one's counseling objectives.

Public safety officials are trained to operate from an incident command center when managing the aftermath of a large-scale disaster. When a mental health provider enters a disaster area, it is important to report to the command center's personnel deployment area, identify one's professional affiliation, provide credentials for working the disaster, and then coordinate fluidly with interdisciplinary trauma response teams already in action (Mendenhall, 2006). In short, someone other than the grief counselor is in charge at the venue, and it is wise to adhere to these existing chains of command (Ritchie, 2003).

Another place-related consideration is privacy. Rarely are there soundproof walls in a disaster area. Often, there may be only a tented area or a curtain providing a visual barrier. As a mental health professional, one's verbal exchange with a survivor or family member could easily happen in an open area, frequently with others nearby. Honoring the person's privacy under these circumstances can be very trying indeed, yet it remains the grief counselors' obligation to try. Temporarily, it may be possible to move away from busier areas in order to converse. Sometimes, modulating one's voice or limiting the amount of personal revelation by the survivor only to that needed to address the question at hand are the only variables the counselor can really control (Rosser, 2008). Some survivors may want family and loved ones present to participate in any exchange. Alternately, individuals may wish for a few moments alone with the grief counselor to express their fears and sorrows. Here, the counselor's clinical acumen and ability to read the situation is invaluable to ensure the maximum possible privacy when counseling disaster survivors.

Problem

The real problem in providing mental health assistance during large-scale disasters is knowing what to do, how to do it, and when to do it. It is beyond the scope of this chapter to present a detailed protocol of how to conduct grief counseling and trauma therapy following large-scale disasters. Instead, we outline some of the basic principles and methods used in emergency fieldwork. Grief counselors seeking to volunteer during public emergencies should note that there are several competing (and overlapping) models described in the literature on disaster response: crisis intervention or early psychological intervention (National Voluntary Organizations Active in Disaster, 2005; Young, 2001); critical incident stress management (Everly & Mitchell, 2003; Everly, Phillips, Kane, & Feldman, 2006; Mendenhall, 2006); evidence-based treatments (Marshall, Amsel, Neria, & Jung Suh, 2006; National Institute of Mental Health, 2002); and psychological first aid (Ritchie, 2003; Ruzek et al., 2007; Young, 2006).

Three powerful existential questions dominate the psychological landscape following mass catastrophe: Will I survive? Will my loved ones survive? Will I have a place to be? (Raphael, 2007). In response, Ruzek et al. (2007) identified five general principles to guide intervention practices with survivors in the immediate to short term after disasters: promoting a sense of safety, promoting calm, promoting a sense that affected persons and communities can help themselves, promoting connectedness, and instilling hope.

Psychological first aid is an umbrella term defining a set of core actions to perform in the early phases of disaster response (National Institute of Mental Health, 2002; Ritchie, 2003; Ruzek et al., 2007; Young, 2006). Because physical care is fundamental, grief counselors and mental health personnel must help ensure survivors' safety, security, and freedom from further harm. Providing food, clothing, and shelter comes next in the hierarchy of needs. Also, orienting survivors to what is known about the event, helping with communication, and reuniting families and loved ones are critical. Maintaining a supportive, comforting presence and listening empathically during these ministrations is a key aspect of psychological first aid (Ritchie).

Survivors who are emotionally overwhelmed may need calming and reassurance. Young's (2006) work features many practical tips for talking with survivors exposed to violent death and traumatic events in ways that comfort and calm. Sometimes an individual's acute distress level—for example, crying uncontrollably, hyperventilating, shaking, or trembling—interferes with their ability to comprehend the situation or respond to directives. If this occurs, mobilizing additional support for the individual or using arousal reduction methods, such as breathing exercises, may be needed (Ruzek et al., 2007).

Other important aspects of psychological first aid include providing information about recovery operations and ensuring that communication flows in a two-way manner between the survivors and rescue personnel. Also, educating survivors about available resources and teaching them how they can help themselves out of the crisis—including education about stress reactions and coping—is important. Some have described such outreach efforts as "therapy by walking around" in an attempt to reach those who have not requested service but yet may benefit from it (National Institute of Mental Health, 2002). All the while, the grief counselor is constantly reassessing needs and identifying high-risk individuals or subgroups that may need additional assistance in order to refer them for more intensive treatment.

Timing is an important aspect of providing psychological first aid. The height of the crisis is a time for supportive presence and reassurance, not psychological counseling. As stated by Ritchie (2003), "if the ambulances are still there, it is probably too early to be asking [individuals] how they are coping" (p. 45). As weeks and months progress after the disaster, follow-up interventions may increasingly resemble more traditional trauma or grief therapy for those who need it. However, applying the reframing techniques of cognitive behavior therapy too soon or too insistently imposing a strategy of retelling and revisiting can be counterproductive.

Ongoing controversy exists over the benefits and risks of group-debriefing methods for helping survivors and first responders after a large-scale disaster (Gamino, 2003; National Institute of Mental Health, 2002; Ruzek et al., 2007; Weisaeth, 2000). These methods derived from practices with emergency personnel such as firefighters and police officers exposed to situations involving gruesome death and destruction. Group formats designed for debriefing, cathartic ventilation, stress reduction, and psycho-education may be most appropriate for cohesive groups who have trained together prior to the event (Ritchie, 2003) or who were briefed beforehand about what to expect or what they might encounter (Weisaeth). Although there is no one-size-fits-all formula for group psychological intervention after large-scale disasters, potential applications of these methods are described in the literature (cf. Everly et al., 2006; Weisaeth). Clearly, these methods are not the solution for everyone. Appropriately trained, field savvy, and ethically conscious grief counselors apply group interventions judiciously in the aftermath of large-scale disasters.

Person(s)

Who are grief counselors and mental health professionals trying to help after a large-scale disaster? Who really needs assistance, and who may be naturally resilient? These questions attempt to identify the persons who are the designated recipients of the counseling interventions described in the previous section. Grief counselors who are experienced in disaster field work and trusted by the public safety personnel with whom they collaborate recognize that both victims and rescue workers themselves are potentially in need of mental health services. Of course, no matter who the person is, the grief counselor is ethically obligated to identify and respect the individual differences that make that person unique (see Chapter 2 on ethical decision making).

Marshall et al. (2006) summarized the arguments that large-scale disasters generate a surge in mental health needs among those affected, based on epidemiological data gathered after the World Trade Center attacks in 2001 that showed a high incidence of psychological disorders such as PTSD and depression in the weeks following (Galea et al., 2002; Silver, Holman, McIntosh, Poulin, & Gil-Rivas, 2002). Astute readers will note that even though the incidence rates may increase twofold or fourfold over typical base rates, the percent of affected persons reporting psychological disorders remains relatively low. However, considering densely populated areas such as greater New York City or taking into account a national population exposed via mass media, this could translate into hundreds of thousands of cases. Many mental health professionals embrace these findings because the data resonate with their intuitive convictions that psychopathology may be quite widespread following large-scale disasters.

Conversely, others argue that most psychological responses to trauma are immediate, mild, and transient and that the appropriate stance for mental health providers during disaster relief is to promote the expectation that most survivors will withstand the trauma involved and emerge intact (Raphael, 2007; Ritchie, 2003; Young, 2006). Embedded in the concepts and procedures of psychological first aid is a working assumption that providing such support will enable the majority of disaster victims to regain their emotional equilibrium within a relatively short period of time. Even the epidemiological studies cited in the previous paragraph indicate that most individuals exposed to a large-scale disaster will not demonstrate enduring psychological symptoms.

Thus, careful screening can help identify those individuals in need of follow-up care or more intensive treatment (Galea et al., 2002; Norris, Friedman, & Watson, 2002; Silver et al., 2002). Several scholars recommend use of risk-factor profiles to make screening less haphazard and more accurate in targeting potentially vulnerable disaster victims (National Institute of Mental Health, 2002; Raphael, 2007; Ritchie, 2003; Young, 2006). This strategy is similar to the one recommended in Chapter 10, on ethical controversies, for identifying those individuals most in need of grief counseling after the death of a loved one. Following is a list of some of the key risk factors associated with adverse mental health outcomes in the aftermath of large-scale disasters:

- Female gender
- Preexisting psychiatric problems
- Socioeconomic disadvantage
- Ethnic minority status
- Intentional mass violence (e.g., terrorist attacks) versus natural disasters (e.g., floods) or technological disasters (e.g., plane crashes resulting from mechanical failure)

- Bereavement as a result of the disaster
- Physical injury as a result of the disaster
- Greater severity of trauma exposure (e.g., more intense, longer duration)
- Exhibiting extreme distress stemming from disaster
- Loss of home/property and displacement/relocation
- Deterioration in social support network, including separation from family members
- Disengagement from coping efforts (e.g., giving up, denial, distraction)

Additionally, Young (2006) lists other warning signs, such as sleep disturbance or spiritual/existential despair, that indicate an individual may warrant psychological intervention following large-scale disaster. Rosser (2008) incorporated many of these risk factors when devising unobtrusive screening questions to assess survivors' mental health needs. For example, the question, "When did you get out [of the disaster area]?" elicits narrative information about exposure level, injuries, losses, displacement, and other clues.

When it comes to identifying rescue workers who may need counseling after a major disaster, there are other factors to consider. Psychological follow-up may be needed when units experience direct exposure to danger with a high rate of mortality, or when difficult rescue operations go wrong and there is a perception of individual or team failure (Weisaeth, 2000). Supervisor or peer referral often will target those individuals having trouble coping or those resorting to maladaptive modes of stress reduction, such as aggression or misuse of alcohol or drugs. Then there are the "super helpers" who insist on working long hours or become over-involved in the helper role to the exclusion of practicing good self-care. They, too, may need professional intervention (Mendenhall, 2006; Raphael, 2007). Ethical dilemmas can arise when boundaries shift from a horizontal relationship as fellow team members to a more vertical relationship as provider–recipient when one counsels a fellow rescue worker. The cautions discussed in Chapter 7 on multiple relationships should be heeded in these situations.

Process

It should be abundantly clear to the reader at this point that predisaster anticipation and training is perhaps the most important process undertaken to ensure ethical practice during disaster relief work. Grief counselors motivated to fulfill a societal obligation to assist in public emergencies need appropriate training or experience in disaster response, psychological first aid, and mental health field work. Compassion in the moment is not enough. Specific professional competencies are required.

Conventional graduate curricula in counseling and mental health services do not routinely include training in disaster relief. Typically, specialized postgraduate continuing education is necessary in order to gain the specific skills for working a large-scale disaster. So how does one obtain such training to become competent in emergency mental health care? Actually, there are many possible avenues.

Mental health providers such as grief counselors generally move into disaster areas as part of an integrated emergency response team (Ritchie, 2003), such as the Medical Reserve Corps (MRC) sponsored by the Office of the U.S. Surgeon General (MRC, 2008). Or volunteers may be part of an authorized relief or aid organization, such as the American Red Cross (ARC), the National Organization of Victims Assistance (NOVA), or the International Critical Incident Stress Foundation. Many of these nongovernmental organizations sponsor education and training in emergency mental health services and maintain databases of appropriately trained professionals available to respond to large-scale disasters. In addition, many local, state, and national professional associations have developed disaster response networks consisting of a subset of their members who undergo disaster response training. This training often occurs in collaboration with Community Emergency Response Teams (CERT) in partnership with the Federal Emergency Management Agency (FEMA), or in conjunction with the ARC Disaster Services Human Resource Network. Those association members who complete the training protocol may be called upon during public emergencies and, because of their geographic proximity, may play a pivotal role in providing counseling services in the immediate aftermath of a disaster.

Some highly experienced grief counselors have been overheard grumbling that ARC or CERT training is too elementary for their expertise level and implying that they have more than enough skills to work a disaster without it. Although it is probably true that advanced practitioners will find instruction in psychological first aid something easily mastered, the training modules of nongovernmental organizations also provide an overview of disaster management needed for coordinating emergency workers from many sectors and promoting effective team collaboration.

Grief counselors must be willing to participate flexibly in disaster relief, even performing roles outside the spectrum of strictly mental health interventions (Mendenhall, 2006; Raphael, 2007). We believe the saying "By their fruits, you will know them" applies here. If willing grief counselors undergo the prescribed training and join an established team or network—thereby earning the respect of that peer group—their special talents in thanatology will be recognized and used accordingly.

Besides issues of training and competency, another crucial process variable is motivation. Ethically conscious grief counselors drawn to disaster work should ask themselves, "Why am I doing this?" (Rosser, 2008). The honest answer should be about helping and not about inflating the counselor's ego. Beresford (2003) raised some soul-searching questions about why so many grief counselors and mental health professionals converge at large-scale disaster sites such as Columbine. Unfortunately, this phenomenon contributes to a perception among some members of the public that grief counselors are intrusive and self-seeking rather than altruistic and self-sacrificing. A telling question to put to oneself is this: "Would I be just as satisfied playing a behind-the-scenes role, perhaps providing follow-up care, even though it is outside the limelight of the emergency's front lines?" An affirmative answer indicates the grief counselor's heart is probably in the right place. Practically speaking, not every grief counselor is in a position, professionally or personally, to deploy as part of a disaster response team. For those who are able to do so, appropriate training and a selfless attitude are essential.

Finally, self-care for the grief counselor doing disaster relief work is critical. Disaster work is uniquely demanding and requires careful attention on the part of the grief counselor to take care of self (Mendenhall, 2006; Osofsky, 2008) in order to avoid the compassion fatigue so common in trauma work (Figley, 1995). Strategies for counselors' self-care are addressed elsewhere in this text (see Chapter 3, "Death Competence").

SUPPORT GROUPS

Turning to public service opportunities less dramatic and more common than large-scale disasters, we now consider support groups. Generally, grief counselors become involved in support groups in one of two ways: ongoing leader or guest consultant. Each of these roles carries with it potential ethical challenges.

By their nature, support groups consist of individuals linked by a common denominator (e.g. bereavement or chronic illness) who gather for the purpose of helping each other through caring and sharing. Support groups afford participants many benefits similar to those accrued during group psychotherapy: instilling hope; finding out that one is not alone in having the problem; imparting information about the disease, treatments, remedies, or strategies; learning from others' successes and failures; experiencing the group's cohesive bond; and venting of emotion (cf. Yalom & Leszcz, 2005).

In the United States, there are many support groups for bereaved persons. Some are based on cause of death (e.g., groups for those whose loved ones died of cancer or Survivors of Suicide). Some are founded on the relationship to the deceased (e.g., sibling groups or groups for bereaved parents such as the Compassionate Friends or Bereaved Parents of the U.S.A.). Some groups are program based (e.g., those whose loved ones died while on a particular agency's hospice service). Some are location-based (e.g., groups for those whose loved ones died in a specific hospital or for bereft members of a church congregation). Support groups are either open or closed. Open groups accept anyone interested in being there, for as many sessions as they care to attend. Closed groups restrict attendance to designated individuals and may meet only for a time-limited duration (e.g., six sessions in 6 weeks). Most support groups are careful to disavow providing therapy or professional counseling.

Ongoing Leader

There are different reasons that a grief counselor might assume an ongoing commitment to lead or facilitate a support group. Sometimes, the reason is altruism—fulfilling a professional obligation to provide some form of public service pro bono, that is, for the common welfare and without charge. However, mixed motives can enter the picture. For a grief counselor just beginning practice in a new community, leading a support group may be part of an effort to become better known and more visible. Or the grief counselor's employer, such as an agency, hospital, or funeral home, may want the counselor to conduct a support group as a form of advertising the institution's services or stimulating referrals to the grief counselor. In these instances, the protocol of informed consent requires that the grief counselor make clear to participants that their attendance is elective and in no way linked to any professional service for which a charge is levied (see Chapter 4, "Consent").

Comments or observations made by the grief counselor during the support group must not include suggestions or recommendations that the person needs to come for formal grief counseling. This can be construed as direct solicitation that potentially preys on the relative vulnerability of the support group member, who may be unduly swayed by the counselor's social influence or prestige (Koocher & Keith-Spiegel, 2008). Should participants spontaneously inquire about the counselor's availability for follow-up care, the grief counselor is certainly free to see those individuals for counseling. However, professional integrity and personal graciousness demand that the counselor clarify that trolling for business is not the reason for leading the support group.

Generally, a professional practitioner's primary role in leading a support group is to stimulate, and sometimes guide, the interactions among the members so that spontaneous helping processes, such as those identified by Yalom and Leszcz (2005), occur. Providing psycho-education about grief and normalizing the participants' subjective experiences are also important (cf. Worden, 2009). Although these roles certainly overlap with therapeutic processes in formal grief counseling, the crucial difference is the lens through which the grief counselor views the participants and the process. Support groups are people with a common experience (not clients with problems) gathered for the purpose of helping each other (not seeking the expertise of the counselor/facilitator). The counselor's position, procedurally and ethically, is in the background, not the foreground. As one esteemed colleague said, "in support groups, those who have lived the experience are the 'experts,' not us."

Is it ever ethical for a grief counselor's active client to attend concurrently a grief support group facilitated by that counselor? Although we know of instances where this has been done, such an arrangement poses several dilemmas inherent in multiple relationships (see Chapter 7) and should be discouraged. Great care would have to be taken to preserve the client's confidentiality by not disclosing privileged information or even the person's status as a client. This means not drawing special attention to the client or steering attention away from the client but treating the client just like any other participant. This may prove quite challenging over the course of an ongoing support group. It would be preferable for one's client to attend a different support group, to attend the support group only after the grief counseling is concluded, or to see a different provider for grief counseling while attending the support group. These alternatives prevent possible boundary violations. Practitioners who deliberately promote both grief counseling and concurrent participation in a support group facilitated by the counselor may have a blind spot in regard to the possible risks associated with maintaining such dual roles (see Chapter 1). Clients who insist on exercising such an option may have unacknowledged transference issues with the counselor that need to be explored.

Guest Consultant

Frequently, a grief counselor may be invited to address a support group as a guest consultant because the group is interested in hearing from a professional about concerns or issues pertinent to their experiences. Consider the following example.

A local support group for patients with Alzheimer's disease and their families invites the grief counselor to attend one of their monthly meetings. Because several members consider themselves to be grieving the many losses attendant to Alzheimer's, they want the counselor to make a short presentation on the nature of grief and then hold a question-and-answer period to enable participants to gain some much-needed perspective on their particular situations. Such invitations constitute a commendable way for a grief counselor to perform public service. The endeavor can be very beneficial for members of the support group and augment the grief counselor's reputation as a consequence.

So where are the ethical landmines in such a scenario? One example is covert agendas embedded in such invitations. Informal leaders of a support group may feel that certain members are too emotionally distraught and really need professional intervention. Or perhaps a certain member is perceived as disruptive or polarizing, and there is an implicit wish for the guest consultant to upstage, quiet, or correct that individual. The best strategy for ferreting out the presence of any covert agendas is to ask beforehand, "Are there any specific issues the group is wrestling with that would be important for me to know?" or "What would you like each member to come away with from my presentation?" This allows the grief counselor to better understand the interpersonal terrain of the support group and clarify what is realistic to accomplish as a guest consultant. At no time should the grief counselor allow an appearance at a support group meeting to become an exercise in group therapy or counseling someone in public. Such boundary violations are not ethically defensible.

Just as group counseling can generate casualties (see Chapter 10 on ethical controversies), some individuals may have a negative response to support group meetings. We have known clients who attended a support group session too early in their grieving when feelings were too raw or their emotional equilibrium too tenuous. Hearing the stories of others' grief was overwhelming and left them only further devastated. Similarly, some grievers need to focus away from their grief onto restoration-oriented activities (Stroebe & Schut, 1999) rather than immerse themselves further in the vicissitudes of grief work. When the grief counselor is a guest consultant to a support group, constant vigilance for such potential casualties is necessary.

Should a support group member emotionally melt down or otherwise decompensate when a grief counselor is a guest consultant, the counselor has an ethical duty to participate in crisis management. Practically, this may mean mobilizing support from family or friends (e.g., taking the person home or companioning the person). In extreme situations, an individual may require transport to a hospital emergency department. Sometimes, the techniques of psychological first aid discussed earlier in this chapter may be employed. Even though the grief counselor is not responsible for the individual in the same sense as for a client who is suicidal, homicidal, or breaking down, there is a professional obligation to act purposefully to render or secure aid. Never should such unfortunate developments be exploited in order to secure a referral for grief counseling (i.e., ambulance chasing).

Another potential pitfall with serving as a guest consultant to a grief support group concerns self-disclosure by the counselor. As mentioned in Chapter 3, "Death Competence," some grief counselors enter the field as a result of their own losses. Also, some grief counselors are quite open about their bereaved status when working with clients. Psychotherapy outcome studies suggest that self-disclosure by the counselor during treatment should occur selectively and only in the interest of helping the client (Orlinsky, Rønnestad, & Willutzki, 2004), not for serving the emotional needs of the counselor (cf. Wogrin, 2007). Ethical propriety demands that the grief counselor have sufficient self-awareness to know the difference.

Some support groups—for example, those organized specifically for bereaved parents or suicide survivors—may recruit a grief counselor as a guest consultant precisely because it is known that the counselor has sustained a similar loss. This may be seen as giving the counselor more credibility by virtue of having been there. In those circumstances, self-disclosure by the grief counselor should be undertaken with caution and only done to promote the adaptation of those attending the support group meeting. The counselor does not want to present a personal story as a model for how grieving should go. Also, sharing personal material should be done only if the grief counselor has sufficiently integrated the loss such that it can be discussed with appropriate poise and objectivity. Otherwise, such disclosures may work in reverse, with the group members feeling sympathy for the consultant or, even worse, attempting to meet the emotional needs of the professional—a clear violation of the rule of abstinence enjoining grief counselors from seeking personal gratification at the client's expense (Simon & Williams, 1999; Wogrin, 2007).

EDUCATIONAL ROLES

Besides assisting with support groups, grief counselors frequently perform educational roles as another form of public service. This might mean addressing civic organizations, groups at places of worship, or other gatherings where people seek information about grieving. Also, it could consist of distributing printed materials, such as pamphlets and books, or maintaining a professionally oriented Web site as teaching tools. Any of these endeavors could pose ethical dilemmas similar to those that occur during involvement with support groups.

Lecturing

Consider the grief counselor who was recruited to give a presentation on grieving during a daylong community workshop for caregivers, sponsored by a local hospital. To illustrate the major points of the presentation, the grief counselor planned to use a few case examples drawn from years of counseling practice. During the introduction to the talk, the grief counselor happened to notice among the audience members a former client—one whose case material was to be cited during the talk! Quickly, the counselor scrapped that plan and substituted another example instead.

This vignette exemplifies some of the confidentiality issues surrounding educational presentations in public forums. Although the case material was to be described anonymously, and the circumstances altered to protect the client's privacy (see the introduction in Chapter 1 and Chapter 5), it would have been highly insensitive on the part of the grief counselor to describe the client's case with that very client in attendance. Most clients do not want to recognize themselves or have others recognize them in case examples given during lectures, seminars, or educational presentations delivered by their grief counselor. Going public to serve the common good is admirable; going public with case material is risky without careful safeguards. This caution is particularly applicable to grief counselors who are college or university professors using case examples in class, grief counselors who are ministers using practice examples in their preaching and teaching, or grief counselors who work in rural communities or smaller towns and cities where individuals are more likely to be acquainted with one another.

As with support group work, grief counselors performing educational roles as public service walk a fine line when it comes to promoting their practice in the process. On one hand, discreet and dignified forms of advertising that accurately portray the provider's credentials and skills are legitimate self-promotion. This may include having one's professional degrees or office location announced during an introduction, making business cards available for interested parties, or even answering questions about the nature and scope of one's practice. On the other hand, unethical self-promotion includes false statements or in-your-face advertising that is pressured or makes unsupportable claims. For instance, tailoring one's talk to drum up business by describing risk factors for complicated grief as "ways you know you need grief counseling" would be a transparent and manipulative ploy. True public service is founded on the ethical principle of beneficence. Exploitation of any kind violates the rule of abstinence and erodes any possibility of establishing fidelity in the professional–consumer relationship.

Educational Materials

Some grief counselors produce educational materials as an adjunctive feature of their practices. Handouts, pamphlets, workbooks, texts, and other printed material or electronic products such as CDs or DVDs may be made available to clients in the course of counseling and do not represent a conflict of interest as long as an exorbitant fee is not associated with them and the clients have a choice about whether to purchase them. It is advisable that such materials be geared to a general reading level and include some disclaimer explaining that there is no single pathway in grief, thereby leaving room for individual differences.

It is a marketing truism that a compelling speaker in the mental health field will create a demand for books or other educational materials authored by that speaker. So, is giving an educational talk a pure form of public service, or is it merely a slick way to sell books and CDs? In our experience, it is rarely either motivation alone. Making books and educational materials available for sale following a public presentation is a legitimate business practice, and the convenience of it will be appreciated by many patrons, as long as such sales are at the discretion of the attendee. Ethically questionable procedures would be actions such as pushing book sales as an implied requirement to gain entry to a free lecture, or teasing an audience by posing difficult questions and problems during one's presentation and then indicating that the answers or solutions are in educational materials for purchase in the lobby. These underhanded variations of the bait-and-switch routine have no place in the ethical practice of grief counseling.

Printed or electronic materials have the advantage of extending the practitioner's ability to help not only clients but also the general public. Many who might not otherwise have access to professional consultation can benefit from reading self-help material or listening to or viewing recorded presentations of an educational nature. From an ethical perspective, a key difference between lectures given in person and educational materials used directly by consumers is that lectures afford at least the possibility for clarifying any misinterpretation or misunderstanding. This is not possible with educational materials. For example, it may not be clear whether the author's assertions and suggestions are based on accumulated counseling experience or on valid scientific studies. Therefore, any printed or electronic educational materials need to be of the highest quality and based on a solid foundation of professional study and scholarship, not pet theories or personal biases.

Web Sites

Many grief counselors now maintain professional sites on the World Wide Web as an adjunct to their practice. These Web sites have multiple purposes: listing the counselor's credentials and work experience; answering frequently asked questions (FAQs) about grief counseling; directing users to educational sources about grief, including the author's own books and materials; or providing office information such as location and hours of service (see Chapter 9 on Internet ethics). Some sites include options for blogging about thanatology-related matters, with the grief counselor commenting on current events or responding to users' observations or questions.

The same cautions enumerated for support group work and other educational roles apply to Web site authorship and maintenance. A Web site is an extension of the grief counselor's professional persona and should accurately and tastefully represent the grief counselor. In particular, blogging is a way to disseminate thanatology-related concepts that readers can expect to have a credible scientific basis, just as would one's comments in a live counseling interaction. Blogging should not be used by the grief counselor as an outlet for ventilating his or her own emotions or promulgating biases, untested assumptions, political opinions, or idiosyncratic worldviews. Justifying this kind of soapbox blogging as simply an exercise in free speech overlooks the professional context in which the exchange takes place and ignores one's obligations as a grief counselor to practice ethically in any public service endeavor.

MEDIA INTERVIEWS AND APPEARANCES

Multiplying media outlets have spawned numerous opportunities for grief counselors and mental health professionals to provide public service through the media. Possibilities include writing newspaper columns or magazine articles, giving interviews to print reporters or radio and television journalists, and taking call-in questions or talking with guests during live broadcasts. Notoriety and fame accruing from media interviews and appearances are seductive siren songs that many grief counselors are hard put to resist. Nonetheless, potential ethical problems exist when working with media, and prudent practitioners need to proceed very carefully when venturing into the world of media.

Koocher and Keith-Spiegel (2008) describe how mental health practitioners have varying degrees of control over what information taken from media interviews and appearances is ultimately published or broadcast. For example, writing one's own column for a newspaper or magazine affords a relatively high degree of control, but something less than final approval over what the public will read. With print media, editors and publishers maintain final authority over what is actually printed. Alterations and deletions based on space constraints or editorial judgment routinely occur, even up to the last minute. Much less control is retained by the professional when giving interviews to journalists or radio and television producers. Because mass media strives not only to inform but also to entertain and sell advertising, market variables may determine the context in which interview information or quotes are used. Legion are professionals who have come away from the experience feeling that they were misquoted or that their statements were taken out of context in order to serve the journalist's purposes rather than the professional's intention.

Fortunately, Koocher and Keith-Spiegel (2008) also offer some helpful tips for how grief counselors and mental health professionals can participate constructively with the media, and still protect their integrity, by maximizing the chances that the contents of their interviews will reach the public ear in a version intended by the professional. Knowing the journalist and the purpose of the anticipated story can go a long way toward helping the professional craft answers that are less likely to be misused or distorted. To that end, it is advantageous to provide interviewing journalists with a brief written synopsis, no more than one or two pages, of major points the professional is trying to make. Later, the journalist can quote directly from these written remarks. Grief counselors should avoid making comments or offering opinions on topics about which they have insufficient knowledge or experience. Although it may be tempting to address a headline-making topic with front-page promise, it is better to decline if the subject matter is beyond the expertise of the grief counselor. It is wise to refrain from making any statements that imply psychological analysis of newsworthy individuals, such as political figures, entertainment stars, or celebrities. Finally, many journalists are adept at plying the egos of professional interviewees by first socializing with them in order to create a more relaxed atmosphere. This kind of chummy association can lead the unsuspecting professional to make inadvertent or offhand comments not intended to be quoted but considered fair game by the journalist. To avoid this problem, prevention is the best medicine.

Consider the following case example. A newspaper reporter wants to do a feature story on holiday grief. Knowing the counselor's reputation in the community as a bereavement expert, the reporter asks for an interview on the topic. To make the story more realistic, the reporter suggests a hypothetical case of a family grieving a recent loss in order to elicit therapeutic recommendations the counselor might make in such a situation. Not sure in what direction the hypothetical case is heading or whether it may represent an actual person or family, the grief counselor declines to engage in the role-playing exercise. However, the counselor provides the reporter with general recommendations for those mourning their losses more acutely during holiday time and includes a one-page handout of key points abstracted from reliable sources. A helpful public service is performed, and potential ethical compromises are avoided by the more conservative interview strategy.

Even less predictable are live broadcast interviews on radio or television. The HFA's annual teleconference on death-related topics is a classic example. These broadcasts require counselors to rapidly formulate responses and think on their feet. Not every grief counselor has the quick reflexes and ready verbal skills needed to articulate adeptly, under time pressure, for an anonymous broadcast audience. A certain degree of showmanship is required as well. Although previewing anticipated questions and rehearsing can reduce uncertainty, they do not eliminate it. Furthermore, some broadcast interviewers cherish spontaneity and like to lead their guests into unexpected territory in order to elicit fresh, unrehearsed comments. This arena of public service is definitely not for the faint of heart.

A significant ethical challenge lurking in live broadcast interviews is the fact that when grief counselors shoot from the hip, there is always a risk that their answers may not be completely thought through. Live broadcasts are fertile ground for omissions, misstatements, ill-advised improvising, glossing over spotty memory in the rush to provide an immediate answer, or delivering comeback lines that may be humorous and witty but that lack a sound scientific foundation. A major difference between a conventional office practice with returning clients and a live broadcast interview is that the latter is totally unforgiving of mistakes. There are no second chances to clarify, correct, or retract something stated in error. One cannot "unring the bell." Therefore, familiarizing oneself ahead of time with the material to be discussed and collaborating beforehand with the interviewer to chart a course for the program can minimize the likelihood of ethical problems.

The ultimate high-wire act of media appearances is live radio broadcasts taking listeners' questions or live television programs with on-air guests as "clients." Such live formats were romanticized in popular culture by the former NBC comedy series *Frasier*, featuring an urbane psychiatrist dispensing advice on a call-in radio show. Because only a select few are able to make their living from such a glamorous position, most grief counselors who get such opportunities for live radio or television appearances do it as a public service. For example, a colleague received an invitation to join a local talk radio host on a program addressing the mental health needs of soldiers returning from war and their families. The counselor agreed to participate with no compensation.

During the call-in segment of the program, the grief counselor first fielded polite questions about PTSD, treatment alternatives, and service-connected benefits for injured soldiers. Then things turned ugly. Some callers began haranguing the U.S. Department of Veterans Affairs for shoddy treatment, while others assailed the country's war policy. Before long, the program was bogged down amid a firestorm of angry protests by argumentative callers with whom the host sparred in kind. The grief counselor's rosy vision of providing free advice to a grateful public was never realized.

This nightmarish episode illustrates how live broadcasts with interactive formats can pose ethical dilemmas. Without restraint, the grief counselor easily could have become embroiled in an on-air debate about political views, the morality of war, or the competence of the U.S. Department of Veterans Affairs, where many of the grief counselor's colleagues worked! Any such discussions are clearly beyond the purview of the grief counselor's professional expertise and therefore to be avoided. The alacrity and intensity with which the on-air brushfire flared could have led to an ill-fated attempt by the counselor to respond to callers as if they were disgruntled clients. Employing individual or group therapy techniques during a radio program that is clearly *not* therapy would be patronizing and inappropriate professional conduct. The counselor in this example learned a hard lesson about the risks associated with live broadcast interviews.

Live broadcasts pose other potential ethical dilemmas for the counselor. Programs vary in the extent to which they seek to entertain rather than to educate the public. Shows emphasizing entertainment, where live guests describing personal problems may be ambushed, misled, or humiliated to titillate the audience, have been dubbed "the modern coliseum" by Koocher and Keith-Spiegel (2008). The best policy is to avoid such venues where professional decorum is lost, and the principle of nonmaleficence is violated. The example of the radio call-in program about soldiers' mental health needs illustrates what can happen when an entertainment agenda supersedes a helping agenda.

On more serious programs where live guests seek advice, a respectful attitude is advised. The guests are not clients in the formal sense, and any advice offered is best prefaced by a disclaimer (e.g., "If I were counseling someone on a matter like this, we'd probably be discussing the following factors. . . ."). Approaching the conversation as an educational exercise rather than a formal counseling session will more likely keep the grief counselor on solid footing. A cautious strategy minimizes any risk of professional liability as a result of extending too far in making definite assessments or prescribing specific solutions for individuals who may construe the situation as an actual therapy session. It is incumbent upon the grief counselor to promote the public welfare while making it clear to producers, hosts, and guests that the on-air discussion is *not* formal counseling.

The Code of Ethics of the ACA (2005a) addresses a practitioner's responsibilities to avoid implying a professional counseling relationship when making media presentations.

> When counselors provide advice or comment by means of public lectures, demonstrations, radio or television programs, prerecorded tapes, technology-based applications, printed articles, mailed material, or other media, they take reasonable precautions to ensure that
> 1. The statements are based on appropriate professional counseling literature and practice,
> 2. The statements are otherwise consistent with the ACA Code of Ethics, and
> 3. The *recipients of the information are not encouraged to infer that a professional counseling relationship has been established* [italics added]. (ACA Code of Ethics, C.6.c.)

SUMMARY

The impulse to put one's grief counseling skills to use for public service is an honorable one. Indeed, most ethics codes mandate public service as an obligation for conscientious professionals. However, a reflexive wish to help the public in need is not enough. Whether it is disaster relief work, support groups, educational roles, or media interviews, grief counselors must be careful only to accept assignments for which they have appropriate training and expertise. Even then, grief counselors must heed the potential ethical pitfalls posed whenever they venture into the domain of public service.

12 Grief Counselor as Expert Witness

Grief counselors are at home in the consultation room, not the courtroom. As members of a broad community of mental health professionals, grief counselors are first and foremost *helpers*, striving to achieve improvement in the mental and emotional well-being of the clients they serve. Inevitably, however, grief counselors may be thrust into the role of expert witness when clients seek legal redress for the losses in their lives or when courts of law compel the grief counselor's participation in adjudication of civil or criminal cases. Juggling the competing demands of professional counselor and expert witness introduces unique ethical challenges. When grief counselors venture into the legal system, even if such forays are relatively rare, they need to be legally informed (Otto & Heilbrun, 2002)—that is, know how to discharge their duty as expert witness without committing an ethical breach and without jeopardizing the counseling relationship that is the basis for their appearance in court. This chapter is intended primarily for grief counselors who are called intermittently to testify as expert witnesses rather than those mental health professionals who deliberately choose the forensic arena as a career subspecialty.

WRONGFUL DEATHS

According to *Black's Law Dictionary* (Nolan, Nolan-Haley, Connolly, Hicks, & Alibrandi, 1990), *wrongful death* refers to deaths attributable to the willful or negligent act of another person. "Wrongful" implies that these deaths could have been avoided by different actions or choices on the part of the person(s) involved. Thus, there is someone to blame or hold accountable in cases of wrongful death. Homicide and manslaughter are classic examples of deaths resulting from intentional harm or negligence. Criminal prosecution and civil lawsuits address grievances over wrongful deaths.

In traditional grief counseling, the term wrongful death is rarely used, probably because its pejorative connotation is inconsistent with a nonjudgmental therapeutic stance. Rando (1993) employed the notion of *preventability* to refer to deaths that could have been avoided. The concept of preventability includes accidental deaths resulting from negligence, carelessness, or engagement in high-risk activities without proper precautions, as well as deliberate deaths due to homicide or terrorism. Preventability also includes medical malpractice that leads to death. Negligence, oversight, and misjudgment are human faults that contribute to preventable deaths and render the actor(s) culpable (Vigilant & Williamson, 2003). That culpability is the basis for wrongful death claims.

Rynearson (1987, 2001, 2006) coined the term *unnatural death* to categorize those resulting from accidents (unintentional injury), suicide, and homicide. Although in the United States the majority of deaths occur naturally (from illness, disease, or old age), unnatural death claims a surprisingly high number of victims among children, adolescents, and young adults (see Table 12.1). Deaths that occur unexpectedly, in a traumatic fashion, or under preventable circumstances are associated with greater complications in grieving (Gamino et al., 2000; Rando, 1993). As a consequence, clients coming into grief counseling may disproportionately report unnatural or violent deaths as the focus of their grief (Gamino et al., 2008). Presumably, such deaths are more difficult to cope with and bear because of the horror, brutality, and calamity involved.

What is considered preventable or unnatural death in the realm of grief counseling may be labeled wrongful death by the legal system. Psychologically, wrongful death breeds anger in the survivors (Lord, 2006;

Table 12.1

PERCENT OF DEATHS BY SELECTED CAUSES PER AGE DECADE, UNITED STATES—2003

AGES	ILLNESS	ACCIDENTS	SUICIDE	HOMICIDE
0–4	90	8	0	2
5–14[a]	54	38	4	5
15–24	27	45	12	16
25–34[a]	46	30	12	11
35–44	70	19	7	4
45–54	86	9	4	1
55–64[a]	95	3	1	<1
65–74[a]	97	2	<1	<1
75–84[a]	98	2	<1	<1
85+[a]	98	2	<1	<1

Adapted from *Statistical Abstracts of the United States: 2007* (p. 85), by U.S. Department of Commerce, Economics and Statistics Administration and U.S. Census Bureau, 2006.
[a]Rounding to two decimal places yields percentages slightly variant to 100% totals per age decade.

Redmond, 1989), and angry victims are more likely to seek retribution and compensation. Legally, retribution is addressed in criminal court, and compensation is addressed in civil court. When working with clients mourning wrongful deaths, the grief counselor may be drawn into testifying as an expert witness regarding the impact of the loss on the clients' mental and emotional health. In such instances, what begins as a well-intended effort to provide grief counseling to the bereaved becomes an exercise in forensic testimony for the grief counselor.

CONFLICTS BETWEEN THERAPEUTIC AND FORENSIC ROLES

Grief counselors and mental health professionals should be wary when treading into the legal system (Koocher & Keith-Spiegel, 2008). For most counselors, this is unfamiliar territory with numerous hazards that can induce ethical lapses. It must be remembered that *any professional activity involving the legal system (e.g., forensic evaluations, depositions, consultations with attorneys, or court testimony) constitutes the practice of grief counseling and is subject to all ethical standards and guidelines governing the profession* (cf. Milunsky, 2003). Appropriate wariness means exercising due caution by thinking twice about statements made and double-checking actions taken. When unsure about the ethics of providing testimony as an expert witness, counselors are well advised to review forensic-specific practice guidelines (e.g., Committee on the Revision of the Specialty Guidelines for Forensic Psychology, 2008) and consult with their own attornies who represent them in professional affairs.

Grief counselors who contemplate giving expert testimony should be advised that there are those *within* the profession who believe testimony from a treating mental health professional (i.e., a psychotherapist or counselor) should be barred categorically from court proceedings (Shuman, Greenberg, Heilbrun, & Foote, 1998) as well as those *outside* the profession dedicated to discrediting such testimony if offered (Ziskin, Faust, & Anderer, 2004). We acknowledge that thorough deliberation of this controversy regarding whether therapists should testify is beyond the scope of this text. Our purpose is to remind the grief counselor providing forensic testimony to do so in an ethically sound manner even while the broader debate over this endeavor continues.

The most common scenario is when a grief counselor providing professional care to a client is called to testify as an expert witness, that is, as someone who possesses specialized knowledge in the field of thanatology and mental health treatment. In legal proceedings involving wrongful death, a properly qualified, competent grief counselor testifies as an expert witness when describing a client's symptoms, mental state, clinical formulation, diagnosis, treatment plan, and prognosis. Such testimony requires specialized knowledge not possessed by an ordinary citizen. In other words, the testimony could not be rendered credibly by a nonprofessional. So how do well-intended grief counselors provide both empathic, effective treatment in the consultation room and dispassionate, objective testimony in the courtroom without compromising loyalty to the client or their own professional integrity?

There are basic differences between therapeutic and forensic roles (Heilbrun, 2001) that carry inherent conflicts for mental health professionals (Greenberg and Shuman, 1997; Strasburger, Gutheil, & Brodsky, 1997). When practitioners attempt to meet clients' needs in both domains simultaneously, a problematic multiple-relationship dilemma results (see Chapter 7, "Multiple Relationships in Thanatology"). After all, counseling is intended to be supportive, accepting, and empathic. It relies heavily on the client's subjective perception of events, often without any attempt at external corroboration of the facts. In counseling, there is great emphasis on the confidential nature of the therapeutic dialogue. The goal is to accomplish something helpful for the client within the framework of the therapy relationship. In effect, the counselor works for the client and maintains loyalty to the client.

Trusting in the confidential nature of counseling, clients tend to be forthcoming because they want the counselor to understand not only the loss events themselves but also the overall context of their experience. Greenberg and Shuman (1997) argue that most people disclose more information, with less self-censorship, in mental health counseling than they do in forensic examinations conducted specifically for the courts. However, once personal and intimate information has been revealed in therapy, and those therapy sessions become the basis for expert testimony by the counselor, it raises the possibility that detailed information may be disclosed in court to the potential detriment of the client. That is the crux of the conflict.

Therapists want to help their clients and are naturally sympathetic to their plights (Greenberg & Shuman, 1997). Yet when entering a court of law, the nature and character of forensic testimony is expected to be neutral, impartial, and detached. The emphasis is on objective discovery of the truth, and disclosure in court is intended to assist the judge or jury in decision making (Shuman & Greenberg, 2003). In the United States, admissibility of expert testimony is based largely on Federal Rules of Evidence 702, Testimony by Experts (Smith, 2004).

> If scientific, technical, or other specialized knowledge will assist the trier of fact to understand the evidence or to determine a fact in issue, a witness qualified as an expert by knowledge, skill, experience, training, or education, may testify thereto in the form of an opinion or otherwise.... (p. 787)

For the most part, state laws governing expert witnesses track this federal standard.

Also, the U.S. Supreme Court clarified in its 1993 ruling in *Daubert v. Merrell Dow Pharmaceutical, Inc.* that scientific evidence presented by experts must meet certain criteria, partly to preclude the admissibility of "junk" science. Specifically, the methods or theoretical principles on which the expert's inferences are based must be considered scientifically valid. A valid method was defined as one that has been or can be tested, has been subjected to peer review and publication, carries a known error rate together with standards controlling its application, and is generally accepted within a relevant scientific community. Although a grief counselor's specialized knowledge in thanatology may not be strictly interpreted by all judges as scientific, practitioners called to testify as expert witnesses are well advised to master the scholarly literature on which their methods or techniques are based in order to address such challenges of inadmissibility based on *Daubert* (Brodsky, 1999). But not every state or jurisdiction has adopted these rigorous *Daubert* standards; therefore, counselors should know whether such standards are applicable in their jurisdiction (Heilbrun, 2001).

When called to be an expert witness in a case pertaining to wrongful death for which the grief counselor is providing treatment to bereaved parties, the counselor may perceive an awkward choice between, on the one hand, advocating for the client(s) and, on the other hand, maintaining professional integrity by testifying truthfully. The ADEC Code of Ethics does not address directly the ethical dilemmas presented when grief counselors testify as expert witnesses. At best, only a general guideline speaks to potential conflicts between therapeutic and forensic roles.

> Members avoid conflicts of interest that interfere with professional discretion and impartial judgment. If a real or potential conflict of interest arises, members take reasonable steps to resolve the issue in a manner that reflects the best interests of the person(s) served. (ADEC Code of Ethics, I. General Conduct, H)

The ACA (2005a) Code of Ethics has a section on conducting forensic evaluations (E.13. Forensic Evaluations: Evaluation for Legal Proceedings). It contains a prohibition on evaluating one's clients.

> Counselors do not evaluate individuals for forensic purposes they currently counsel or individuals they have counseled in the past. Counselors do not accept as counseling clients individuals they are evaluating or individuals they have evaluated in the past for forensic purposes. (ACA Code of Ethics, E.13.c.)

The Specialty Guidelines for Forensic Psychology (Committee on the Revision of the Specialty Guidelines for Forensic Psychology, 2008) clarifies the difference between providing expert testimony and testifying as a forensic expert.

> Providing expert testimony about a patient who is a participant in a legal matter does not necessarily involve the practice of forensic psychology even when that testimony explicitly embraces a psycholegal issue that is before the decision-maker. For example, providing testimony on matters such as a patient's reported history or other statements, mental status, diagnosis, and treatment provided, as well as expert opinion regarding the patient's response to treatment, prognosis, and likelihood of relapse or remission would not ordinarily be considered forensic practice even when the testimony is related to a psycholegal issue before the decision-maker. Rendering opinions and providing testimony about a person on psycholegal issues (e.g., criminal responsibility, legal causation, proximate cause, trial competence, testamentary capacity, the relative merits of parenting arrangements) would ordinarily be considered the practice of forensic psychology. (Specialty Guidelines for Forensic Psychology, 6.02.02 Expert Testimony by Practitioners Providing Therapeutic Services)

These ethical rules and guidelines draw clearly the distinction between therapeutic and forensic roles but offer little pragmatic guidance to grief counselors who find themselves in the position of testifying about their evaluation and treatment of clients whom they serve.

CASE EXAMPLE

The following case example illustrates the conflicts that can arise between therapeutic and forensic roles and provides a platform for discussing how such conflicts can be handled by employing the Five P Model for ethical decision making.

Two teenagers returning home from an all-night, supervised graduation party died when the driver failed to negotiate a turn at high speed and the vehicle flipped and crashed. Both sets of parents, who had a cordial relationship through their children's association, sought help from a licensed grief counselor with a reputation for expertise with parental bereavement. The grief counselor accepted as clients the deceased passenger's parents, who came first for consultation. When the parents of the driver also came for help later, the grief counselor referred them to a counselor-in-training who was working under the grief counselor's supervision, an arrangement that had been used previously with good results in other multiple-death situations. This referral was made because the grief counselor worked in a rural area where there were relatively few choices for mental health treatment and the counselor was the only local professional known for working with grief cases.

After some months, the parents of the passenger decided to sue for wrongful death. In order to file a claim against the driver's insurance company, they had to sue the parents of the driver. Thus, the cordial association between the two families ended with the onset of a civil lawsuit. This development intensified the ethical dilemma for the grief counselor. By virtue of the supervisory relationship, the grief counselor knew of extenuating circumstances that magnified the driver's liability. Besides the all-night graduation party, the driver had attended another party the previous night so that, over a 48-hour period leading up to the crash, the driver had actually slept only about 3 hours. Also, the driver's family had been advised by their mechanic to replace the entire brake system in the vehicle, yet they had delayed the needed repairs for financial reasons. Finally, the driver had been in some trouble with his parents prior to graduation for drag racing. However, this extenuating information was *not known* by the parents of the deceased passenger. According to confidentiality standards, this information could not be revealed to them by the grief counselor because it was privileged within the context of the counseling relationship with the parents of the driver.

For legal purposes, the grief counselor was the counselor of record for both families because the work done by the counselor-in-training was supervised and undersigned by the licensed grief counselor. The grief counselor was called as an expert witness to testify about the pain and suffering incurred by the deceased passenger's family because of their teenager's death. The counselor's testimony made it clear to the passenger's family that the grief counselor had been aware all along of the extenuating circumstances implicating the driver. They were furious, feeling that they had been betrayed and that the fidelity due them from the grief counselor had been violated.

To make matters worse, the opposing attorney for the driver's family seized on the fact that the grief counselor was legally responsible for the treatment rendered to the driver's family as well. Choosing to fight fire with fire, that attorney began asking the grief counselor to speak to the pain and suffering of the driver's family and compare it to that of the deceased passenger's family. Even though the grief counselor declined to compare the two cases by stating, "They've both lost children; they're both hurting terribly," the damage to the therapeutic relationship was done. The day in court ended with near total estrangement between the grief counselor and the parents of the deceased passenger. They terminated treatment shortly thereafter.

THE FIVE P MODEL

This unfortunate case shows how the therapeutic role of grief counselor and the forensic role of expert witness can collide when a mental health professional attempts to discharge both roles. We will now review the case using the elements of the Five P Model.

Person

The difficulties begin with establishing who is the client. Obviously, the parents of the deceased passenger who first consulted the grief counselor are clients. These aggrieved parents lost a child in a motor vehicle crash that was probably preventable. They believed their only recourse for holding someone accountable for their child's death—in effect, speaking for a child who can no longer speak—was to sue in civil court for wrongful death.

What about the parents of the driver? Legally, they are clients as well because the licensed grief counselor is ultimately responsible for their care, even though a counselor-in-training is actually working with them. Pragmatically, they are a step removed from the counselor's direct aegis. However, they also are persons to whom the counselor has a formal responsibility. They, too, are bereaved parents agonizing over loss of a child, and they are additionally burdened with the pressures of defending themselves and their child in a lawsuit.

Then there are the judge, the attorneys, and the jury to consider. Once the court compels the grief counselor to participate in its proceedings, the judge and attorneys, as officers of the court, are persons to whom the grief counselor owes a duty. Likewise, the jurors, who are charged with evaluating the guilt or innocence of their peers, are entitled to an objective description of the counselor's findings about the pain and suffering of the families. The judge, attorneys, and jurors are not clients of the counselor, but they are stakeholders in the outcome of the case and "consumers" of the counselor's professional work via the forensic testimony.

Problem

The ethical dilemma in this case is twofold. At one level, the grief counselor has a fiduciary relationship with multiple parties who have competing agendas. The deceased passenger's parents want grief counseling and help to plead their case in court. The driver's parents also want expert therapy and seek to defend themselves in court. The judge and jurors want truth as objectively as it can be stated. The attorneys on both sides want to bring out that aspect of the truth most advantageous to their clients' positions. The adversarial nature of the legal system pits one of the counselor's clients against the other, yet each party in this drama expects loyalty to their cause from the grief counselor.

At another level, the grief counselor is trying to juggle simultaneously two largely irreconcilable roles—therapist and expert witness. Being a good grief counselor does not readily translate into being a good expert witness. This conflict is the reason Greenberg and Shuman (1997) are so explicit about the abiding differences between therapeutic and forensic roles. In therapy with the bereaved parents, the grief counselor delves deeply into their pain with an attitude of respect and with an unquestioning, nonjudgmental, empathic manner. There are no challenges as to the legitimacy or reality of their suffering. Yet in court, the clients' mental and emotional distress may be viewed more like a physical injury that can be calibrated in its severity and compensated accordingly, like amputation cases where the loss of a whole arm is rated as more severe than the loss of a hand only. But how does one quantify the loss of a child? Interrogation of the grief counselor on this very point can be enough to alienate clients who perceive that their pain has been overlooked, invalidated, or minimized. In the case example, the therapeutic relationship with the parents of the deceased passenger foundered, a casualty to their perception that the counselor betrayed them in court.

Place

Just as there are multiple persons complicating this case scenario, the factor of place is crucial in the ethical dilemma. The consultation room itself becomes a different place once legal action is initiated. Knowing that third parties may later review everything that is spoken or communicated modifies the inviolability of the counselor–client privilege. Privilege is no longer as ironclad as before because an exception now applies. As Greenberg and Shuman (1997) warn, clients may be less forthcoming or may come forth more selectively when aware that the contents of their counseling sessions may be disclosed in court. The grief counselor has an obligation to reclarify the nature of this exception to confidentiality because not every client-litigant may recall that exception from the initial informed consent discussion or understand what it means.

A very different set of contingencies and regulations operates when the action shifts to the courtroom and the grief counselor enters the legal system. Thus, place dictates much about what the counselor can and cannot do. Shuman and Greenberg (2003) remind mental health professionals that expert witnesses are expected to provide the court with impartial information from the expert's field of competence. Feelings of likeability, support, or empathy for clients do not enter into a dispassionate description of their problems and prognoses. Identification with or, alternately, antipathy toward a particular litigation team is proscribed. Although the adversarial system in law is based on partisanship, the expert witness is expected to rise above the fray and avoid taking sides. In the case of the fatal car crash, the grief counselor was the treating professional of record for both plaintiff and defendant and, once in court, expected to champion neither but instead honor truth as the highest ideal.

Principle(s)

More than one ethical principle informs the grief counselor's decisions in this case. Although in hindsight it would have been better for the grief counselor not to be professionally involved with two families now opposing each other in court, the decision to do so was made with the information available at the time, when the priority was delivering services to two parties in urgent need of grief counseling. Beneficence, or attempting to accomplish something helpful and therapeutic with the grieving families, was the rationale that ruled the day. However, some may question whether this exposed a proverbial blind spot on the part of the experienced counselor who let the ego-appeal of being the locale's premier consultant in bereavement sway the decision to treat both parties of the same headline-making crash.

A more conservative policy would have been to avoid any professional involvement with the second family, either by referring them to another licensed professional or by declining a supervisory relationship with the counselor-in-training who treated them. This approach would assign priority to nonmaleficence, or precluding possible harm to clients, as the greater good and invoke Murphy's Law that "if something can go wrong, it will." Contrasting decision-making strategies emphasizing either beneficence or nonmaleficence may reflect dispositional differences on the part of the mental health professionals making the decision. Millon (1994) posited that one of the fundamental personality polarities comprising individual differences is the distinction between a *gain-enhancing orientation* (cf. beneficence) in which calculated risks are incurred in the interest of accomplishing something worthwhile and a *pain-avoiding posture* (cf. nonmaleficence) in which potential gains are sacrificed in order to follow a low-risk or no-risk policy.

Whenever two parties are involved in the same multiple-death scenario, the potential exists for partisan agendas to emerge later and create ethical conflict for a grief counselor who attempts to treat both parties. Certainly, this does not always occur, and some may argue that avoiding this is simply not practical in underserved areas where the expertise of a specialist in grief counseling is not easily duplicated. Suffice it to say that the maxim "no good deed goes unpunished" fits this example. By trying so hard to assist both families, the grief counselor inadvertently set up a situation in which the original intent to help was thwarted by the deceased passenger's family dropping out of counseling once they felt alienated by the grief counselor's court testimony.

Fidelity to the client in the professional relationship is another key principle in this case. Fidelity in action means proving to be trustworthy by faithfully following through with one's professional obligations—demonstrating competence, maintaining confidentiality, keeping one's word, and advocating when necessary. The fact that the family of the deceased passenger felt abandoned by the grief counselor's attempt toward equanimity in court indicates a problem with fidelity. The family's expectations of loyalty were not met, and in this scenario, under the circumstances, perhaps there was no way they reasonably could be met.

One extension of fidelity is client education. When providers learn that their clients are involved in legal action pertaining to their grief counseling, such as a wrongful death suit, the judicious practitioner begins immediately to educate the clients about the machinations of the legal system and how that can impact the therapeutic relationship if the counselor is called to testify. Such anticipation can forestall or reduce damage to the carefully cultivated fiduciary relationship between the grief counselor and the client(s).

Process

Once the parents of the deceased passenger filed suit, events cascaded until the grief counselor was left in a largely reactive position: answering a summons to court, responding to opposing attorneys' questions, and complying with rules of evidence that shape the admissibility of what may be said (cf. Gutheil, Hauser, White, Spruiell, & Strasburger, 2003). "Playing defense" in legal proceedings is never a comfortable position and does not enhance the ability to make sound ethical decisions. Even so, the grief counselor in this example could take some specific steps to prepare for the many decisions embedded in how expert testimony is given, such as familiarizing oneself with literature specific to how mental health professionals may testify effectively (Brodsky, 1991, 1999; Heilbrun, 2001). Also, in a situation such as this, consultation with an independent attorney who can advise the counselor on how to handle potential hazards would be helpful.

A steady, modestly confident style during court testimony is a safe strategy. Excessive equivocating or undue circumspection imply uncertainty or lack of knowledge and can undermine one's credibility. Oppositely, arrogance, cockiness, and blatant partisanship are risky. Instead, Greenberg and Shuman (1997) recommend that mental health professionals give straightforward answers in plain language and acknowledge frankly the limits of what they can accurately and reliably assert based on the therapeutic relationship. When certain legal questions are raised, such as asking the counselor to quantify the client's pain and suffering or to pose suppositions as to causal relationships between life events and subjective distress, grief counselors may deflect such questions to avoid taking a position on an issue that was not the focus or purpose of their work with the client. For instance, one might aptly respond to such inquiries with a statement such as, "In my role as grief counselor to the parents, I can only tell you what I observed during the course of counseling." By not overstepping the limits of one's knowledge or extrapolating from one's contacts with the client to answer speculative questions, the grief counselor avoids untoward outcomes.

Two very helpful books by Stanley Brodsky (1991, 1999) address how a counselor or psychotherapist can keep from being marginalized or discounted as an expert witness. For example, should one's role as grief counselor be characterized as inherently partisan or biased, and therefore questionable in relevance, Brodsky recommends the admit–deny strategy to handle such hostile interrogatives concerning one's credibility. It starts with admitting the limitations of one's knowledge in a *dependent* clause (e.g., "Although I did not perform an independent forensic evaluation of my clients...") followed by an *independent* clause strongly denying the untrue part of the assertion that one has nothing of substantive value to contribute (e.g., "I can say, based on several hours of in-depth psychotherapy interviews with the clients, that I understand well their pain and suffering"). As a final caveat to grief counselors called to testify as expert witnesses, Brodsky reminds practitioners that their testimony can be strengthened by emphasizing the value of the participant-observer role in psychotherapy (cf. Sullivan, 1954) and the extended opportunity to interact over time with the client rather than relying on a single evaluation interview.

THE CONCEPT OF JUSTICE

Consider another case in which the grief counselor testified as an expert witness.

A couple and their three young children were returning to the city from a Sunday afternoon visit with grandparents who lived in the country. The mother was driving while the father dozed in the passenger seat. Topping a hill on the two-lane rural highway, only a split second separated them from a drunk driver passing illegally. The mother instantly veered to the shoulder to avoid a collision. Inexplicably, so did the oncoming driver. The two vehicles crashed at high speed on the grassy embankment. The driver's side of the family car was torn away, critically injuring the mother and killing the two boys in the backseat. The father, and the daughter seated directly behind him, survived.

Categorically, these were wrongful deaths that were clearly preventable and never should have happened. Raphael (1986) refers to such tragic events as *personal disasters* in the lives of those affected. Catastrophes such as this completely rewrite the personal histories of those involved. In this case, once the mother's survival was assured after several surgeries, the couple sought grief counseling to deal with their multiple losses. Grappling with the gruesome nature of the crash and the devastating loss of their sons generated intense grief and rage. Certainly, this required that their grief counselor possess the ability not only to tolerate their trauma and pain but also to guide them toward a recovery process (cf. Balk, 2008)—the very epitome of death competence described in Chapter 3.

Hearing out the aggrieved parents' story of loss and affording them the opportunity to express their innermost thoughts and feelings about the deaths of their sons was all part of good counseling practice, predicated on the ethical principle of beneficence—helping those who are hurting. Phenomenologically, it was extremely important for the parents to narrate their loss experience to the counselor as part of the therapeutic collaboration. Particularly when constructivist (cf. Neimeyer, 1998, 2001) or narrative therapy (cf. Angus, Levitt, & Hardtke, 1999) approaches are used, formulating a coherent understanding of the loss events and their meaning is central to the cognitive work in grief counseling. Justice in a therapeutic setting requires that the parents be heard, thoroughly and completely.

However, this kind of "therapeutic justice" is very different from the operation of justice in the legal arena, where trying facts, finding fault, and meting out consequences follow a meticulously codified rule of law. A grief counselor must recognize the differences between therapeutic justice and legal justice to maintain ethical integrity when testifying as an expert witness. Understanding this distinction also enables the grief counselor to educate clients in preparation for trial by judge or jury.

In the case of the parents who lost both sons in a drunk-driver crash, the driver at fault was charged by the district attorney with negligent homicide. In the criminal trial, only the father was called as a witness. The mother, who had been severely injured, was placed on the defendant's witness list but was never called to testify—a transparent move designed to keep the grieving mother out of the courtroom and beyond view of the jury. The grief counselor helped prepare the father for the fact that the defense attorney's questions might well be designed to circumvent a comprehensive account of the crash, in stark contrast to the ethic of thorough retelling that prevailed in their grief counseling sessions.

Indeed, the defendant's attorney sought to divert the jury's attention from the father's tearful description of finding his dead sons on the roadside by focusing rebuttal questions only on peripheral facts, such as the make, model, and color of the cars involved. These deft moves by the defendant's attorney constituted precisely the kind of vigorous defense to which an accused person is entitled in the tradition of American and English jurisprudence. The strategy also enraged the parents, who felt muted in their attempt to represent their deceased sons who could not speak for themselves, an important psychological task for bereaved parents whose generativity strivings are otherwise stymied by the deaths of their children (Klass, 2001; Klass & Marwit, 1988–1989). However, timely preparation of the parents about the differences between therapeutic justice and legal justice softened the sting of what seemed to them to be a travesty of justice in a court of law.

Once the driver was convicted of a lesser charge, vehicular manslaughter, the grief counselor was called by the prosecution during the penalty phase of the trial to testify about the parents' emotional pain and suffering. The defense attorney never directly challenged any of the grief counselor's statements regarding the parents' grief. In fact, the topic was avoided altogether upon cross-examination. Instead, cued by the grief counselor's exhaustive history documented in the initial evaluation session, the attorney for the defense focused on two other problems dating back to the months immediately preceding the wreck: the father's employment trouble resulting in near termination and the heartbreaking estrangement that occurred between the mother and her cherished older sister that created a family crisis. The implication of this line of inquiry was clear to all—any distress experienced by the bereaved parents was multiply determined and not easily reduced to a simple cause-effect relationship with the deaths of the sons. The grief counselor felt handcuffed by the attorney's strategy, which precluded any elaboration about the impact of the fatal crash on the parents' emotional and mental health. Again, legal justice differed from therapeutic justice, and from the broader principle of justice that underlies an ethical approach to grief counseling.

TRUTH TELLING

The grief counselor's frustration in the prior example arose from a perception that the whole truth about the bereaved parents' emotional pain was never told in court. Gutheil et al. (2003) explore how truth is always in tension with admissibility in a court of law. That is, even though expert witnesses take a time-honored oath "to tell the truth, the whole truth and nothing but the truth," the adversarial nature of the legal system often makes this ideal difficult or impossible to achieve. Opposing attorneys seek to shape the testimony of an expert witness to reveal only those aspects of the professional's findings that support their view of events. In the case example, the defense attorney highlighted stressors affecting the parents *other than* the loss of their sons in order to diminish the degree of pain and suffering that the jury might assign directly to the fatal crash. Instead of the whole truth, only partial truth was admitted into evidence, in the eyes of the grief counselor and the bereaved parents. According to Gutheil et al., testifying as an expert witness carries with it the ethical challenge of honoring the truth first. But how does one maintain professional integrity in an adversarial arena where there are winners and losers and the truth is frequently shaped by omission?

Shuman and Greenberg (2003) exhort expert witnesses to remember that credibility derives from impartiality. Impartiality comes from fearless truth telling and from candid presentation of the results of one's evaluation or treatment of a client. Experts should have the prerogative to explain their complete answer to a question. Gutheil et al. (2003) add that expert witnesses are allowed to be ardent supporters of their presentation of the whole truth, which they hope will be credible and convincing.

Rappeport (1993) reminds practitioners that there is no absolute truth in mental health or medicine. Rather, inferences are made, and conclusions drawn by applying one's best professional judgment. In courts of law, there are different legal standards of proof that apply to different issues. Criteria such as "reasonable [expert] certainty" or "preponderance of evidence" (meaning more likely true than not true, or having at least 51% probability of being true) can confuse counselors unfamiliar with their definitions. The use of such criteria illustrates how the standards of proof for courtroom testimony differ from the "ways of knowing" employed in counseling practice (Greenberg & Shuman, 1997), where one's case formulation and clinical diagnosis develop from a cognitive and intuitive appraisal of the data. One's clinical anamnesis consists of a matrix of working hypotheses constantly subject to revision and refinement as counseling progresses. We recommend that grief counselors consult their attorneys or legal advisers to familiarize themselves with legal standards of proof that may be applied during cases in which they testify as expert witnesses.

Besides external threats to an expert witness's ability to tell the whole truth, such as circumscribed questioning by attorneys that limits admissibility or rules of discovery that preclude certain lines of inquiry, there are inevitable internal threats to objectivity as well. Human biases and partisan preferences can mold one's position in subtle ways by selectively deleting or accenting certain information. Schultz-Ross (1993) cautions mental health providers against overlooking their own biases that may infiltrate their concept of the truth.

> However desirable, objectivity may be elusive . . . even witnesses attempting to be objective are likely to have nascent opinions leaning toward one side. This opinion, even if subconscious, may be transmitted in verbal and nonverbal emphasis. Such testimony may then represent a covertly adversarial approach. Indeed, no expert can explain with equal skill all the available evidence. (p. 389)

The antithesis of objectivity and impartiality in truth telling is the performance of so-called hired guns, expert witnesses who willingly subjugate the truth to align their testimony with the preformed opinions or partisan positions of whichever legal team employs them. *Testimony for hire is not ethical practice of grief counseling.* Unfortunately, this reprehensible practice blackens the eye of everyone in the profession who takes seriously the ethical obligation to testify with honesty and integrity. Many have condemned this practice (Haas, 1993; Heilbrun, 2001; Milunsky, 2003; Mossman, 1999; Rappeport, 1993; Schultz-Ross, 1993). They lament how hired guns stain the credibility of the entire profession by contributing to a public perception that any mental health testimony rendered in court can be dismissed because of its plasticity and phoniness.

In the case of hired guns, all-too-willing, unscrupulous "expert" witnesses collude with attorneys who *dictate* the content and conclusions of the expert's testimony, obfuscating truth in the process. Of course, the adversarial legal system allows for a vigorous presentation of each side's position, and expert witnesses can legitimately disagree about clinical findings and scientific results. However, part of the intention of the U.S. Supreme Court's *Daubert* decision was to eliminate fabricated testimony from transparently biased experts such as hired guns. Heilbrun (2001) advocates a telling method, based on work by Colbach (1981), for uncloaking such professional charlatans by calculating their "contrary quotient," the percentage of times the so-called expert reaches a conclusion *unfavorable* to the referring source. A low percentage suggests that such individuals rarely disagree with the party paying them and thus, indeed, are available for hire. A moderate percentage connotes impartiality.

Finally, sometimes a grief counselor is called to testify in a jurisdiction other than the one in which the counselor is licensed to practice, such as when a wrongful death occurs in one state where the case is litigated, but the counselor practices in another state. In such instances, it is important to know that some jurisdictions prohibit altogether such testimony by visiting experts or that special local requirements may apply to any temporary forensic work done in the alternate jurisdiction (Simon & Guthiel, 2003; Tucillo, DeFilippis, Denney, & Dsurney, 2002). Checking with the disciplinary licensing board in the jurisdiction where one does not hold a professional license is necessary to avoid potential ethical or legal sanctions.

POINTS TO REMEMBER

In closing this chapter on grief counselor as expert witness, we reiterate the major points to remember in order to be adequately prepared to practice ethically should one become involved in legal proceedings in which one's client is a litigant.

1. Remain alert to the possibility that legal action may ensue and that one can be called as an expert witness when counseling clients whose loved ones died a wrongful death.
2. Incorporate into the informed consent dialogue a discussion about the potential negative consequences legal action can have on the therapy should litigation over the loved one's death occur.
3. Remember that any professional activity involving the legal system constitutes the practice of grief counseling and is subject to all ethical standards and guidelines governing the profession.
4. Bear in mind that legal resolution of disputes is an adversarial process and that one side may attempt to discredit the grief counselor's credentials or dismiss any testimony as inherently biased or of little consequence.
5. Become familiar with the role conflicts that arise when a psychotherapist enters the legal system on behalf of clients and be prepared to face those challenges.
6. Focus testimony on what one confidently *knows* from the process of counseling the client, and maintain a circumspect attitude toward legal questions, such as quantifying pain and suffering or positing causal relationships. Those questions are for the court to answer, not the grief counselor.
7. Educate clients about the differences between justice in a therapeutic environment and justice in a legal arena.

8. Never compromise the truthfulness of one's public testimony, even in the face of attorneys' attempts to limit or shade the truth. Pay attention to one's own biases. Testimony for hire is not ethical practice of grief counseling. Integrity is everything.
9. Be ready to substantiate the scientific foundation for one's methods and practices by knowing the scholarly literature on which their efficacy is based, as well as acknowledging any limitations to the methods.
10. Never involve oneself in forensic activity in a jurisdiction where one does not hold a license for professional practice without first investigating any prohibitions or rules governing inter-jurisdictional practice in that locale.

13 Moving or Closing a Practice

Moving or closing a professional practice is inevitable in every grief counselor's life. Career opportunities, geographic pulls, health changes, yearnings to do something different, relocations for family reasons, or planned retirement are common examples of why a counseling practice may be moved or closed. Some practitioners, once they have completed their career in counseling, may even consider selling their practice to another professional. Moving, selling, or closing a counseling practice is a transition that constitutes a loss of sorts, both for the clients and for the counselors. Managing that sense of loss is part of the challenge. Yet the distinguishing feature of these transitions is the deliberate *planning* with which they are carried out. Planned retirement contrasts sharply with unexpected death or incapacitation of the grief counselor—contingencies for which the Professional Will was developed (see Chapter 3). How to meet one's ethical obligations during an orderly transition of moving or closing a practice is the subject of this chapter.

MOVING A PRACTICE

Moving or relocating one's counseling practice can be contemplated for a variety of professional and personal reasons. Professional considerations may include seeking a better practice opportunity, leaving or joining a group practice, adding or changing affiliation with a college or university, a wish to increase or reduce practice demands, or even involuntary termination of employment. Personal considerations for moving a counseling practice may include better climate; better housing; better schools; better cultural, community, or social offerings; better lifestyle; shorter commutes; or closer proximity to extended family or friends. Moves may be as short as across town to a better office location or as long as across the country to another state or jurisdiction.

A responsible, ethical approach to moving a counseling practice requires exercising primary concern for client welfare in all phases of the process. When anticipating and planning a move, ethically conscientious grief counselors first ask themselves some questions. What will be best for the clients? How and when should clients be informed of the impending move? Would the move allow clients to follow the counselor and continue care in the new location? Or do factors such as distance, economics, or insurance coverage prevent such continuity? What about continued counseling over the telephone or on the Internet via e-mail? (See Chapter 9 on Internet counseling.) Should termination of counseling be influenced by the counselor's decision to relocate? How does the counselor make referrals for clients who need additional help? Koocher (2003) stresses thoughtful planning as the best strategy for avoiding potential ethical problems associated with practice transitions such as moving.

To make our exploration of these assorted questions more practical, we describe two scenarios of colleagues who moved their practices. In one case, the counselor moved to a nearby city approximately 70 miles from the original practice location. This meant a shorter-range move. In the second case, the counselor relocated to a different state almost halfway across the continental United States. This was a longer-range move. Similarities and differences in the ethical dilemmas posed by these two examples of moving a professional practice are considered in succession.

Shorter-Range Move

The first grief counselor moved the practice to a nearby city largely for personal considerations. In mid-career and with adult children pursuing their own lives, the counselor began to give thought to eventual retirement, projected for about 10 years in the future. The size and offerings of the new metropolitan area made it seem an ideal retirement venue.

In fact, the counselor had already purchased a smaller home in the new community and decided to move sooner rather than later. This short-range move required no changes in professional licensure or malpractice insurance and no change of membership in state professional associations. Only notification of the change in business address was needed. Records of active and inactive clients would be transferred, in whole, to the new office. It was anticipated that some, but certainly not all, of the counselor's clients would transfer their care to the new location. As moves go, this one was relatively uncomplicated.

Showing primary concern for clients' welfare and respecting the counselor–client relationship demanded that the counselor inform active clients of the planned move with enough notice to allow clients to make appropriate arrangements in response. This process of giving notice began approximately 6 months in advance of the scheduled move. For some clients, the counselor's relocation meant mostly logistical adjustments to continue counseling in the new location. For others, the distance posed genuine obstacles to continuing, and if additional care was needed, transfer to another counselor was recommended. Usually, two or three referral names were provided. Finally, a small number of clients opted for termination within the 6-month timeframe, deciding that their therapeutic work was finished, or mostly finished, and they did not desire to transfer to another counselor.

Some clients requested the option of telephone consultation should they find themselves in the midst of a crisis or decide later that they needed more help. The counselor agreed to "telephone triage" on a case-by-case basis but declined to maintain an ongoing long-distance counseling relationship by telephone. The counselor believed it was healthier for clients ending care to address actively any loss-related feelings or issues pertaining to the termination rather than avoiding them (Fieldsteel, 2005) or maintaining a fantasy that unrestricted access to the counselor could continue via telephone consultation. This illustrated one of the ways the counselor attempted to process the termination event with active clients. The counselor communicated that the termination, because of its deliberate nature, constituted a normal life change or natural ending rather than an abandonment (Bauer & Kobos, 1987). The ADEC Code of Ethics addresses this very issue connected with termination of care.

> If members determine that they are unable, or no longer capable of providing a particular service, they carefully prepare the client and assist in

> making appropriate arrangements for continuing care when necessary. The client's well being is of primary concern; therefore, every attempt is made to ensure that the client does not feel abandoned and that possible adverse effects are minimized. All efforts to this end should be documented. (ADEC Code of Ethics, GC-I. Responsibility to Those Served, J)

Regarding the question of inactive clients, the counselor reviewed cases in two ways. First, any clients seen in the preceding 2 years were contacted by letter apprising them of the location change, in the event they wished to contact the counselor in the future for treatment, referral, or any matters pertaining to their counseling records. Second, the counselor searched further back in the case files for clients with whom there had been either a significant working relationship or who had indicated a possible wish to return to counseling in the future. As a courtesy, these inactive clients received the same letter of notice.

Likewise, colleagues and referral sources at the existing practice location were given notice of the counselor's intention to relocate. The counselor identified colleagues who agreed to accept referrals of clients who needed continuing care but for whom it was not feasible or advisable to travel to the new city. In this way, the counselor imparted goodwill among community colleagues who could continue to spread the word regarding the counselor's relocation and provide a contact phone number to interested parties, if needed. A positive relationship with clerical staff in the original office location helped ensure that subsequent callers seeking the grief counselor would be redirected to the telephone number at the new practice venue and that surface mail would be forwarded.

As one of many steps involved in setting up practice in a new community, the grief counselor began early the process of establishing professional contacts in the new city. This ensured that essential aspects of responsible counseling practice, such as providing psychiatry backup for clients needing medication or hospitalization and arranging for weekend call coverage, would be in place before actual service provision began in the new location.

Longer-Range Move

The second grief counselor was part of a dual-career couple, and the counselor's spouse accepted a promotion with an out-of-state university nearly halfway across the continental United States. As a result, the counselor was in a position of closing the existing practice in the home state and moving or restarting practice in a brand new city and state. Although this move was made primarily for the spouse's professional advancement, it was not an unwelcome change for the grief counselor, who saw the relocation as a chance to grow professionally by virtue of closer proximity to major health care facilities with end-of-life programs. At the same time, it meant closing what had been a professionally and personally rewarding practice of grief counseling, with an established client pool and a favorable reputation in the local community.

The spouse's new position was administrative rather than academic, so the move was scheduled with only 4 months' lead time, conforming primarily to the children's school calendar. This timeline left the grief counselor with only a brief interval to manage everything involved with closing one practice and preparing to open another. Even though a move had been contemplated for well over a year, the option of a comparable promotion for the spouse at a local university made all contingencies tentative until the best offer was accepted. For this reason, the grief counselor had not revealed to current clients any plans of an impending move. However, the counselor had been accepting new referrals on a more judicious basis (i.e., either declining or limiting involvement with clients requiring long-term intervention).

Needless to say, this move was relatively complicated because of time constraints and the number of changes involved. Because the out-of-state move involved closing a practice in the home state, the grief counselor faced important matters of how to protect the welfare of clients in the existing practice. The counselor believed it was essential to discuss the move in person with each active client, including the reasons for it and the impact on that client as far as remaining therapeutic work and possible transfer of care to another professional. For active clients whose next appointment was considered too distant to give reasonable notice of the move, telephone contact was made to apprise them of the move in a timely manner and to alert the client of the necessity to process this development in the next session. Some elected an earlier appointment to do just that.

Whether or not additional services were needed beyond the grief counselor's remaining tenure, each client faced the prospect of termination of care with *this* counselor. The counselor took special care to allow for processing of emotion, including any negative feelings generated by the counselor-initiated termination (cf. Gabbard, 2000; Warren, 2000).

An accepting, nonjudgmental therapeutic attitude was especially important, given that some clients were hesitant to disclose hostile feelings in deference to the counselor as authority figure, fearing reprisal such as a more precipitous ending or loss of goodwill on the part of the counselor. In these discussions of termination, the counselor was careful to affirm clients by acknowledging any expressions of gratitude and appreciation for the counseling work accomplished (Manosevitz & Hays, 2003) and by declaring that the therapy work was uniquely valuable and involved a type of parent-like sadness for the counselor who was invested in the growth and development of the client (Fieldsteel, 2005).

Similar to the previous example, some clients chose to finish counseling in the remaining timeframe. Those who needed to continue counseling longer were given two or three referrals to consider. Different from the previous example, the counselor extended to a small handful of clients the opportunity to finish their therapeutic work via telephone consultation (Manosevitz & Hays, 2003; Warren, 2000). This option was restricted to those meeting two specific criteria. First, the counselor had to know the client well enough to feel secure in relying on voice stylistics and nuance alone to really hear what was being conveyed over the telephone without benefit of visual cues. Second, there had to be a realistic prospect that the counseling work could be completed in a time period of 4 to 6 weeks. The counselor viewed telephone therapy as a time-limited, adjunctive extension of the face-to-face counseling already accomplished, rather than a suitable medium for indefinite continuation of care (cf. Haas, Benedict, & Kobos, 1996). Any efforts to persist longer than that in a telephone therapy relationship were perceived as unwise and taken as an indication that transfer to a local colleague for continuing care was needed. Furthermore, the counselor's familiarity with emergency services in the home community allowed effective response to any crisis situation that might present itself during these telephone consultations. The counselor was not accustomed to using Internet modalities for psychotherapy and declined requests by some clients to continue counseling online via e-mail exchanges or chatting (see Chapter 9 on Internet counseling).

Providing for confidential storage and management of existing client records was a major focus of the second counselor's efforts during the 4-month transition period. The counselor decided to transfer all records to compact electronic media that would travel with the counselor to the office location in the new state, in part because of the plans for continuation of care via telephone for some clients. This way, records would be available for those clients or in the event of future contact or inquiries from any other clients from the former practice.

At the same time, it seemed imprudent to rely exclusively on such an arrangement for maintaining client records given the geographic distance involved, the transfer beyond state lines into a new jurisdiction, and the low probability that clients from the existing practice, active or inactive, would ever be treated again by this counselor. Therefore parallel arrangements were made to transfer all existing client records to a local custodian, an esteemed colleague with an established practice who agreed to take on this duty and who was paid a consignment fee by the counselor to do so. The ADEC Code of Ethics emphasizes the grief counselor's obligation to ensure viable protection of confidential client records.

> Members take reasonable precautions to protect the confidentiality of clients/students in the event of the member's termination of practice, incapacitation or death. (1) Members insure confidentiality of client/student records; (2) Members either transfer client/student records to another professional, or assure secure storage of the records; (3) Clients/students or their legal guardians are informed about the termination of practice and about the transfer/storage of records. (ADEC Code of Ethics, III. Responsibilities to Those Served, F)

Also, the ACA Code of Ethics (ACA, 2005) speaks to the necessary disposition of records associated with termination of practice.

> When counselors leave a practice, they follow a prepared plan for transfer of clients and files. Counselors prepare and disseminate to an identified colleague or "records custodian" a plan for the transfer of clients and files in the case of their incapacitation, death or termination of practice. (ACA Code of Ethics, C.2.h.)

In this example, significant issues arose regarding licensure, professional affiliations, and liability insurance coverage. Immediately upon confirming the spouse's position in the new state and deciding to make the move, the grief counselor applied for licensure in the new state. Happily, the fact that the grief counselor held board certification credentials in that respective professional discipline accelerated the process of obtaining a license to practice in the new state (cf. Koocher, 2003). For the time being, the counselor chose to maintain a license in the home state as well. However, membership in the home state's professional association was discontinued, and application was made to join the new state's professional association. Affiliation in national organizations was unaffected, save for notice of change of address.

The decision to maintain dual licensure, at least temporarily, was made for two reasons. First, it was a hedge against a possible return to the home state in the future. Second, it was to provide a basis for continued counseling by telephone with some clients residing in the home state. When a counselor changes jurisdictions yet continues to provide telephone therapy to clients residing in the original jurisdiction, it is not always clear which jurisdiction governs any issues related to malpractice (Koocher & Keith-Spiegel, 2008). The counselor in this example deemed it most prudent to retain licensure in both jurisdictions (Haas et al., 1996; Koocher & Morray, 2000).

Securing professional liability insurance for practice in the new state was not so easy. The grief counselor's current carrier was a firm that had made affordable coverage available for members of the state professional association, and it operated only in the home state. Because the physical move, licensure application in the new state, establishment of new office location, and membership in the new state's professional association were all proceeding on independent timelines, the counselor sought malpractice insurance through a major carrier affiliated with one of the national professional organizations. This allowed the counselor to obtain coverage sooner without having to wait on all the other relocation factors. It also provided for greater mobility in the future should there be another move.

Fortunately, the counselor's policy with the current carrier in the home state was occurrence-based (i.e., one providing protection against any claims pertaining to services rendered while the policy was in force, even if not filed until a later date after the policy was discontinued). This is opposed to less expensive claims-made policies that cover only claims in which *both* the triggering event and the filed complaint occur while paid coverage is in force. Having the luxury of occurrence-based coverage precluded the grief counselor from purchasing additional *tail coverage* from the prior carrier to cover claims filed after the original policy ended or *nose coverage* from the next insurer to cover acts prior to the purchase of a new policy (Koocher, 2003).

The grief counselor would not be established immediately and ready for practice in the new state until sometime after the actual move, so clients could not be furnished with a forwarding address. Instead, they were provided with the name, address, and phone number of the colleague who was to become the records custodian. Letters of notice about the practice closing were sent to inactive clients from the last 3 years, and they too were given that same colleague's contact information. The colleague also agreed to facilitate the referral process should inactive clients seek further care. The few clients who planned to continue in time-limited telephone counseling were given a cell phone number that the counselor kept active as a business phone for a few months beyond the move, while obtaining another cell phone in the new state for ongoing personal use. The entrusted colleague was charged with screening calls or inquiries about the counselor's new location and with making the cell phone number available only to those with a legitimate reason for contacting the counselor. Eventually, when the new practice office was operational, address and phone information was conveyed to the colleague in the home state.

These two case examples illustrate many common factors involved in moving or closing a grief counseling practice. Making client welfare a priority means giving timely notice of the move, showing respect for bereaved clients who may be especially sensitive to endings, processing termination, facilitating referrals, ensuring proper storage and maintenance of confidential counseling records, and arranging for a professional representative to serve as a proxy in handling future business matters when needed. Licensure, credentialing, professional affiliations, and liability insurance coverage also figure prominently in moving or closing a grief counseling practice.

Special Considerations for Clergy

An additional caveat to the discussion of moving or closing a practice is in order for grief counselors who are ordained ministers or pastoral counselors. Like the military, clergy can be reassigned or called to new locations with some regularity. That may be the reason for moving or closing a practice. Generally, clients may be more understanding at a cognitive level of the reasons for clergy relocation, although the emotional upheaval created by such reassignments may be no less painful. Also, for ministers, requests may come from former clients asking them to return to preside at significant life events such as funerals or weddings. Even though a professional goodbye has occurred, continuing bonds may operate that pull the grief counselor back into a relationship with former clients, even for brief periods. Typically, the familiarity of the old connection provides comfort for clients who are reassured by the presence of their esteemed counselor-minister at emotional life events.

Accepting such requests is not inherently problematic, but it raises certain ethical questions for the grief counselor who is a minister. Is the counselor obligated to fulfill such requests, if practically feasible, or is the counselor free to decline? Is the prospect of beneficence (i.e., doing some good) a sufficient basis on which to decide? Or does the prospect of nonmaleficence (i.e., avoiding potential harm from not agreeing) figure into the decision? When some requests are accepted and some declined, are countertransference feelings a determining factor? Does returning for funerals and weddings create a situation of multiple relationships? If so, the principles discussed in Chapter 7 on multiple relationships in worship settings apply. Secular grief counselors who move or close a professional practice rarely face such questions of postmove contact, but ministers and pastoral counselors need to be aware of the ethical issues involved in making these decisions.

SELLING A PRACTICE

Some grief counselors who are moving or closing a practice may consider the option of selling their practice to a qualified colleague. This possibility may seem like an attractive alternative when the grief counselor has built a successful practice, cultivated a good reputation, and created a demand for services in the form of referral volume and a waiting list for appointments. However, in light of clients' autonomy—their freedom of choice regarding which professionals with whom they consult—there is no guarantee that clients treated by the seller will want to continue counseling with the colleague who is the buyer. Thus, the notion of selling a practice raises several questions. What exactly is being sold? How does one assign a monetary value to something as ephemeral as a grief counseling practice? Is selling a practice an ethically sound proposition?

Part of the problem lies in the nature of the counseling endeavor. Grief counselors cannot clone themselves. Much of their success relies on personal, idiosyncratic factors in the counselor–client relationship, phenomena referred to generically as *therapist variables* in research on psychotherapy outcome (Beutler et al., 2004), as opposed to technique-specific methods (Lambert, 2004). Any counselor who has accepted a referral from a departing colleague or treated a client formerly counseled by another professional is well aware that every pairing of counselor and client is unique and cannot be replicated. Sometimes, different can work and a viable counseling relationship can be developed with a new counselor, but even where successful, it is never the same as it was with the prior practitioner. In this sense, a psychotherapy practice is substantively different from a medical, dental, or legal practice (Koocher, 2003). With the latter specialties, there is a greater reliance on the professional's technical skill to achieve success—a success that can always be augmented by a caring bedside manner or a winning personality. However, in grief counseling, the person of the counselor is the chief tool, and it is almost impossible to separate the counselor from the counseling.

So just what is being sold when a grief counselor sells the practice? According to Woody's (1997) careful inventory of the theoretical assets of a mental health practice, what is really being sold is goodwill created by the seller. Presumably, such value may be conveyed to a buyer through lists of client names, both active and inactive, identification of referral sources, and any ongoing contracts. However, neither clients nor referring professionals can be bought and sold, and one cannot presume that either will necessarily continue doing business with the buyer of the practice. The Ethics Committee of the American Psychological Association (1986) opined that *selling lists of clients' names as part of a practice is not ethical, unless prior agreement from the clients to do so is obtained.* Otherwise, their confidentiality is violated. Also, selling a professional endorsement of the buyer could be interpreted as receiving remuneration for referrals and, therefore, is considered unethical.

On the other hand, purchase of a physical location (i.e., real estate) and tangible assets such as furniture and office equipment carries market value that is more easily appraised. In Koocher's (2003) view, these physical assets are the primary thing being sold when a counselor sells the practice. So how much is a grief counseling practice worth to a buyer? Woody (1997) estimates there is really a rather bleak sale potential for the typical mental health practice. Aside from real estate and tangible assets, there is really not much actual monetary value in the goodwill aspects of the business. In short, practitioners wanting to develop a grief counseling practice could probably do just as well by simply setting up shop and developing a clientele and referral base on their own efforts.

The one exception to this wisdom may be the case in which the sale of a practice takes place over a matter of months with the buyer first joining the seller's practice and becoming known to the existing clients (Koocher, 2003). This could occur by providing coverage during vacation periods or absences, by introducing new services (e.g., eye movement desensitization and reprocessing [EMDR; Shapiro, 1995] for clients exposed to traumatic death) or by conducting cotherapy with the seller when treating couples or families. This way, when the seller moves or retires, there is a higher likelihood that at least some clients would stay on with the counselor purchasing the practice. Should the seller designate the buyer as records custodian and referral facilitator, the probability of clients transferring care to the new counselor is further enhanced.

Is it an ethically sound idea to sell a grief counseling practice? Our discussion should make the reader wary of any simplistic scheme to buy a mental health practice. There may be some merit to the idea when the physical location and furnishings of the practice are sold, or when the purchase is structured more like a transfer as in the preceding example. In any consideration of selling a practice, it is ethically imperative always to respect the dignity and worth of clients as people rather than commodities. As decision makers with full autonomy, clients decide whom to consult for grief counseling, and their choice must be honored in any transaction such as the sale of a professional practice. Buildings and equipment can be bought and sold; people and goodwill cannot.

RETIRING FROM PRACTICE

A familiar saying goes, "All good things must come to an end." Barring sudden, untimely death or incapacitation, most grief counselors will face retirement and the ending of their professional career at some point. The practice of grief counseling itself is about endings and dealing with the sense of loss left in their wake. As thanatologists, grief counselors claim expertise in addressing loss-related problems and in caring clinically for the bereaved. Will that expertise be applied to the counselor's own ending of a professional career at retirement? Certainly, "practicing what you preach" means the grief counselor makes a planned, responsible, graceful exit from professional work when the time comes. Ideally, the grief counselor's retirement should serve as a model not only to one's clients but also to one's colleagues, family, and friends. The last section of this chapter is devoted to the process of professional retirement and cites ethical considerations to keep in mind when contemplating a final closing of one's professional practice of grief counseling.

Is Retirement Mandatory?

Throughout this book, we espouse client welfare as a cardinal virtue to employ in ethical decision making. A principal question to ask when a grief counselor is contemplating retirement is, "What is good for the clients?" Because counseling is a skill that generally improves with age and experience, retirement would not appear to be mandatory if the grief counselor wishes to keep working, and clients continue to benefit. Of course, diminution of skill as a result of health problems or aging physiology could lead to the opposite conclusion that, indeed, retirement is required. As in all aspects of professional practice, self-awareness is the key. Should grief counselors be in doubt about whether their skills are still sharp, they would be well advised to consult a trusted colleague for a more objective viewpoint and visit with their personal physician about whether to continue with the rigors of a counseling practice.

A second perspective to consider in deciding whether retirement is mandatory is the wishes of the grief counselor. Does one want to retire or keep working? Writing from a psychodynamic angle, Kelly and Barratt (2007) discuss how a mental health professional's identity may be so closely tied to work, *laboro ergo sum* (my work is me), that retirement is difficult to contemplate. Without one's work, what would one be? The allure of being needed, of helping put things right for others, of having a daily dose of intimacy in relationships that many other people only read about—these things are among the most compelling rewards of a psychotherapist's life. According to Kelly and Barratt, these alluring payoffs are the reason many mental health professionals choose *not* to retire but, instead, to "die in the saddle." Loss of power, prestige, and a sense of importance or even of omnipotence that come from professional practice is hard to relinquish (McGee, 2003). Especially for grief counselors in private or solo practice, retirement may not be that appealing, for both identity and financial reasons.

We have no argument with those who choose not to retire. At the same time, we remind those postponing retirement that death-competent grief counselors realistically face the prospect of their own mortality and prepare for it, in part, by having a Professional Will as described in Chapter 3. Succumbing to the denial of death (Becker, 1973) so prevalent in a youth-oriented culture by continuing to practice as if one could simply go on forever, without making responsible provision for an eventual closing of practice, is folly and blatantly unethical. Continuing the cowboy metaphor, if a grief counselor figures to die in the saddle, that counselor had best leave detailed instructions with someone riding close by for what to do with the horse, the saddle, and any other possessions as well as for how to manage the cattle left untended.

The decision of whether to retire does not have to be an all-or-none categorical one. There are transitional approaches to retirement, sometimes called *scaling down* (Kelly & Barratt, 2007). Scaling down means the grief counselor gradually retires from professional activity by reducing commitments or practicing only part-time. For example, some grief counselors may continue indefinitely with an independent, part-time practice after official retirement from an agency or institution. We know personally some older professionals who opt for such a low-volume, simplified practice by maintaining licensure and liability coverage and then seeing clients in their private study at home and accepting only direct payment.

Calo (2005) advocates for a paradigm shift in society's thinking about retirement and describes the notion of a *generativity track* for older professionals who wish to continue working in response to a need to feel productive and intellectually stimulated. This is a qualitatively different mindset compared to younger professionals typically more focused on career advancement and financial gain. He suggests three variations to the generativity track: *mentor* to newer or younger professionals; *ambassador* for the profession in social and political arenas; and *flex-timer* who works a reduced or part-time schedule, as do some working parents who are also raising children.

An interesting commentary on the idea of transitional retirement came from a study by Draper, Winfield, and Luscombe (1997), who conducted a cross-sectional comparison of the attitudes of working psychiatrists *anticipating* retirement and the actual lifestyles of older, retired psychiatrists. The authors found that the retired professionals were significantly less active in writing, consultation, mentorship, and attendance at professional meetings than estimated by working professionals *imagining* how to spend their time during retirement. When the choices that retirement offers actually come to pass, mental health professionals may find the scaled-down version of retirement less attractive than they would have thought!

Certainly many, if not most, grief counselors *want* to retire, and they look forward to entering a stage of life in which new priorities can be pursued and enjoyed. They not only embrace the concept of retirement but would feel cheated without it. Those who work for agencies or organizations that have a mandatory retirement policy have less choice in the matter. Yet often, working toward retirement with an accumulated pension was an important reason for selecting that employment in the first place. So we now turn our attention to that cohort of grief counselors who fully intend to voluntarily and completely retire. Like other important aspects of one's professional practice, retiring takes preparation. McGee (2003) cautions psychotherapists that experience in helping clients with their retirement-related concerns is inadequate preparation for one's own retirement. Personal, legal, and ethical challenges of retirement require study and careful planning in order to ensure that retirement is implemented in an orderly and ethically principled manner.

Process of Retiring From Practice

One of the first decisions facing the retiring grief counselor is determining *when* and *how* to inform clients and colleagues of one's intentions to retire. Robbins (2006) explained poignantly her thoughts on the matter of retiring from a 40-year private practice of psychotherapy.

> Mulling this over I realized I wanted to give my clients—several of whom had been in therapy with me for many years—a year to prepare for this important change. I was also aware that I wanted to give myself a year to work out my own feelings. Retiring from my practice was a momentous life transition. (p. 190)

McGee (2003) suggests the optimal time to inform clients and colleagues about one's retirement is when a definite retirement schedule has been completed. Ordinarily, giving notice anywhere from 3 to 12 months in advance may be appropriate, depending on the nature of one's counseling practice. Those in office settings who may work with a client over a period of several years need to give earlier notice. Those whose involvement with clients is briefer in duration, such as a hospice counselor who typically works only a matter of weeks or perhaps months with a family, may give notice later in the process. For McGee, the time when the practitioner begins notifying clients about retirement should be linked to a simultaneous decision to stop accepting new clients. In colloquial terms, "When it's time to start stopping, it's time to stop starting." He also suggests informing clients and colleagues within a delineated time period (e.g., 1 month). Notice should be given to clients both orally and in writing to minimize confusion or denial. Table 13.1 displays a sample letter giving clients notice of the counselor's intention to retire from practice, based on McGee's work. Grief counselors may peruse this model and then customize something similar to fit their particular circumstances.

In addition to notifying current clients, there is the question of whether to notify former or inactive clients as well. The finality of retiring from professional practice should prompt a case review of files going back 5 years or more to identify inactive clients who deserve notification of the grief counselor's intention to retire. McGee (2003) believes this list may include long-term clients from the past, those who returned for counseling more than once over the years, and those who had especially strong transference feelings toward, or attachment to, the grief counselor. A letter similar to the one given to active clients should be mailed to these selected former clients, some of whom may want to schedule a session prior to the retirement date as a symbolic coda to their work with the grief counselor. The ethical obligation embedded in the notification process is giving clients sufficient time to adjust themselves to the counselor's retirement, to work out any difficult feelings, and to make reasoned decisions about the need for continued counseling.

Not abandoning clients at the time of retirement means providing names of other practitioners available for transfer or follow-up care, if needed. McGee (2003) argues that the counselor owes each client a clear, clinically based recommendation on whether additional therapy is indicated. Of course, clients are not required to agree with the counselor's assessment. Some clients who are struggling emotionally with the counselor's retirement may make a precipitous decision to forgo transfer to another counselor, not because there is no further need, but because they cannot envision working with someone else while they are absorbed in grieving the loss of their cherished counselor (Warren, 2000). Therefore, we recommend that referral names be given, even if the client demurs, in the event that the client decides later to pursue additional counseling after reconsidering.

Grief counselors are legally obligated to provide for secure storage and maintenance of confidential counseling records. Relevant state laws and regulations as well as the applicable professional discipline's ethics code should be followed, particularly with regard to mandated time requirements for record retention (Barnett, 1997). Records that are not likely to be needed in the future *and* that have been inactive beyond the

Table 13.1

SAMPLE LETTER INFORMING CLIENTS OF GRIEF COUNSELOR'S INTENTION TO RETIRE FROM PRACTICE

[YOUR OFFICE LETTERHEAD]

Dear _________:

As you know from our recent conversation, I plan to retire from the practice of counseling on _________. This letter serves as written confirmation that, as of that date, I will no longer provide grief counseling services. Additionally, in light of my impending retirement, I am no longer accepting any new referrals for counseling.

Until my retirement date, I will be available to continue your counseling, and I will be happy to respond to any questions or comments that you have about my plans to retire.

I also wish to discuss your plans, if any, to continue in counseling after my retirement. If you believe that you will need further help after that date, I will be glad to discuss potential new counselors with you so that we may identify the practitioner most likely to be suited to your needs and personality.

If you are not certain whether you may require additional help after my retirement, I will be happy to provide you the names of two or three colleagues in the event that you decide to seek additional counseling at some future date.

If you select a new mental health provider to whom you will transfer your care after my retirement, I will ask you to sign a Release of Information to enable me to forward your pertinent counseling records to the new provider.

Following my retirement, all client records of mine will be transferred to and maintained confidentially under the custody of [Dr. Best Friend]. In the future, should copies of your counseling records be needed for clinical or administrative purposes, you may contact [Dr. Friend, address, telephone number] for retrieval.

In closing, I would like you to know how personally important and professionally meaningful it has been for me to provide grief counseling services to you. Your diligent efforts at personal change and growth have impressed me. I know you may find it somewhat awkward for your counselor to retire, but I trust that you will understand that I have reached the end of my professional career. Please know that I wish the very best for you in all your future endeavors.

Sincerely yours,
Signature

Based on "Observations on the Retirement of Professional Psychologists," by T. F. McGee, 2003, *Professional Psychology: Research and Practice, 34,* p. 390. Adapted with permission from the American Psychological Association, January 5, 2009.

mandated time requirements for retention may be disposed of through secure means (i.e., shredding).

The procedure for records maintenance is similar to that described in the earlier section of this chapter on moving a practice. A trusted colleague needs to serve as records custodian. It could be the same individual designated in one's Professional Will to discharge this duty. The custodian must be capable of responding to subsequent requests from clients for transfer of counseling records to a new therapist or to legitimate requests for copies of records for medical, legal, or educational purposes. The custodian is entitled to be compensated for such services, and some understanding in this regard should be reached before the grief counselor's retirement.

Another procedural matter to address is making a decision about one's professional license. Some retiring grief counselors may prefer to keep their license active and participate willingly in continuing education programs that meet the requirements for annual renewal. Others are content to let their license renewal lapse and do not wish to pay any more fees, given that they never plan to practice again. Many state licensing boards offer the option of a retired status for one's license, which for a nominal fee deactivates the license. Then it may be reactivated in the future should the counselor ever wish to practice again, provided that one can demonstrate evidence of staying current in the field. Given the significance and meaning of professional licensure as a credential, some grief counselors see retiring their license as a fitting end to their career and find that their commensurate identity as a retired counselor is more satisfying and ego-sustaining than relinquishing their ties to the profession altogether.

Similar decisions need to be made about memberships in professional societies, journal subscriptions, and professional liability coverage. As with licenses, some professional associations will grant emeritus status to retiring professionals at a greatly reduced fee. The decision whether to go emeritus or simply drop one's membership may hinge on whether the retiring counselor still plans to attend annual conferences, in which case reduced conference fees for emeritus members will usually more than offset any associated costs. Also, continued fraternization at meetings with long-time professional colleagues may be an excellent way to continue some degree of professional identity. Likewise, reading journals may be one of the most common and practical ways to remain connected to the field or stay abreast of new developments for those so interested (Draper et al., 1997). Continuing to read professional literature can enhance one's mental mastery of the environment, known to be one avenue to healthy aging (Neugarten & Datan, 1996). Regarding professional liability insurance, it is important for the retiring counselor to arrange for tail coverage for any claims filed against the counselor after retirement based on events that occurred prior to retirement, unless one held an occurrence-based policy during the years of active practice (Koocher, 2003).

Psychological Aspects of Retiring

Retirement may be thought of as the ultimate practice transition. As such, it is a demanding time both for the retiring grief counselor and for the clients. Adequate self-care is essential in order for the grief counselor to maintain the emotional poise necessary to help clients through their termination or transfer processes. Manosevitz and Hays (2003) compare this to the self-care instructions given to passengers on airplane flights in the event of an emergency—adults are instructed to place the oxygen mask on their own faces before attending to their children's needs. Thus, retiring counselors need to remain healthy themselves before they can help clients handle the stresses associated with the counselor's projected retirement. The same self-care methods recommended in Chapter 3, "Death Competence," apply to grief counselors in the preretirement transition phase of their practices.

An all-important aspect of providing ethically sound grief counseling services in the weeks and months leading up to retirement is understanding carefully how clients' unique loss histories impact their response to termination or transfer (McGee, 2003).

> The client's actual and perceived history of losses, including how recent and severe they have been, as well as the type and level of a client's reactions to them, are critical in understanding potential reactions to the retirement. Indeed, this factor often plays a central role in unexpected, at times extreme, reactions to therapist terminations, including retirement. (p. 392)

Thus, losses of other significant figures in the client's life, including terminations with previous psychotherapists, if any, are grist for the mill when working through the client's reactions to the impending retirement of the counselor. Bauer and Kobos (1987) explain that managing termination in psychotherapy often includes focusing profitably on variants of some common themes: relationships come to an end; not every ending is logical; and ending a relationship is not an abandonment.

Although the bereavement literature confirms that an individual's loss history and attachment style are important determinants of the grief response (cf. Worden, 2009), the planned retirement of the grief counselor offers an opportunity rich with possibilities for helping clients learn how to deal with life losses. After all, are not losses the very purview of grief counseling? Because it involves coping with a stressful upcoming event whose occurrence is certain, like death, the methods of anticipatory grieving encouraged among family members of terminally ill hospice patients apply especially well (Rando, 2000). The retiring grief counselor gently guides the client into an exploratory discussion of the spectrum of interior thoughts and feelings triggered by the prospect of retirement. All the while, the counselor keeps an eye open to presenting alternatives to the client for how to tolerate, minimize, or safely discharge any negative affect. The counselor emphasizes active coping in the form of cognitive reframing, or taking concrete behavioral steps to master the situation or navigate through the most difficult aspects.

Successfully helping clients with termination issues related to the retirement requires grief counselors to engage in a parallel process of monitoring and managing their own feelings and attributions along the way. Retirement being the momentous transition that it is for many career grief counselors, they grieve too, just as the clients are grieving (Fieldsteel, 2005; Robbins, 2006). In this sense, preparing clients for one's retirement differs significantly from the bereavement work that makes up the bulk of the grief counseling endeavor—client's responses to the deaths or losses of unrelated third parties. Here, the retiring counselor is both the "dying person" and the "grief facilitator" to the client. Tricky indeed is the therapeutic balancing act demanded by this juxtaposition of roles. One of our retired colleagues reflected that it had taken everything that had been learned and synthesized over a full career as a grief counselor to execute this successfully. It was much like Ginger Rogers's dance steps "backwards and in high heels" complementary to Fred Astaire's moves. The counselor not only had to process the personal grief experienced over retirement but also had to stay a half-step ahead of the clients in helping them to adjust to their grief over the practice closing. For this reason, some may choose to obtain supervision focused on countertransference issues involved with leaving a practice (Warren, 2000).

Case Vignette

We conclude this section of the chapter with a case vignette that illustrates many of the points raised in the preceding pages.

The retiring grief counselor was a mature woman in her late 60s who decided the time had come to close her professional practice and, with only a modicum of ambivalence, reinvest her energies in activities beyond the consultation suite she had occupied for so long. One of her active clients was a young adult man in his early 30s who had consulted her for assistance in resolving grief related to the untimely death of his mother when he was a teenager.

Because of the tragic car crash in which his mother was killed, the client never had the chance to say goodbye, nor was he emotionally able to derive much comfort from the funeral with a closed casket. Among the therapeutic interventions the grief counselor used was directing the client to compose a eulogy for his deceased mother and, amid tears flowing, read it aloud during a counseling session. This intervention was employed to help the client honor his mother's role in his early upbringing and, at the same time, say goodbye symbolically and let go of the grief he internalized.

Clearly, there was a maternal quality to the transference relationship that developed over the course of the counseling. The grief counselor was acutely aware that she represented a mother figure to the client, who actively sought her advice and insight much as he might from a parent, particularly in matters related to partner relationships with women. This transference did not have an unhealthy dependency associated with it and had even been the subject of some good-natured humor between them.

Predictably, when the counselor informed the client of her plans to retire in a few months, he was initially distraught and engaged briefly in some regrieving over the death of his mother so many years before. The counselor assiduously turned the discussion to the topic of her retirement, and they processed its meaning for the client on several occasions. He admitted that he felt somehow orphaned by her decision and even expressed some anger toward her for electively leaving. At the same time, he was enormously grateful for her help and viewed her as a pivotal person in his life.

On the day of their final session, the client announced that he had written a "eulogy" for the grief counselor, meant to be a tribute to her formative influence and positive impact on his life. With a steady resolve and a calm voice, he insisted on reading it aloud to the counselor, who perceived accurately that listening and receiving this accolade was the most important thing she could do therapeutically at that moment. This time, the tears were hers, not his! It was a tender farewell and effectively completed their relationship (cf. Byock, 2004) so that their mutual departure that day, while bittersweet for both, was as much about growth for the client as it was about loss.

SUMMARY

Moving or closing a practice as a result of relocation or retirement presents several ethical challenges for the grief counselor. Protecting client welfare in the process requires fastidious attention to notification, referral, records management, licensure, professional liability coverage, and many other practice details. Careful planning makes possible moving or closing a practice with minimal hazards for the grief counselor and the clients. Therapy terminations associated with the grief counselor's relocation or retirement represent a recapitulation of other losses sustained by clients in grief counseling. It brings the loss experience full circle, so to speak, into the therapeutic encounter itself. As such, moving or closing a professional practice is replete with opportunity to achieve something uniquely beneficial for clients—teaching and showing them how leave-taking can occur in a healthy rather than harmful fashion and helping them realize that endings can be an occasion for growth as well as pain.

14 Reporting a Colleague or Facing a Complaint

Over the course of one's career, a grief counselor may face a situation of noticing unethical or unprofessional behavior by a colleague. Because all mental health professionals, whether novices or masters, are subject to blind spots (see the introduction in Chapter 1), mistakes may occur because practitioners do not even realize that the actions taken, or omitted, are a problem. In other cases, ethical misconduct may be intentional. Uncomfortable as these situations may be, grief counselors have an ethical obligation to respond to misconduct by another health care professional through informal peer monitoring (Koocher & Keith-Spiegel, 2008) or, when necessary, through formal reporting.

On the other hand, every counselor will make mistakes even with good intentions, adequate training, careful practice procedures, expert counseling skills, responsible business management, continuing education, and conscientious efforts to follow a credible model of decision making when facing ethical dilemmas, such as the Five P Model. A colleague may bring to the grief counselor's attention some ethical concern about the counselor's professional activity and seek to resolve the matter informally. Or the grief counselor may face a situation where a client files a formal complaint and the counselor becomes the object of an investigation by a licensing board or an ethics committee or is the subject of a lawsuit. In this chapter, we review the fundamental steps to follow when there is an ethical obligation to confront or report a colleague, as well as what to do when a charge of misconduct or an ethical complaint is filed against the grief counselor.

REPORTING A COLLEAGUE

Applying the Five P Model for ethical decision making is a useful way to conceptualize the issues involved when the grief counselor has to confront or report a colleague for a potential ethical infraction. As with any ethical dilemma, proceeding in a systematic fashion that accounts for the key variables is important.

Person

Who is the colleague in question? Is it someone known to the grief counselor? Is the colleague a casual acquaintance, a close associate, a business partner, a friend, an employee, or a supervisor? What if the colleague happens to be a personal nemesis or a professional competitor? Obviously, the relationship between the grief counselor and the colleague has much to do with how the ethical dilemma is interpreted and handled (Koocher & Keith-Spiegel, 2008). When one has an ethical concern, it may be easier to approach a colleague who is a friend compared with someone who is an antagonist. However, more is at stake when the colleague is a friend. As a result of confronting or reporting a colleague, friendships may be strengthened or strained, business relationships may be altered or severed, and research collaborations may be ruptured or lost. If the colleague under suspicion is someone for whom the counselor has little respect, the counselor must be careful not to let personal vendettas influence judgment about the situation.

When encountering unethical behavior or misconduct by another health care professional, an important consideration is identifying the *source* of the information. Who is the informant? Was the ethical impropriety something that the reporting counselor observed directly or discovered firsthand through documents and other evidence? Was the problem disclosed unwittingly by the colleague in question who happened to mention the situation without realizing that an infraction was involved? Or is the information coming from a secondhand source, such as a disgruntled client or a concerned coworker of the colleague in question? It is helpful for a concerned grief counselor to ask, "How do I know what I know?" because this is one of the first questions he or she can expect to be asked, either by the colleague whom he or she confronts or by the licensing board or ethics committee whom he or she contacts.

The time-honored adage "consider the source" applies to secondhand reports about a colleague's potential misbehavior. When receiving a secondhand report of a colleague's ethical misconduct, one must ask whether it comes from a credible source and whether that individual may have an agenda beyond legitimate reporting of an ethical impropriety. When a secondhand informant appears credible and seems to have a legitimate ethical complaint about a colleague, such as a client describing mistreatment by a previous provider, it may be possible to assist the client with developing an appropriate plan of action that will not require direct involvement by the grief counselor—for example, coaching the client on where and how to lodge a formal complaint (Koocher & Keith-Spiegel, 2008).

Problem

Before embarking on the road of confronting or reporting a colleague, one must be certain that the issue at hand constitutes an ethical problem. Koocher and Keith-Spiegel (2008) propose two criteria for deciding whether one should go forward with confronting or reporting a colleague for a suspected ethical breach. First, one should be able to identify the overarching moral principle involved or the specific ethics code provision or professional standard being violated. Second, one should be convinced that the alleged conduct may undermine the integrity of the profession or harm one or more of the consumers served by the colleague. Otherwise, one may be facing a situation where there are disagreements about therapy approaches, practice styles, or even personal views, but there is no actual ethical violation occurring. In the latter case, one is free to express feelings on such matters to a professional colleague, but the conversation should not be characterized as a professional duty to report.

Ethical misconduct runs the entire gamut of possibilities: misrepresenting one's credentials; practicing in an area for which one does not have sufficient competence; bypassing or undermining informed consent; breaching confidentiality; mishandling client records; engaging in compromising multiple relationships; using deceptive or fraudulent billing methods; mistreating clients, staff, or trainees; advertising falsely; prevaricating during expert testimony; tampering with research data;

plagiarizing publications; and so on. The list is endless. Pope and Vetter's (1992) survey study of ethically challenging or troubling situations faced by American psychologists showed five areas most frequently mentioned: confidentiality, multiple relationships, payment problems, dilemmas in educational environments, and forensic issues.

More recently, Pope and Vasquez (2007) reported unpublished data compiled by the Association of State and Provincial Psychology Boards on reasons that licensed psychologists were disciplined. Topping the lists for both the United States and Canada were "sexual/dual relationships" with clients and "unprofessional, unethical, negligent" practice. An earlier summary by Kirkland, Kirkland, and Reaves (2004) clarified that the first category reflected exclusively *sexualized* dual relationships. Kirkland et al. argued for a more specific and descriptive classification system for unprofessional conduct, such as sexual misconduct, conviction of crimes, fraudulent acts, or breach of confidentiality, in order to track more clearly specific infractions and related sanctions. Greater specificity is needed because many plea bargains result in a formal finding of unprofessional conduct as a way of providing sanctioned practitioners with a more innocuous or benign description of their unethical behavior.

Place

Place can be quite important in determining when and how to confront or report a colleague suspected of unethical behavior. For example, when the professional relationship between the reporting counselor and the suspected colleague is determined in part by an agency's organizational structure or hierarchy, this structure directly affects the resolution process.

If the colleague in question is subordinate to the reporting counselor (e.g., an employee or supervisee in the same clinic or department), the counselor bears administrative responsibility for confronting, correcting, and remediating any ethical misconduct perpetrated by that subordinate practitioner. This co-responsibility usually heightens the urgency of dealing with the problem. Internal agency policies for handling unethical or unprofessional behavior may be followed, raising questions of whether and when a colleague's behavior would be reported externally to a licensing board or an ethics committee of a professional association.

We believe that many instances of ethical impropriety are never reported to licensing boards or professional associations because they are handled internally by agencies or institutions as disciplinary actions or terminations. If the offending colleague's inappropriate behavior has been stopped or corrected, or the colleague has been dismissed from employment and thus effectively prevented from continuing the problem behavior *in that setting*, then the agency may consider the matter resolved. Institutional employers may be reluctant to report the incident(s) for two reasons. First, reporting the colleague to a licensing board or an ethics committee of a professional association may invite unwanted scrutiny of the institution's policies and procedures by that regulatory body. Second, reporting may prompt a countersuit by the dismissed colleague alleging defamation of character or wrongful termination. Most health care institutions and agencies prefer to avoid the cost and trouble involved in such legal disputes. These private resolutions to instances of ethical misconduct beg the question of what impact the offending colleague's future behavior may have on the profession or the public. Yet, one cannot be prosecuted for what one *might do* in the future. Welfel (2006) argued that resolution at the agency level is probably the preferred method for handling infractions of minor or moderate severity. However, serious infractions, such as sexual impropriety with a client or billing fraud, warrant formal reporting to a licensing board or ethics committee.

We are aware of a case where the grief counselor was the division director of mental health services with administrative responsibility for several mental health providers on staff in a large agency. One counselor employee was observed to follow inadequate record-keeping practices, such as failing to file evaluation reports and progress notes for sessions billed to third-party payers. The offending practitioner was reprimanded repeatedly and even placed on unpaid leave at one point. When the unethical behavior continued, the practitioner was terminated "for cause." The matter was never reported to the practitioner's licensing board because the supervising grief counselor believed that the agency had discharged its professional obligation to protect its clients from a lax provider and because the supervisor refused to recommend the dismissed individual for employment elsewhere.

On the other hand, what if the suspected colleague is a supervisor or superior of the reporting counselor in the same agency or institution? Then, concerns about job security, administrative reprisal, or whistleblower status may introduce hesitation and doubt about confronting or reporting. The inferior position in a vertical relationship is a very difficult place from which to address or confront potential ethical misconduct on the part of a colleague who is higher on the organizational chart. Agency policies for reporting unethical behavior may favor upper-level personnel. Going outside the agency to report ethical impropriety by a colleague holding superior rank could mean losing one's position. This threat leaves the counselor who is concerned about ethical impropriety on the part of a superior with the classic dilemma of "voting one's conscience" versus "voting one's pocketbook." It is also possible that an errant superior may intend for the grief counselor to participate in an unethical practice or activity. Maintaining one's ethical integrity means that the grief counselor does not knowingly violate the ethical codes and principles of the profession. The ADEC Code of Ethics addresses the situation of unethical employer demands.

> When employer demands require members to violate ethical principles, members clarify the nature of the conflict between the demands and the principles, inform all parties of members' ethical responsibilities, and take appropriate action consistent with prevailing ethical standards. (ADEC Code of Ethics, V. Responsibility to Employers, I)

Another way that place affects ethical decision making about confronting or reporting a colleague is consideration of the local professional community or one's professional association, of which both practitioners may be members. Reporting can have a detrimental effect on the suspected colleague's professional reputation and standing. In the same fashion, the counselor who reports the colleague may be viewed differently, perhaps as a hero by some and a rat by others. Polarized relationships, altered referral patterns, and shifting allegiances can result.

Principles

The ethical principle of justice is crucial in situations of confronting or reporting a colleague. Following the reasoning of rule deontological ethics (i.e., doing what is right), confronting or reporting a colleague's misbehavior means standing up for clients or the public who may be harmed and protecting the integrity of the profession. The preceding discussion illustrates how promoting the principle of justice can be an uncomfortable and unpopular stance, particularly if it entails negative consequences for the counselor confronting or reporting the colleague.

Aligned with a sense of justice are the dual principles of nonmaleficence and beneficence. The counselor willing to confront or report ethically problematic behavior in a colleague is acting to prevent harm to any parties at risk from the unethical behavior and promote a good outcome for all. Hopefully, the colleague may be persuaded to rectify the faulty behavior as a result of the experience. Thus, present and future clients may be protected, and other colleagues and members of the profession can retain an unsullied reputation.

The ADEC Code of Ethics addresses the issue of confronting or reporting a colleague whose behavior is errant or unethical:

> Ethical behavior among members and their associates, both members and nonmembers, is expected at all times. When a member becomes aware of another person's violation of ethical standards, the member attempts to rectify the situation. If the situation continues without a satisfactory ethical resolution, the member pursues the issue through appropriate channels. (ADEC Code of Ethics, I. General Conduct, C)
>
> If the member is unable or unwilling to remedy personal conditions that may jeopardize the welfare of the member's clients, it is ethical for another member or other professional person to intercede and assist the member in taking remedial action. (ADEC Code of Ethics, II. Competence, E)

Although these provisions certainly make it clear that a grief counselor with knowledge of a colleague's ethical misconduct has an obligation to intercede by taking some corrective action, the specific steps to be taken remain somewhat vague. The implication is that if the situation cannot be resolved satisfactorily between the confronting counselor and the errant colleague, additional action "through appropriate channels" is required. Presumably, this additional action means reporting the colleague.

The ACA Code of Ethics (ACA, 2005a) provides more specific guidance on dealing with suspected ethical violations by peers and outlines the ethical obligations of counselors confronting or reporting a colleague.

> When counselors possess knowledge that raises doubts as to whether another counselor is acting in an ethical manner, they take appropriate action. (ACA Code of Ethics, H.2.a.)
>
> When counselors have reason to believe that another counselor is violating or has violated an ethical standard, they attempt first to resolve the issue

> informally with the other counselor if feasible, provided such action does not violate confidentiality rights that may be involved. (ACA Code of Ethics, H.2.b.)
>
> If an apparent violation has substantially harmed, or is likely to substantially harm, a person or organization and is not appropriate for informal resolution or is not resolved properly, counselors take further action appropriate to the situation. Such action might include referral to state or national committees on professional ethics, voluntary national certification bodies, state licensing boards, or to the appropriate institutional authorities. This standard does not apply when an intervention would violate confidentiality rights. (ACA Code of Ethics, H.2.c.)
>
> When uncertain as to whether a particular situation or course of action may be in violation... counselors consult with other counselors who are knowledgeable about ethics... with colleagues, or with appropriate authorities. (ACA Code of Ethics, H.2.d.)

Process

The process of responding to a suspected ethical violation by a colleague starts with informal efforts at confronting and resolving the situation. Both the ADEC Code of Ethics and the ACA Code of Ethics encourage informal remedies as a first step in addressing ethical misconduct (cf. Welfel, 2006). Koocher and Keith-Spiegel (2008) offer tactical advice on how to approach the delicate task of confronting a colleague about an ethical concern. Consistent with the directive from the ACA Code of Ethics quoted previously, Koocher and Keith-Spiegel suggest first getting consultation from a trusted colleague to make sure that one is on the right track with the concerns that have been identified. They recommend talking to the offending colleague in person, where there is the best opportunity for a back-and-forth exchange conducive to settling matters of this kind, rather than giving in to the temptation to write an e-mail or call on the telephone to avoid a face-to-face confrontation. An educational attitude rather than an accusatory one is more constructive—state the concern directly, note the aspirational principle or ethics code provision in question, and present the evidence on which the concern is based. One should allow time for the colleague, who is likely to be caught off guard, to react and respond. Positive outcomes include an acknowledgment of the error by the offending colleague, together with openness to correction or remediation, or clarification by the colleague indicating that an ethical violation has not occurred.

Another way to approach one's colleague is to take a "one-down" position in order to give the colleague the benefit of the doubt: "John, I've received some information that says you have been overbilling Medicare and insurance for counseling services. As you know, these charges are very serious. Do you have any idea where these accusations may have originated? We need to go to the source and provide accurate information about how you are billing." A comment such as this one is not meant to set up a collusion of denial but to provide an opportunity for the colleague to clarify the situation. Because the one-down approach is not a direct accusation, the colleague may feel less need to respond defensively.

Unfortunately, attempts at informal resolution of an ethical concern may not go well or be received gracefully. If informal efforts to address potential ethical misconduct by a colleague result in denial, intransigence, or other responses that leave the grief counselor convinced that an ethical violation has or is occurring, it is necessary to take further appropriate action, that is, formally reporting the errant colleague. As stated in the ACA Code of Ethics (2005a), reporting a colleague might mean notifying agency or institutional supervisors, jurisdictional licensing boards, or state or national committees on professional ethics. According to Welfel (2006), professional associations commonly forward any complaint about a member to the licensing board in the state or jurisdiction where that member holds a license. Whichever reporting mechanism is used, the grief counselor who formally reports a colleague can expect a subsequent request to submit in writing the nature of the concern and the evidence on which it is based (ACA, 2005b). Accordingly, it is important to secure permission from disaffected clients or parties to include their confidential information in any formal report. Once a formal report has been made to a licensing board or an ethics committee, the reporting counselor has an ethical obligation to see the process through by cooperating with any investigation. The ACA Code of Ethics (ACA, 2005a) stipulates this requirement.

> Counselors cooperate with investigations, proceedings and requirements of the ACA Ethics Committee or ethics committees of other duly constituted associations or boards having jurisdiction over those charged with a violation. (ACA Code of Ethics, H.3.)

In the United States, clients who believe they have been injured or harmed by a mental health professional's unethical behavior have the option of filing a civil lawsuit. Ethical violations of a serious nature, such as sexual impropriety with a client or fraudulent billing practices, may result in criminal prosecution as well. Thus, there are multiple avenues of accountability when formally reporting a colleague for an ethical violation: reports to agency or institutional superiors, complaints to licensing boards or ethics committees, or lawsuits by the aggrieved clients themselves. Grief counselors may find themselves in the position of helping clients sort through the options for reporting and redressing grievances against a previous provider whose unethical behavior has harmed them (Welfel, 2006).

Grief counselors should be aware of the National Practitioner Data Bank (NPDB) maintained by the U.S. Department of Health and Human Services (2008). NPDB is a resource intended to encourage licensing boards, hospitals, and professional societies to identify and discipline health care professionals who engage in unprofessional behavior or ethical misconduct, especially when violators attempt to move from state to state without disclosure or discovery of previous unethical behavior. Physicians, counselors, nurses, psychologists, and social workers are reported to the NPDB when malpractice payments are made because of a claim or judgment against them or when adverse actions are taken against the practitioner's license, hospital privileges, professional society memberships, or Medicare/Medicaid reimbursement eligibility. This information is then made available when practitioners apply for jurisdictional licensure, hospital privileges, employment with a health care entity, or membership in a professional society, in order to assist in screening their qualifications, professional record, and character.

FACING A COMPLAINT

Grief counselors who are devoted to their careers as helping professionals and dedicated to accomplishing something beneficial for their clients do not want to think that an ethical complaint might ever be lodged against them. Although there is a low likelihood of facing a complaint over the course of one's career (cf. Pope & Vasquez, 2007), the possibility must be acknowledged. As with other potential hazards of professional practice, such as responding to suicidal clients in crisis or having a Professional Will in place in the event of the counselor's incapacity or sudden death, contingency planning is necessary to anticipate a dilemma such as facing a complaint and to ensure an ethical response on the part of the grief counselor. What happens to the grief counselor against whom a colleague, client, employer, or third-party payer registers a complaint, either informally or formally? How do grief counselors facing a complaint defend themselves and their actions if they believe they have acted with integrity? What is the best redemptive strategy if the counselor comes to recognize an ethical error as a result of the complaint? What is the appropriate relationship between the counselor and the party who initiated the complaint? What are the implications for a counselor's career after an ethical complaint has been settled?

If it is a colleague confronting the grief counselor about a potential ethical impropriety, Koocher and Keith-Spiegel (2008) suggest listening carefully and considering seriously the colleague's concern. Listening reflectively means quelling temporarily any shock, distress, and anger that may arise naturally when encountering constructive criticism from a peer. Perhaps clarification can demonstrate that no ethical violation has occurred. Alternately, if an ethical problem is verified, then corrective action can be initiated by the errant counselor to address the issue, begin making needed changes, and preclude a more protracted problem. Koocher and Keith-Spiegel even suggest that one can be grateful for the informal approach, which provides an opportunity to resolve the matter without the embarrassment of a full review by outside evaluators or more public forms of censure.

We are not so naive as to believe that such instances of informal peer monitoring always have a tidy, happy ending and that cool heads prevail. Grief counselors, too, are subject to human frailties such as defensiveness, bruised egos, confusion, resentful jealousy, rationalization, blind spots, or competitive counterattacks. It may take some time for one to work through difficult emotions before matters can be evaluated more clearly and resolved as a result of informal peer monitoring. Sometimes the matter may not be resolved at all.

When a grief counselor faces a formal complaint brought to a jurisdictional licensing board or an ethics committee of a professional association, Pope and Vasquez (2007) stress how important it is to avoid a state of panic that may lead to impulsive reactions or may undermine one's ability to respond thoughtfully. Additionally, Pope and Vasquez outline a series of steps designed to promote a sensible, well-reasoned response to serious charges of malpractice or ethical misconduct. Consulting one's attorney first and taking to heart the lawyer's counsel can prevent needless missteps such as trying to talk a client into withdrawing a complaint, venting one's frustrations to colleagues who later may be compelled to testify about those conversations, firing off an indignant e-mail, or contacting the opposing attorney. Any temptation to forgo or delay consulting one's own attorney leads Pope and Vasquez to remind practitioners that those who insist on self-representation "have a fool for a client."

Additional steps recommended by Pope and Vasquez (2007) include notifying one's professional liability carrier. It is important to understand if one's attorney actually works for the insurance carrier rather than directly for the grief counselor. This important distinction may influence how vigorously the case is investigated or defended. Some carriers may want to minimize costs by settling claims quickly rather than contesting them, even if the practitioner believes the claim is bogus. Probably the most challenging step in responding to a formal complaint is a searching, honest self-inventory regarding the behavior in question. Pope and Vasquez suggest counselors ask themselves, "Is there any truth to the allegation?" If there is validity to the claim, one needs to consider, in consultation with one's attorney, apologizing and accepting responsibility to set things right. Furthermore, one should be aware whether the complaint was inadvertently fostered by one's own faulty or arrogant communication style in counseling that left the client feeling there was no recourse other than a complaint or lawsuit to address a grievance.

Consider the case where the grief counselor was working with a bereaved mother and father whose only daughter died of a sudden heart attack at age 22. The daughter had been rebellious during her teenage years, and her wayward behavior had created a major rift with her parents. However, the daughter settled down, finished school, got married, and left her unsavory friends behind. The young woman was rebuilding a close bond with her parents and, when she became pregnant, drew even closer to her mother. This rapprochement seemed only to add to the tragedy when the daughter collapsed and died at a baby shower when she was 8 months pregnant. The baby was taken by caesarean section and survived but was hopelessly brain-damaged from lack of oxygen for a critical period. The young woman's bereft father demanded to talk to the obstetrician, believing that the doctor had mismanaged his daughter's congenital heart condition and, in effect, caused her death. The doctor refused any contact with the parents. After several failed attempts to communicate with the physician, the parents filed a malpractice lawsuit because they felt it was the only way they could hear from the doctor and have their questions answered.

Even though this tragic case example is about alleged medical malpractice, it illustrates two important points to remember about responding to client complaints. First, risk managers are quick to remind practitioners that a compassionate communication style, or a warm bedside manner, will go a long way toward ameliorating client dissatisfaction with an adverse treatment outcome and may engender a more forgiving attitude by clients toward practitioner mistakes or even ethical misjudgments. In the case example, if the physician had agreed to meet with the young woman's father, offered condolences for the daughter's tragic demise, and attempted a sincere explanation of medical factors beyond his control that led to her death (assuming that permission was given by the son-in-law for protected health information to be disclosed to the father; see Chapter 5 on confidentiality in postmortem circumstances), it is possible that a lawsuit may never have been filed.

Second, even though communicating with clients in a sincere, straightforward manner that demonstrates genuine caring may compensate for a multitude of counselor shortcomings, including ethical lapses, the time for talking is over once a colleague lodges a formal complaint or a client files a lawsuit. After a formal complaint or legal action is initiated, it is inappropriate for the grief counselor to contact directly the client or any individuals who are party to the action. Instead, grief counselors facing formal complaints should communicate only through their attorneys. Yet some counselors persist in believing that if they could just talk to the disgruntled client, the misunderstanding could be settled amicably and the problem dispatched. Appealing directly to disaffected parties who have filed a complaint is not only unwise strategically, but also prohibited legally. The formal complaint or lawsuit is a signal that the opportunity for informal resolution of the problem has expired.

In the final analysis, when a grief counselor is the object of a formal complaint or the subject of a lawsuit alleging unprofessional or unethical conduct, the counselor has an ethical obligation to see the process through to its conclusion. The guidance of an attorney is irreplaceable during the process of responding to a formal complaint. Cooperation with investigating bodies such as licensing boards or ethics committees is necessary. Timely responding to judges and courts is required. As in all things, it is important to tell the truth, even if that means acknowledging one's shortcomings or ethical failings and living with the consequences of one's actions (or inaction). Professional integrity demands no less. Yet when facing serious complaints that may stain one's professional reputation or jeopardize the future of one's counseling career, some practitioners may be tempted to rewrite history by altering client records to remove incriminating information or by fabricating a more favorable version of events to tell investigators. Paradoxical as it may seem, being truthful remains the best policy. Truthfulness does not sacrifice one's integrity on the altar of expediency when facing a complaint of ethical misconduct or a lawsuit alleging malpractice or unprofessional behavior, and that integrity may be the key to one's chances for future practice after an ethical error.

SUMMARY

Our fondest hope is that readers will never need personally the material explained in this final chapter on reporting a colleague or facing a complaint. Although no grief counselor can take complete responsibility for the actions of a colleague, there may be occasions where one has an obligation to step forward and confront or report a colleague who is violating the ethical standards of the profession. Reporting takes courage and leadership. Ethically conscientious grief counselors exercise moral leadership every day when they model sound ethical practice in their treatment of clients, trainees, support staff, and fellow professionals. Careful adherence to the guidelines and recommendations included throughout this text can minimize the probability that grief counselors will make unintentional, or intentional, ethical mistakes leading to a complaint or a lawsuit filed against them.

15 Epilogue

Our purpose in writing this book has been to provide grief counselors and mental health professionals the domain-specific information needed for sound ethical practice when caring for the dying and bereaved. Ethical practice begins with mastering the basic triad of death competence, consent, and confidentiality. Careful attention must be paid to the unique needs and challenges of caring for people at the end of life. Clearly, specialized knowledge in thanatology is a prerequisite for understanding various ethical dilemmas that can arise in grief counseling. In our exposition of the content areas covered in chapters throughout the book, we have strived to inform grief counselors about the issues and variables that create professional or ethical dilemmas when one works with grief- and bereavement-related problems in mental health.

Familiarity with at least one credible model of decision making enables the grief counselor to work through ethical challenges in a thoughtful, reflective manner rather than relying solely on an immediate intuitive response or falling prey to impulsivity. We propose the Five P Model as a vehicle for ethical decision making that is especially applicable to the domain of grief counseling: A *person* with a challenging ethical *problem* in a particular contextual *place* applies appropriate ethical *principles* in a deliberate decision-making *process*. By incorporating traditional, overarching ethical principles borrowed from the fields of medical ethics and psychology—autonomy, beneficence, nonmaleficence, justice, and fidelity—the Five P Model provides a systematic method for analyzing ethical dilemmas and charting a course for professional behavior that is therapeutically effective and ethically sound. Sound ethical practice is good counseling practice, and good counseling practice requires sound ethical practice. Our goal is that grief counselors practice their profession with uncompromising professional integrity that makes them a credit to themselves, an asset to the profession, an example to the community, and a sensitive, compassionate agent of healing for their clients.

Appendix A
Association for Death Education and Counseling (ADEC) Code of Ethics

INTRODUCTION[1]

Membership in ADEC commits members and student affiliates to comply with the standards of the ADEC Code of Ethics. A lack of awareness or a misunderstanding of an Ethical Standard is not itself a defense to a charge of unethical conduct.

The Preface and Basic Tenets are explicative and provide aspirational goals to guide thanatologists toward the highest ideals. Although the **Preface** and **Basic Tenets** are not themselves enforceable rules, they should be considered by thanatologists in arriving at an ethical course of action. Most of the Ethical Standards are written broadly, in order to apply to thanatologists in varied roles, although the application of an Ethical Standard may vary depending on the context. The Ethical Standards are not exhaustive. The fact that a given conduct is not specifically addressed by an Ethical Standard does not mean that it is necessarily either ethical or unethical. The Ethics Code applies across a variety of contexts, whether in person or by postal service, telephone, internet, and/or other electronic transmissions.

In the process of making decisions regarding their professional behavior, thanatologists must consider this Code of Ethics in addition to the applicable laws and professional board regulations that they are subject to. If this Code of Ethics establishes a higher standard of conduct than is required by law or other codes, thanatologists must meet the higher

---

Reprinted with permission.

[1] Portions of this Code of Ethics are based on the "Ethical Principles of Psychologists and Code of Conduct" (*American Psychologist,* 2002, 57, 1060–1073), which is the copyrighted property of the American Psychological Association. While the American Psychological Association has given permission to ADEC to utilize the APA Code of Ethics, APA has in no way advised, assisted, or encouraged ADEC to utilize the APA Code of Ethics. APA is in no way responsible for ADEC's decision to utilize the APA Code of Ethics, or for any actions or other consequences resulting from such use by ADEC.

ethical standard. If thanatologists' ethical responsibilities conflict with law, regulations, practice standards, or other governing legal authority, thanatologists make known their commitment to this Code of Ethics and take steps to resolve the conflict in a responsible manner.

PREFACE

The Association for Death Education and Counseling (herein referred to as the Association), founded in 1976, is an international, professional organization dedicated to promoting excellence in death education, care of the dying, and bereavement counseling and support. Based on quality research and theory, the Association provides information, support, and resources to its multicultural, multidisciplinary membership, and, through it, to the public.

The Association envisions a world in which dying, death, and bereavement are recognized as fundamental and significant aspects of the human experience. Therefore, the Association, ever committed to being on the forefront of thanatology, provides a home for professionals from diverse backgrounds to advance the body of knowledge and to promote practical applications of research and theory.

Recognizing the impact that death education and/or grief counseling can have upon the lives and well-being of people, the following is the Code of Ethics of the Association for Death Education and Counseling, adopted by the membership of the Association, and subscribed to by all who hold membership in the Association.

BASIC TENETS

1. Death education and grief counseling are based upon a thorough knowledge of valid death-related data, methodology, and theory rather than stereotypes or untested hypotheses. Thus, the practice of death education and/or grief counseling requires knowledge of current thanatological literature.
2. The member strives to understand his or her death-related feelings and experiences and the ways in which these may impact his or her thinking and work in the field.
3. The member takes care to know the student or client. Good education and counseling are based upon an understanding of, and a respect for, the student's or client's cultural background,

developmental status, perceptions, and other individual differences and needs.

4. The member neither exploits nor deceives others, but strives to improve the health and well-being of the individual and society. Fees, if charged, conform to an available schedule, consistent with comparable services. Research conforms to standards for human participation (as the Commission on Rights of Human Subjects has currently established).
5. The member serves in an advocacy role to assist the individual or society to cope with death-related issues. The member intervenes to prevent exploitation of the student or client and is obligated: (a) to be available to the student or client; and (b) to educate or counsel regarding rights, responsibilities and options with their possible consequences.
6. The member strives to present various views of a death-related question, indicating the member's own values if appropriate, and respecting the student's or client's choice among alternatives.
7. Recognizing that conflicts over the needs of the individual, family, institution, community, or society might arise, the member includes in his/her ongoing relationship, when appropriate, discussion of confidentiality and primary responsibility to the individual, to the family, to the institution, to the community, or to society.
8. The member recognizes his/her own limitations in meeting individual needs, and has available adequate consultation and referral resources. The member assesses the efficacy of his/her referral system by obtaining feedback from the referee, the referral resource, and knowledgeable consultants.
9. The member works to promote greater understanding among lay persons and professionals of dying and death so that each member of society can achieve a more satisfying life and personal acceptance of death.

ETHICAL STANDARDS

I. General Conduct

A. The Association is committed to defining and maintaining high standards of professional service and conduct. Members are responsible for keeping the Association informed about developments of new knowledge and improvements in skill development.

B. Members continually strive to improve themselves, their professions, and the Association through diligent efforts to improve professional practices, services, teaching, research, and the preparation of professionals.

C. Ethical behavior among members and their associates, both members and nonmembers, is expected at all times. When a member becomes aware of another person's violation of ethical standards, the member attempts to rectify the situation. If the situation continues without a satisfactory ethical resolution, the member pursues the issue through appropriate channels.

D. Members provide their professional services to anyone regardless of race, religion, gender, sexual orientation, socio-economic status, or choice of lifestyle. When the member cannot render service, the member makes an appropriate referral.

E. Members do not use their professional relationships to further their personal, political, religious, or business interests.

F. Sexual relationships with clients, students, and/or their significant others is unethical.

G. Members refrain from multiple relationships if (1) such relationships could reasonably be expected to impair the objectivity, competence, or effectiveness of the member in performing his/her responsibilities; or if (2) such relationships otherwise risk exploitation or harm to the person(s) with whom the professional relationship exists or formerly existed.

H. Members avoid conflicts of interest that interfere with professional discretion and impartial judgment. If a real or potential conflict of interest arises, members take reasonable steps to resolve the issue in a manner that reflects the best interests of the person(s) served.

I. Members neither offer, seek, nor accept payment of any kind for referrals.

II. Competence

A. Members continually strive to attain higher levels of competence. Each member is obliged to pursue continuing education and professional growth in all possible and appropriate ways, including participating in the affairs and activities of the Association and pursuing learning activities that lead to professional certification and licensure when available.

B. When called upon to deliver professional services, members accept only those positions and assignments for which they are professionally qualified.

C. Members are aware of the limits and boundaries of their professional competence and in no way represent themselves as having qualifications beyond those which they possess. Each member is responsible for correcting any misrepresentation other persons may make regarding that member's professional qualifications.

D. Members provide only those services and utilize only those techniques for which their training and experience qualifies them.

E. Members do not engage in professional activities when it is likely that personal problems or impairment may prevent them from performing such activities in a competent manner. In such situations, members seek appropriate professional consultation and assistance toward resolution of the situation. If the member is unable or unwilling to remedy personal conditions that may jeopardize the welfare of the member's clients, it is ethical for another member or other professional person to intercede and assist the member in taking remedial action.

III. Responsibilities to Those Served

A. The primary obligations of members are to respect the integrity of and to promote the welfare of clients and students.

B. When members believe that a client's or student's condition indicates that there is a foreseeable, serious, and imminent danger to the client, to the student, or to others, members take immediate, reasonable, and prudent action and/or inform appropriate authorities in accordance with applicable legal mandates. Consultation with other knowledgeable professionals is highly encouraged.

C. Members are free to consult with other professionals about clients and/or students provided that the consultation does not place the consultant in a position of conflict of interest and providing that all concerns of privacy, informed consent, and confidentiality are met appropriately.

D. In providing professional services to clients or students, members neither violate nor diminish their legal and civil rights.

E. Members who offer services, products or information via electronic transmission inform their clients and students of the risks to privacy and the limits of confidentiality.

F. Members take reasonable precautions to protect the confidentiality of clients/students in the event of the member's termination of practice, incapacitation or death. (1) Members insure confidentiality of client/student records; (2) Members either transfer client/student records to another professional, or assure secure storage of the records; (3) Clients/students or their legal guardians are informed about the termination of practice and about the transfer/storage of records.

IV. Responsibility to Others

A. Ethical, respectful and considerate behavior is expected of members at all times among and between professional associates, whether they are members or nonmembers.
B. Members respect the confidences colleagues share with them during the course of their professional relationships and transactions unless confidences transgress legal and ethical mandates to disclose.
C. Members who have responsibility for employing and/or evaluating the performance and achievements of others fulfill those responsibilities in a timely, fair, considerate, and equitable manner on the basis of clearly enunciated criteria. Members share their evaluation of a person with the person evaluated.
D. Members maintain familiarity with the network of professional and self-help systems in the community and assist clients to avail themselves of those resources as appropriate.
E. Members know and take into account the traditions and practices of other professional groups with whom they work and cooperate fully with those groups.

V. Responsibility to Employers

A. Members clarify and establish interpersonal relations and working agreements with supervisors and subordinates especially in matters of professional relationships, confidentiality, distinctions between public and private material, maintenance and use of recorded information, and work load accountability.
B. Members inform employers of conditions that may limit their effectiveness.
C. Members submit regularly to professional review and evaluation.

D. Members accept only those assignments that are within their competency.
E. Members are responsible for on-going continuing education and development of their expertise and the expertise of their subordinates. Continuing education and staff development should address current knowledge and emerging developments in the field.
F. Members work to improve the employer's policies, procedures, and effectiveness of services.
G. Members use employer resources only for purposes for which they were intended.
H. Members neither engage in nor condone illegal or discriminatory practices.
I. When employer demands require members to violate ethical principles, members clarify the nature of the conflict between the demands and the principles, inform all parties of members' ethical responsibilities, and take appropriate action consistent with prevailing ethical standards.

VII. Responsibility to Society

A. Members work to prevent and to eliminate discrimination against any person or group on the basis of age, color, race, gender, sexual orientation, lifestyle, religion, national origin, marital status, political belief, or mental or physical disability.
B. Members act to ensure that all persons whom they serve have access to the resources, services, and opportunities they require.
C. Members clarify whether they speak as individuals or as representatives of an organization.
D. Members provide their appropriate professional services in public emergencies.
E. Members interpret and share with the public their professional expertise regarding issues affecting the welfare of the society.

VIII. Confidentiality and Privacy

A. Members regard as confidential all information arising in the course of the professional relationship. Consideration for the client welfare is an abiding concern of members.
B. Members inform clients about the limits of confidentiality in a given situation.

C. Members obtain informed client consent prior to recording or allowing third party observation of their activities. Members inform clients about the purpose of recording/observing, who will have access to the recording and under what conditions, and the disposition of the recording. Client consent for one purpose is not valid for another or different purpose.
D. Members shall disclose confidential information when members believe there is clear and imminent danger to the client or to others, and that the danger can be alleviated or avoided by disclosing the information. In such circumstances, members are encouraged to consult with other knowledgeable professionals.
E. When members disclose confidential information without client consent, they do so only with appropriate others and only for compelling reasons.
F. Members safeguard written and recorded information about clients and are alert to potential threats to confidentiality in duplications processes, in use of computer equipment, and in electronic mail and facsimile transmission.
G. In those rare instances when members may disclose information, they disclose only that which is relevant within the context of the incident.
H. Members adequately disguise clinical and other material they use in teaching, writing, and public speaking in order to preserve client anonymity; an alternative is to obtain adequate prior client consent.
I. Members who have professional relationships with minor children assure them proper confidentiality. Members exercise careful judgment and respect applicable laws when discussing those children with their parents or guardians.
J. Client information received in confidence by one agent or agency is not forwarded to another without the client's written consent.
K. Members take into account an individual's capacity to give consent[.]

DEATH EDUCATORS AND TRAINERS

This section addresses those thanatologists who, on either a full-time or part-time or an occasional basis, function as a death educator or provide death education or training in any way to others.

DE-I. Responsibility to Others

A. Members in charge of programs establish learning experiences that integrate academic study and supervised practice. Such programs develop student skill, knowledge, and self-understanding.

B. Members orient students to program or learning expectations, basic skills development, and, when appropriate, to employment prospects prior to admission.

C. When a program or learning experience has a focus upon self-disclosure, self-understanding or growth, members ensure that potential students are made aware of this fact before they enter the program or begin the experience.

D. Members who employ exercises and simulations which draw upon participant thoughts, feelings, and memories must ensure that appropriate professional assistance is available to participants during and following those learning experiences.

E. When a student is expected to disclose relatively intimate or personal information about themselves as part of their learning experience, educators and supervisors shall not evaluate the student based upon such self-disclosure. The degree of self-disclosure will be respected without coercion or punitive measures.

F. When a program or learning experience has a focus upon self-disclosure, self-understanding or growth, members ensure the confidentiality and privacy of information shared in this setting.

G. Members make students aware of professional ethical responsibilities and standards.

H. When members function as educators, they maintain high standards of scholarship and objectivity. Members present information fully and accurately, and they provide appropriate recognition of alternative viewpoints.

DE-II. Standards of Professional Competence

A. Members assuming educative functions do so within their professional competence.

B. Members teach only in areas in which they have received professional preparation.

C. Members engage in continuous study and professional development in order to insure that they provide instruction based on the most current information available in the profession.

D. Members accurately cite or credit those authors and researchers whose work the member is presenting.

GRIEF COUNSELORS/THERAPISTS

This section refers to those thanatologists who, either on a full time or part-time or an occasional basis, function as grief counselors/therapists providing thanatology-related clinical services to others.

GC-I. Responsibility to Those Served

A. When members receive a referral, they actively seek all available, pertinent information from the client, legal guardian, or referral source, with appropriate written consent.
B. When a member is contacted by an individual who is receiving services from another agency or colleague, the member carefully considers the client's needs before agreeing to provide services. Members should (1) discuss with potential clients the nature of the client's current relationship with the other service provider and the possible risks and benefits of entering into a new professional relationship; (2) seek consent for exchange of information when it would be beneficial to the client. All resources utilized by the client should be documented appropriately.
C. Before members enter into professional relationships with potential clients, members inform clients/legal guardians about their expertise, techniques and other practices that may be used and that may affect the client's well being. Members clarify client/legal guardian goals and the purpose and expectations of the services they provide.
D. Clients/legal guardians are informed verbally and in writing at the time of the first interview about the limits of confidentiality as stipulated by law, regulation, or organizational process.
E. Prior to initiation of services, members notify clients/legal guardians of all financial responsibilities assumed by client/guardian or counselor. Fees for services, and any changes, must be identified and agreed to prior to services rendered. As a portion of their professional activities, members are encouraged to provide pro-bono or reduced fees to clients who experience financial constraints/difficulties.

F. Members make appointments with relatives or collateral[s] of clients only when clients have given their permission, unless an emergent situation requires another course of action. In this case, members consider legal and ethical implications and seek consultation before proceeding.

G. When members agree to provide services to clients at the requests of third parties, the nature of each of the relationships of the involved parties is clarified, accepted by all, and documented as such. Any limitations to confidentiality will be noted as well.

H. Members keep records and other information related to clients confidential for at least the number of years determined by laws in the member's state, province or country of practice.

I. Members should seek professional consultation whenever such consultation is in the best interests of those served.

J. If members determine that they are unable, or no longer capable of providing a particular service, they carefully prepare the client and assist in making appropriate arrangements for continuing care when necessary. The client's well being is of primary concern; therefore, every attempt is made to ensure that the client does not feel abandoned and that possible adverse effects are minimized. All efforts to this end should be documented.

GC-III. Responsibility to Others

A. Grief counselors/therapists do not solicit the clients of others.

B. Grief counselors/therapists fully cooperate with professionals who treat former clients of that provider.

C. Grief counselors/therapists are encouraged to offer their expertise in the geographical community in which they live and to take part in collaboration and interdisciplinary teamwork when working in a hospital or school environment.

RESEARCHERS IN THANATOLOGY[2]

This section refers to those thanatologists who, either on a full time, part-time or an occasional basis, function as researchers in thanatology-related subject areas.

---

[2] Ibid.

RT-I. Responsibility to Institutions

A. When institutional approval is required, members provide accurate information about their research proposals and obtain approval prior to conducting the research.

B. Members conduct research in accordance with approved research protocol.

RT-II. Responsibility to Research Participants

A. When obtaining informed consent, members inform participants about the purpose of the research, expected duration, and procedures; and about their right to decline to participate and to withdraw from the research study without penalty.

B. When members conduct research with clients/patients, students, or subordinates as participants, members take steps to protect the prospective participants from adverse consequences of declining or withdrawing from participation.

C. When research participation is a course requirement or an opportunity for extra credit, the prospective participant is given the choice of equitable alternative activities.

D. Members may dispense with informed consent only (1) where research would not reasonably be assumed to create distress or harm and involves (a) the study of normal educational practices, curricula, or classroom management methods conducted in educational settings; (b) the use of anonymous questionnaires, naturalistic observations, or archival research for which disclosure of responses would not place participants at risk of criminal or civil liability or damage their financial standing, employability, or reputation, and confidentiality is protected; or (c) the study of factors related to job or organization effectiveness conducted in organizational settings for which there is no risk to participants' employability, and confidentiality is protected or (2) where otherwise permitted by law or federal or institutional regulations.

E. Members provide a prompt opportunity for participants to obtain appropriate information about the nature, results, and conclusions of the research, and they take reasonable steps to correct any misconceptions that participants may have of which the members are aware. If scientific or humane values justify delaying or withholding this information, members take reasonable measures to reduce the risk of harm.

F. When members become aware that research procedures have harmed a participant, they take reasonable steps to minimize the harm.

RT-III. Responsibility in Reporting and Publishing Data

A. Members do not fabricate data.

B. If members discover significant errors in their published data, they take reasonable steps to correct such errors in a correction, retraction, erratum, or other appropriate publication means.

C. Members do not present portions of another's work or data as their own, even if the other work or data source is cited occasionally.

D. Members take responsibility and credit, including authorship credit, only for work they have actually performed or to which they have substantially contributed.

1. Principal authorship and other publication credits accurately reflect the relative scientific or professional contributions of the individuals involved, regardless of their relative status. Mere possession of an institutional position, such as department chair, does not justify authorship credit. Minor contributions to the research or to the writing for publications are acknowledged appropriately, such as in footnotes or in an introductory statement.
2. Except under exceptional circumstances, a student is listed as principal author on any multiple-authored article that is substantially based on the student's research. Faculty advisors discuss publication credit with students as early as feasible and throughout the research and publication process as appropriate.

E. Members who review material submitted for presentation, publication, grant, or research proposal review respect the confidentiality of and the proprietary rights in such information of those who submitted it.

Updated: March 3, 2006

ADEC is professionally managed by The Sherwood Group, Inc.,
111 Deer Lake Road, Suite 100, Deerfield, IL 60015 USA
telephone 847-509-0403 fax 847-480-9282
www.adec.org

Appendix B
Five P Model for Ethical Decision Making

"A *Person* with a challenging ethical *Problem* in a particular contextual *Place* applies appropriate ethical *Principles* in a deliberate decision-making *Process*."

1. ***Person:* Who is this person?**
   Age _____ Education _______ Economic background ________________________
   Single, Married or Partnered __________ Friends ______________________
   Home/Family (location) ____
   Ethnicity, Culture, Religion ____________________________________
   Community/Civic activities ____________________________________
   Strengths/Resources ____
   Other personal history (e.g., losses, decision-making style) ______________

2. ***Problem:* What is the specific ethical challenge to be resolved?**
   Statement of the problem ______________________________________
   ____
   Who is formulating the problem? ________________________________
   Who else has an interest in the problem? ________________________
   Is the problem properly stated? Other variables? ___________________

3. ***Place:* Where does the ethical dilemma occur?**
   Physical location ____
   Requirements of the setting? ___________________________________
   Agency/Institutional considerations? ____________________________

4. ***Principles:* What ethical principles are the focus of the problem?**
   Ethical principles: **(autonomy, beneficence, nonmaleficence, justice, fidelity)** ____
   ____
   Federal/State law ____
   Ethics of the profession/ADEC __________________________________
   Other considerations (e.g., personal narrative) ____________________

5. ***Process:* How will the decision be made?**
   How will information be gathered?_______________________________
   How will all voices be heard? ___________________________________
   What are the time limitations? __________________________________
   What ethical theory will be used? _______________________________
   Resolution: ____

Appendix C
Professional Will: Guidelines, Sample Template, and Instructions for Professional Executors

GUIDELINES FOR PREPARING YOUR PROFESSIONAL WILL

These guidelines for preparing a Professional Will are for information purposes only. This document does not provide legal advice and these suggestions are not equivalent to or a substitute for advice from an attorney. The authors offer no warranty regarding this sample Professional Will. Grief counselors should consult an attorney in order to draft a Professional Will appropriate to the unique demands of their professional situation.

The incapacitation or death of a counselor is an event with profound ramifications for families, friends, and clients. There are many legal, ethical, clinical, and personal issues for the practicing grief counselor to consider. When there is advance warning of serious health problems, one can plan ahead for the benefit of one's clients, help them get through it with as little trauma as possible and, sometimes, with further growth.

Sometimes there is no advance notice. Unexpected incapacitation or death is a real possibility for any grief counselor. Clients can perceive this as the ultimate abandonment. Overcoming denial means not waiting until retirement age to think about it. Responsible practitioners who really care about their clients' welfare will plan ahead against the possibility of unexpected incapacitation or death.

The completion of a Professional Will is a good way to ensure that, in such catastrophic scenarios, the most important bases are covered. This

---

The sample Professional Will provided is a composite of many different versions. It is modeled closely after one crafted by the San Diego Psychological Association's Committee on Psychologist Retirement, Incapacitation or Death (www.sdpsych.org or sdpa@sdpsych.org). It has been adapted for grief counselors and is used here with the permission of their Executive Director (S. J. Farrar, personal communication, March 29, 2008).

involves naming a professional executor, naming one's attorney, specifying the location(s) of one's records and anything necessary for access. It means providing a list of clients to be contacted and their phone numbers. For active clients, a Professional Will allows the smoothest possible transition of care under such difficult circumstances. It enables access to the grief counselor's voice mail and e-mail. It specifies one's malpractice carrier. It indicates the practitioner's wishes about client involvement in memorial services, if any. It specifies anything to be conveyed to clients after one's death.

Completing a Professional Will makes it much easier and less stressful for the grief counselor's family and personal executor to take care of what needs to be done with the practice in the event of sudden death or disability. Having a Professional Will is sound ethical practice. However, more than anything, completing a Professional Will communicates to clients a genuine concern about their welfare.

Disclaimer

First, it should be understood clearly that this document, even though it is called a "will," is not a substitute or replacement for one's personal last will and testament. It is intended only to give authority and instructions to the professional executor regarding one's counseling practice, in the event of incapacitation or death. Neither these guidelines nor the Professional Will should be construed as legal advice. Grief counselors should consult an attorney and anyone helping with estate planning to see if this Professional Will meets the need and is consistent with any other documents already in place.

Guidelines Only

This version of a Professional Will is only one of many possible ways of planning for what is to be done in the event of the grief counselor's incapacitation or death. These guidelines are designed to facilitate the process of thinking through the nature of one's professional practice and to suggest possible options and issues to consider in providing instructions for the professional executor.

Professional Executor

The designation of a professional executor may be the single most important function of this document. This designation will greatly facilitate the process of what needs to be done in the event of incapacitation or untimely death. The professional executor should be a fellow mental health professional whom the grief counselor respects and trusts. It is recommended to meet with this colleague as part of the process of writing a Professional Will in order to familiarize the colleague with one's practice and discuss what is envisioned. A Professional Will is most likely to be executed effectively if the professional executor is involved in the planning process. The professional executor needs the counselor's authority to take appropriate actions and to delegate activities to others so that no single person becomes overwhelmed by the magnitude of the task.

Backup Professional Executor

If for any reason the designated professional executor is unavailable or unable to perform this function, it is wise to have a backup. This backup may also be the best person to assist the professional executor in the event assistance is needed.

Attorney

The grief counselor should discuss with a knowledgeable attorney the details of how one's professional affairs will be handled. A final copy of the Professional Will should be filed with that attorney. The Professional Will should specify the attorney's name and contact information in order to expedite the professional executor's task.

Executor of Personal Will

Including the name and contact information of the executor of one's personal will allows the professional executor to reach this person quickly. There will be a number of things that the two of them will need to discuss and coordinate.

Client Records

The Professional Will should specify the location(s) of current and past client records. If not already so organized, the grief counselor should sort client records into these two groups and arrange them alphabetically. Specifying the date first seen and the date when the case was closed will also be helpful to the professional executor. If records are kept in a paper format, legibility is essential. Special care should be taken to ensure that demographic information (i.e., the client's name, phone number(s), address, and e-mail) is easily accessible.

Billing and Financial Records

The Professional Will should specify the location of billing and financial records. This information will allow the professional executor to assist the executor of one's estate in an orderly completion of any outstanding billing and financial transactions related to one's practice.

Appointment Book and Client Phone Numbers

This information will be one of the first items needed by the professional executor. Ready access to this information will allow clients for whom appointments have been scheduled to be contacted personally, rather than have them arrive at the office only to find the counselor not there. If appointment and treatment records are maintained electronically, the professional executor needs passwords and log-in information to access them.

E-mail Address Password and Voice Mail Access Code

Having this information readily available will allow one's voice mail or e-mail messages to be answered in a timely fashion. The voice mail greeting can be changed to reflect the new circumstances and indicate whom to contact if there are questions. If preferred, passwords and access codes can be specified in the Professional Will and the document kept with one's professional liability insurance information.

Keys

The professional executor should either maintain a duplicate set of keys or be able to locate easily the keys to one's office, filing cabinets, or storage facility.

Further Assistance in Locating/Accessing Records

Listing any other people who might be helpful in locating or accessing confidential counseling records, billing and financial records, appointment book, and telephone numbers is helpful. This might be a spouse, relative, secretary, office assistant, billing clerk, friend, or suite mate.

Location of Copies of Professional Will

It is suggested that the original Professional Will be filed with one's personal will and copies be given both to one's attorney and to the professional executor. In addition, it is recommended to file a copy with one's malpractice insurance policy. This step ensures that it will be seen annually and creates a regular opportunity to consider any changes that need to be made. Otherwise, it could be filed away and forgotten long past the time when much of the information is outdated.

Notification of Current and Past Clients

A list of current and selected past clients to be notified about one's death and any planned memorial services, along with their phone numbers, will allow this to be done smoothly. Notifying clients about incapacitation or death of the grief counselor can be done in a number of ways: by telephone; in writing; and/or through a notice in the newspaper. This can be left up to the discretion of the professional executor or specified in the Professional Will. It should be expected that some clients will want to talk to someone about the details of what happened to their counselor, much as they would if a family member had died. Some may require additional counseling. Ideally, one would identify fellow professionals to whom clients needing additional care could be referred.

Professional Liability Insurance

One's malpractice carrier should be notified as soon as possible after death. This step will allow arrangements for any additional coverage, if needed, to be made immediately. Such timely action can help protect one's estate.

Client Records

Record-keeping guidelines specified by state law and one's professional discipline should be followed by the professional executor. This process includes arrangements for storing, releasing, and disposing of confidential client records as may be appropriate. With authorized Release of Information, copies of a client's records may to be sent to the new therapist.

Reimbursement of the Professional Executor

The professional executor may spend considerable time discharging the duties required by one's Professional Will. It is reasonable to reimburse the professional executor for time spent and expenses incurred, particularly for later record maintenance. A reasonable reimbursement rate can be specified in one's Professional Will and provided for in one's estate. The professional executor needs some discretion in this matter and may consider some of the duties performed to constitute "grief work" for which no remuneration is required.

SAMPLE TEMPLATE

Professional Will

I, ________________________________, a resident of the County of ______________, State of __________, being of sound and disposing mind and memory, do hereby declare this to be my Professional Will. This supersedes all prior Professional Wills, in the event there are any. This is not a substitute for a personal last will and testament. It is intended to give authority and instructions to my professional executor regarding my counseling practice in the event of my incapacitation or death.

First

I am a licensed professional in independent practice. My _________ (specify discipline) License # is ________.

My office address is: ______________________________________

____

I also maintain an office at: __________________________________

____.

Second

In the event of my death or incapacitation, I hereby appoint _______ ________________, whose phone number is _____________ and whose office is located at: _______________________________

____

as my professional executor.

In the event that _________________ is unavailable or unable to perform this function, I hereby appoint ___________________ whose phone number is ______________ and whose office is located at: ____

__________________________________ as a backup professional executor.

I hereby grant my Professional Executors full authority to:

a. Act on my behalf in making decisions about storing, releasing, and/or disposing of my confidential client records;

b. Carry out any activities deemed necessary to properly administer this Professional Will;
c. Delegate and authorize other persons determined by them to assist and carry out any activities deemed necessary to properly administer this Professional Will.

Third

My attorney for my Professional Will is ____________________, whose phone number is ____________ and whose offices are located at: ____
____.

Fourth

The executor of my current personal will is __________________, whose phone number is __________________, and who is located at: ____
____.

Fifth

A. My current client records are located at: ____________________
____
__________________________________.

B. My past client records are located at: ________________________
____.

C. Billing and financial records related to my counseling practice are located at: _______________________________________
_____________________________.

D. Some or all of my client, billing, and financial records are on a computer, located at: ___________________________________
_____________________________________.

E. My appointment book and client telephone numbers are located at: ____
______________________.

F. My e-mail address is ________________________, and the password is ______________.

G. My office phone number is ____________________, and the voice mail access code is __________.

H. Any keys needed for access to my office, filing cabinets, or storage facilities are located at: ______________________________________

____

____.

I. For assistance in locating/ accessing my records, you may contact _______________, whose phone number is _____________, and whose address is: ____

____.

In addition, the following person(s) may be helpful in locating/ accessing my records:

____

____.

Sixth

My specific instructions for my professional executor are:

A. First of all, I would like to express my deep appreciation for your willingness to serve as the professional executor for this will.

B. There are four copies of this Professional Will. They are located as follows:
   a. One is in your possession.
   b. One is in the possession of my attorney.
   c. One is with my personal will.
   d. One is with my professional liability insurance policy.

C. A list of current and selected past clients and their phone numbers who are to be notified about my death and any planned memorial services is located with the copy of my Professional Will, in my professional liability insurance file. This file is located at: ____

____

____.

   a. Please use your professional judgment and discretion in deciding how you want to notify current and past clients and whether or not to publish in the newspaper a notice of my death and identifying whom to contact for further information.

b. If indicated in your judgment, you may wish to offer a face-to-face meeting with some clients. Please provide clients needing additional counseling with three referral names, which can, of course, include your own.

D. My professional liability insurance is currently provided by ___ ____, whose phone number is ____________, and whose address is: _________ ____.

My policy # is _________________.

Please notify my professional liability carrier of my death, in writing, as expeditiously as possible and arrange for any additional coverage that may be needed.

Please also notify the state licensing board at ________________.

E. Please arrange for copies of referred clients' records to go to their new therapists.

All remaining records, active and inactive, are to be maintained securely for the duration of time stipulated by state laws and by my professional code of ethics governing the storage of mental health records. Access is needed should records be requested for legitimate uses. When disposing of outdated records, please ensure it is done in a manner that destroys all materials that could identify the client (e.g., burning or shredding). It is also suggested that any records of individuals where there has been or is likely to be legal action(s) should be retained indefinitely.

F. If you need any further information or an update of requirements, you can contact the ______________________ (state professional association) at ______________________, or the Association for Death Education and Counseling, www.adec.org.

G. You may bill my estate for your time and any other expenses that you may incur in executing these instructions. Unless otherwise ordered by the court, the hourly rate of ___________ is acknowledged to be reasonable.

I declare under penalty of perjury and under the laws of the State of _________________ that the foregoing is true and correct.

Executed at (location) ________________, on (date) __________.

____
Signature

Witnesses

Printed Name: __________________ Signature: ________________
Residing at: ____

Printed Name: __________________ Signature: ________________
Residing at: ____

INSTRUCTIONS FOR THE PROFESSIONAL EXECUTOR

The professional executor serves an extremely important role when a colleague dies or becomes incapacitated. These guidelines are intended to facilitate this work, yet it is quite likely that some situations will arise that are not covered in these guidelines. Accordingly, it is essential to use professional judgment when discharging the duties of a professional executor and to seek consultation from others as needed. It is particularly important to cooperate with the executor of the colleague's estate. The professional executor has authority to delegate tasks and activities to others who may be in a position to assist with the many duties involved.

The following guidelines are organized by time periods, because immediate action is usually required surrounding a colleague's sudden death or incapacitation. Ultimately, duties continue for an extended period of time, up to a year or longer.

Immediate (Same Day/Next Day)

Welfare of Patients (Primary Concern)

1. Contact the family and/or executor and explain the role of the professional executor. Describe any assistance needed and attempt to coordinate with them. Naturally, it is important to remember that family members will be affected by shock, grief, and loss, requiring sensitivity to their condition.
2. Review the guidelines and directives of the Professional Will, if there is one.
3. Gain access to the deceased colleague's appointment calendar and phone records to prepare for contacting clients. Access the office computer or personal digital assistant (PDA), if records were kept electronically.
4. Gain access to the colleague's office and post a notice with a phone number to call. A sample note on the door might read: "Dr. ____________ is unavailable. For further information, please call me: (name) (area code) (phone number). Thank you. (Your signature)". It is important that any communication regarding a grief counselor's demise be communicated in person, not through a recorded phone message, a note taped to the door, or an e-mail blast. Such impersonal methods might

appear brutal and unkind, having a negative or traumatizing effect.

5. Gain access to the colleague's voice mail and change the greeting; leave a phone number to call. A sample greeting is similar to the note above: "Dr. ______________ is unavailable. I am Dr. ___________ and I am taking calls for him/her. Please leave a message with your phone number and a good time for you to receive a call, and I will return your call as soon as possible. Thank you."
6. Call the clients with same day/next day appointments to cancel. At that time, explain that the grief counselor has died or been incapacitated. Continue with cancellation of the current week's, and then the current month's, appointments.
7. In all contacts with clients, offer telephone triage, if needed, or offer to schedule an appointment or make referrals to other colleagues, as appropriate.

Related Professional Practice Issues

Inform office staff, colleagues, and building management.

Short-Term (First Week and Following Weeks)

Welfare of Patients

1. Form a liaison with the colleague's family regarding their wishes for funeral or memorial services, and whether they wish clients to attend.
2. If appropriate, notify all clients listed in the grief counselor's appointment records for the past year to apprise them of service plans.
3. Continue contact needed with current clients in order to address their needs, e.g., providing appointments or making referrals.
4. Confidential files should be placed in storage and released to another mental health provider upon receipt of an appropriately documented request. When records are in a handwritten format, it is strongly recommended that they be released only to another mental health professional in order to avoid any harm that might occur upon reading random notes which cannot be processed because the writer is not there.

Related Professional Practice Issues

1. Notify the state licensing board of the colleague's death or incapacitation and send needed documentation.
2. Inform the malpractice carrier within the first month following the colleague's death or incapacitation. It is necessary to do this in writing to ensure the addition of "tail" coverage to the insurance, if needed.
3. Advise the family or executor of the colleague's estate, as needed, regarding the dismantling of the colleague's office and its contents. Collection of outstanding bills is ultimately the responsibility of the family or the estate executor.

Long-Term (First Few Months and Beyond)

Welfare of Patients

1. Keep the colleague's telephone and voice mail active, ideally for up to a year. Update the greeting as appropriate, check weekly for messages, and respond as needed.
2. Continue to facilitate referrals and handle appropriately documented requests for transfer of records.
3. Arrange for permanent storage and disposition of confidential counseling records.

Related Professional Practice Issues

1. Inform ADEC, and any other international, national, state, or local professional organizations of which the grief counselor was a member.
2. Inform certification boards or any other credentialing bodies requiring annual renewals.
3. Cancel journal subscriptions.
4. Continue to be available to discuss the grief counselor's death or incapacitation with professional colleagues who learn of it at a later date.

Appendix D
Sample Client Information Brochure for Informed Consent for Grief Counseling

YOUR OFFICE'S LETTERHEAD

Your Name, Degree(s)
Special Certifications or Academic Affiliations
(e.g., CT, Certified in Thanatology, or
Associate Professor of Psychology, State University)
Address
Phone/Fax/E-mail

INFORMATION YOU NEED TO KNOW
ABOUT GRIEF COUNSELING...

PURPOSE

Grief counseling consists of a guided conversation with a professionally trained counselor about your loss experience. It is different from a social conversation. The purpose of grief counseling is to help you reach a better understanding of your loss-related problem and to work toward resolving the problem or finding a way to cope with it.

METHODS

Typically, grief counseling begins with you "telling your story" and describing the problems or dilemmas associated with your loss. Often, the counselor will ask you some questions to clarify things or better understand all dimensions of a problem before offering advice or suggesting alternatives. Thus, grief counseling is a joint effort between you and the counselor, and your active participation is a key element in its success.

DURATION

The initial session of grief counseling usually lasts 60–75 minutes in order for the counselor to fully evaluate your concerns and get to know you better by asking about your background and personal history. Follow-up meetings, if needed, are 45–50 minutes in length. The frequency of follow-up appointments can vary from weekly to monthly, depending on the nature and urgency of the problem.

Short-term grief counseling may be concluded in just a few sessions or in a matter of weeks. Other times, more lengthy counseling is needed and follow-up meetings may extend for a matter of months, or longer.

RISKS AND BENEFITS

Grief counseling can be a powerful experience with many potential benefits. While results cannot be guaranteed, most clients find grief counseling helpful. Progress depends on many factors such as the complexity of the problem, the motivation of the client, life circumstances, and the skill of the counselor.

Sometimes, simply confiding in the counselor helps relieve pressure and tension. Many clients feel unburdened by sharing their difficulties and their pain with a nonjudgmental, objective listener. Grief counselors use their expert knowledge and training to make recommendations, pose alternatives, and suggest possible solutions to loss-related problems.

However, there may be risks. Strong emotions or unpleasant memories may be stirred up. Because problems are addressed rather than avoided or postponed, your distress level may increase at first. Your personal relationships may be affected as a result of grief counseling if your family or friends do not understand the changes you are making. Generally, by the end of the initial meeting, most clients have a pretty good idea whether or not they think grief counseling will work for them.

ALTERNATIVES

Grief counseling is not for everyone. Some people find different ways to deal with their losses *without* consulting a grief counselor. For example, some simply "let time heal." Some may resolve to "pick themselves up and go on with their lives" as best they can. Others choose to take medicine to ease their emotional pain. Others may prefer to read self-help books, write in a journal, or practice alternative therapies like yoga or meditation. Support groups are available for bereaved persons as well.

WITHDRAWAL

Grief counseling is voluntary. You have the right to withdraw from grief counseling at any time if you do not wish to continue. Withdrawing from grief counseling carries no penalty or loss of benefits and does not prevent you from receiving health care services [at this institution] for any other conditions or problems.

COMPLAINTS

If grief counseling is not going well from your perspective, the first step is to tell the counselor that things are not satisfactory. If the difficulty cannot be worked out between the counselor and you, you have the right to request a transfer to another counselor.

If you believe the counselor has acted in an inappropriate or unprofessional manner, a complaint can be made by contacting [the Director of This Agency, Dr. First Surname, telephone number]. A complaint may also be lodged with the [State] Board of Examiners of [Professional Discipline, telephone number].

CONFIDENTIALITY

The information you convey to the grief counselor during a professional visit is confidential and will not be revealed to anyone without your consent. Knowing your session is confidential gives you the freedom to talk about whatever you choose in the grief counseling. If you wish someone else to receive information about your counseling, you will be asked to sign an Authorization to Release Information, which permits your counselor to communicate with that person.

Confidentiality is the basis of trust between you and your counselor. The grief counselor is bound to protect your privacy and will not reveal to anyone that you are even receiving counseling. Should the grief counselor ever ask for a colleague's opinion about how best to help you, no information is shared that would identify you personally.

If you wish to discuss the contents of your grief counseling with another person, that is your right. You may even wish to invite a family member or friend to attend a grief counseling session with you. In that case, you and the counselor work together to determine what will be discussed during the session for that person to hear.

It is important for you to know that there are *some exceptions to confidentiality* based on ethical principles followed by grief counselors as well as certain state laws. Here is a list of the situations that would require your grief counselor to break confidentiality.

- If the grief counselor believes you are *in danger of harming yourself,* such as planning to attempt suicide, the counselor is obligated to notify authorities or other appropriate persons to intervene.
- If the grief counselor believes you *intend to harm someone else,* or if you make threats to harm someone else, the counselor will notify the police to intervene. The person you have targeted or threatened will be notified as well.
- If the grief counselor receives information that *a child, an elderly person, or a disabled person is being abused or neglected,* either by you or by someone else, the counselor is obligated to contact Child Protective Services or Adult Protective Services.
- If a *court order, legal proceeding, or statutory law* requires the grief counselor to disclose information about your counseling, confidentiality cannot be maintained.
- Some *insurance companies or health maintenance organizations* require the release of certain counseling information (e.g., diagnosis, severity of the condition, or expected length of counseling) in order to determine the extent of benefits that will be paid for grief counseling services. If such information is required for insurance payment, it will be released.

Your privacy is also protected by the Federal Health Insurance Portability and Accountability Act (HIPAA). This law ensures the confidentiality of all electronic transmission of information about you, such as faxes or electronic billing. In these cases, special safeguards are used to protect your privacy. Please remember that *e-mail communications sent from your computer to the grief counselor are never completely confidential* because they are retained in the logs of your, or the grief counselor's, Internet service provider.

RECORDS

Good professional practice requires that counselors keep written records to document grief counseling services. Generally, such records consist of the date and time duration of your session, a summary of what was discussed, and, when necessary, a mental health diagnosis of your condition. The grief counselor is required to maintain such records in a secure manner so that no one else has access to them.

You are entitled to know what is in your counseling records. When grief counseling is ongoing, the counselor can discuss with you what information is in your records and explain in clear language what it means. Once grief counseling is concluded, you may request a copy of your counseling records or a written summary of what is recorded there.

In the event the grief counselor becomes sick and is unable to practice, or dies unexpectedly, custody of all professional records and billing information will pass to a designated colleague, [Dr. Best Friend, telephone number].

FEES

The grief counselor's professional charge for an initial evaluation lasting 60–75 minutes is [$ dollars]. The charge for follow-up visits lasting 45–50 minutes is [$ dollars]. Payment is due at the time of service.

When you require other services from the grief counselor that cannot be billed to your insurance, such as reviewing personal documents, reading e-mails, or talking on the telephone longer than [10] minutes, these services are charged at an hourly rate of [$ dollars]. The grief counselor will calculate this fee on a prorated basis, using 15-minute increments. In other words, every 15 minutes of time spent delivering these services will be billed at the rate of [$ dollars].

Feel free to ask the grief counselor any questions you may have about professional fees. However, it is your responsibility to clarify with your carrier any questions you have about your health insurance coverage or health plan benefits. Many plans require co-payments or pay only a percentage of billed professional charges. Any difference between the grief counselor's professional charge and amounts covered by your insurance carrier remain your responsibility to pay. Also, some plans limit the number of sessions they will reimburse.

If your account has not been paid for more than 60 days and arrangements for payment have not been made, the grief counselor retains the option of using a collection agency or other legal means to recover payment.

OFFICE HOURS

Appointments for grief counseling are scheduled during regular office hours from 8:00 a.m. to 5:00 p.m., [Monday through Friday]. Evening appointments are available on [Weekday] evening from 6:00 p.m. to 9:00 p.m. If you cannot keep a scheduled appointment, it should be cancelled at least 24 hours in advance. Otherwise, you may be assessed an administrative fee of [$ dollars].

Should you need to reach the grief counselor by telephone, please leave a message with [the office staff]. Every effort will be made to return your telephone call on the same day, usually at the end of ordinary office hours. If you need help after hours or on the weekends, please be aware that a rotating team of mental health professionals handles those calls so that you will probably not be speaking directly with your grief counselor.

If you have an emergency or crisis that requires immediate attention, you should call [the local crisis center, telephone number] or go directly to [Hospital] Emergency Department, [address, telephone number].

When the grief counselor is unavailable for an extended period due to professional travel, vacation, or other personal reasons, you will be provided with the name of a reputable grief counselor who may be contacted in the event that a need occurs while the grief counselor is away.

CREDENTIALS

[First name, Surname, degree] is licensed to practice grief counseling by the [State] Board of Examiners of [Discipline]. [Title, Surname] is

Certified in Thanatology (CT) by the Association for Death Education and Counseling (ADEC). This designates special knowledge in the areas of dying, death and bereavement.

[Title, Surname] earned [his/her, terminal degree] at [name] University and completed an [internship/supervised practicum] at [place, city, state]. [Title, Surname] has practiced grief counseling since [date]. [His/her] style of counseling is called [descriptive designation] and [brief explanation].

STATEMENT OF CLIENT CONSENT AND AUTHORIZATION

The process of grief counseling has been explained to me by the counselor. I have had an opportunity to read this client information brochure and have all of my questions answered. My signature below indicates that I understand and agree with what this document defines and limits. I freely consent to proceed with grief counseling.

I understand that I can discuss any of the provisions mentioned above with the grief counselor at any point in our meetings. I understand that I may withdraw my consent for counseling at any time, without penalty. A signed copy of this informed consent authorization will be given to me.

Signature of Client	Printed Name	Date

STATEMENT OF COUNSELOR WITNESSING CONSENT

I have carefully explained to the client the process and methods of grief counseling and have reviewed with the client the provisions of this informed consent authorization. I have responded to all questions. I believe the client fully understands the nature, demands, benefits, and possible risks involved with grief counseling. I can attest that I have witnessed the client's signature above and provided the client with a copy of this informed consent authorization.

Signature of Counselor	Printed Name	Date

References

Abbott, K. H., Sago, J. G., Breen, C. M., Abernethy, A. P., & Tulsky, J. A. (2001). Families looking back: One year after discussion of withdrawal or withholding of life-sustaining support. *Critical Care Medicine, 29,* 197–201.

Abt, P. L., Fisher, C. A., & Singhal, A. K. (2006). Donation after cardiac death in the US: History and use. *Journal of the American College of Surgeons, 203,* 208–225.

Adams, F. (Trans.). (2005, November 29). The Oath by Hippocrates: Written 400 B.C.E. In *Internet Classics Archive.* Retrieved March 26, 2008, from http://classics.mit.edu/Hippocrates/hippooath.html

Agarwal, P. (1991). *Passage from India: Post-1965 Indian immigrants and their children—Conflicts, concerns, solutions.* Palos Verdes, CA: Yuvati.

Aging With Dignity. (2007). *Five wishes.* Tallahassee, FL: Author. Retrieved September 14, 2008, from http://www.agingwithdignity.org

Ainsworth, M. (2002). My life as an e-patient. In R. C. Hsiung (Ed.), *e-Therapy: Case studies, guiding principles, and the clinical potential of the Internet* (pp. 194–215). New York: Norton.

Ainsworth, M. D. S., Blehar, M. C., Waters, E., & Wall, S. (1978). *Patterns of attachment: A psychological study of the strange situation.* Hillsdale, NJ: Erlbaum.

Allumbaugh, D. L., & Hoyt, W. T. (1999). Effectiveness of grief therapy: A meta-analysis. *Journal of Consulting Psychology, 46,* 370–380.

American Association for Marriage and Family Therapy. (2001). *AAMFT Code of Ethics.* Retrieved September 1, 2007, from http://www.aamft.org/resources/LRM_Plan/Ethics/ethicscode2001.asp

American Association of Retired Persons. (2005, December). Where there's a will, there's not always a way. *AARP Bulletin Today.* Retrieved September 22, 2008, from http://www.aarp.org/family/lifeafterloss/articles/where_will.html

American Counseling Association. (2005a). *ACA code of ethics.* Retrieved April 13, 2006, from http://www.counseling.org

American Counseling Association. (2005b). *ACA policies and procedures for processing complaints of ethical violations.* Retrieved October 22, 2008, from http://www.counseling.org/Resources/CodeOfEthics/TP/Home/CT2.aspx

American Medical Association. (2002). *Code of medical ethics: Current opinions.* Chicago: Author.

American Medical Association Council on Ethical and Judicial Affairs. (2000). *Confidentiality of health information postmortem* (Rep. No. 5-A-00). Available from the American Medical Association Ethics Standards Group. Chicago: Author.

American Nurses Association. (2001). *Code of ethics for nurses with interpretive statements.* Washington, DC: Author.
American Psychiatric Association. (2000). *Diagnostic and statistical manual of mental disorders* (4th ed., text rev.). Washington, DC: Author.
American Psychological Association. (1993). Guidelines for providers of psychological services to ethnic, linguistic, and culturally diverse populations. *American Psychologist,* 48, 45–48.
American Psychological Association. (2002). *Ethical principles of psychologists and code of conduct.* Retrieved April 13, 2006, from http://www.apa.org/ethics/
American Psychological Association. (2003). Guidelines on multicultural education, training, research, practice and organizational change for psychologists. *American Psychologist, 58,* 377–402.
Anderson, H. (1989). After the diagnosis: An operational theology for the terminally ill. *Journal of Pastoral Care, 43,* 141–150.
Anderson, S. K., & Kitchener, K. S. (1996). Nonromantic, nonsexual posttherapy relationships between psychologists and former clients: An exploratory study of critical incidents. *Professional Psychology: Research and Practice, 27,* 59–66.
Angus, L., Levitt, H., & Hardtke, K. (1999). The narrative processes coding system: Research applications and implications for clinical practice. *Journal of Clinical Psychology, 55,* 1255–1270.
Annas, G. J. (1991). Sounding board: The health care proxy and the living will. *New England Journal of Medicine, 324,* 1210–1213.
Ardelt, M. (2003). Physician-assisted death. In C. D. Bryant (Ed.), *Handbook of death and dying* (Vol. 1, pp. 424–434). Thousand Oaks, CA: Sage.
Associated Press. (2007, June 14). *Evangelist Billy Graham's wife dies at 87.* Retrieved June 19, 2007, from http://www.msnbc.msn.com
Association for Death Education and Counseling. (2006). Code of ethics. Retrieved April 13, 2006, from http://www.adec.org/about/ethics.cfm
Association of Professional Chaplains. (2000). *Code of ethics.* Retrieved April 13, 2006, from http://www.professionalchaplains.org
Aulisio, M. P., DeVita, M., & Luebke, D. (2007). Taking values seriously: Ethical challenges in organ donation and transplantation for critical care professionals. *Critical Care Medicine, 35* (Suppl. 2), S95–S101.
Balk, D. E. (2008). A modest proposal about bereavement and recovery. *Death Studies, 32,* 84–93.
Balk, D., Wogrin, C., Thornton, G., & Meagher, D. (2007). Certifications in thanatology: How the *Handbook of thanatology* can assist. In D. Balk, C. Wogrin, G. Thornton, & D. Meagher (Eds.), *Handbook of thanatology: The essential body of knowledge for the study of death, dying and bereavement* (pp. vii–xii). Northbrook, IL: Association for Death Education and Counseling, the Thanatology Association.
Ballou, M., Hill, M., & West, C. (2008). *Feminist therapy theory and practice: A contemporary perspective.* New York: Springer Publishing.
Barnett, J. E. (1997). Leaving a practice: Ethical and legal issues and dilemmas. In L. VandeCreek, S. Knapp, & T. L. Jackson (Eds.), *Innovations in clinical practice: A source book* (Vol. 15, pp. 181–188). Sarasota, FL: Professional Resource Press.
Barnett, J. E. (2007, September/October). Professional will is ethical and legal necessity. *National Psychologist,* p. 12.

Barnett, J. E., & Johnson, B. (2008). *Ethics desk reference for psychologists.* Washington, DC: American Psychological Association.

Barnett, J. E., & Scheetz, K. (2003). Technological advances and telehealth: Ethics, law, and the practice of psychotherapy. *Psychotherapy: Theory, Research, Practice, Training, 40,* 86–93.

Barnett, J. E., & Yutrzenka, B. A. (1994). Nonsexual dual relationships in professional practice, with special applications to rural and military communities. *Independent Practitioner, 14,* 243–248.

Bauer, G. P., & Kobos, J. C. (1987). *Brief therapy: Short-term psychodynamic intervention.* Northvale, NJ: Jason Aronson.

Beauchamp, T. L., & Childress, J. F. (2008). *Principles of biomedical ethics* (6th ed.). New York: Oxford University Press.

Beck, A. T., Rush, A. J., Shaw, B. F., & Emery, G. (1979). *Cognitive therapy of depression.* New York: Guilford.

Becker, E. (1973). *The denial of death.* New York: Macmillan.

Becvar, D. S. (2003). The impact on the family therapist of a focus on death, dying and bereavement. *Journal of Marital and Family Therapy, 29,* 469–477.

Begley, S. (2007, June 18). Get shrunk at your own risk. *Newsweek,* p. 49.

Bendiksen, R. (2001). Aftercare programs and ethical awareness: A first step in quality care to the bereaved. In O. D. Weeks & C. Johnson (Eds.), *When all the friends have gone: A guide for aftercare providers* (pp. 43–56). Amityville, NY: Baywood.

Beresford, L. (2003). Looking back at Columbine. In M. Lattanzi-Licht & K. J. Doka (Eds.), *Living with grief: Coping with public tragedy* (pp. 41–51). Washington, DC: Hospice Foundation of America.

Berg, J. (2001). Grave secrets: Legal and ethical analysis of postmortem confidentiality. *Connecticut Law Review, 34,* 81–122.

Bernat, J. L., D'Alessandro, A. M., Port, F. K., Bleck, T. P., Heard, S. O., Medina, J., et al. (2006). Report of a national conference on donation after cardiac death. *American Journal of Transplantation, 6,* 281–291.

Bernsen, A., Tabachnick, B. G., & Pope, K. S. (1994). National survey of social workers' sexual attraction to their clients: Results, implications, and comparison to psychologists. *Ethics and Behavior, 4,* 369–388.

Bersoff, D. N. (2002). Some contrarian concerns about law, psychology, and public policy. *Law and Human Behavior, 26,* 565–574.

Bersoff, D. N. (2003a). Confidentiality, privilege and privacy. In D. N. Bersoff (Ed.), *Ethical conflicts in psychology* (3rd ed., pp. 155–156). Washington, DC: American Psychological Association.

Bersoff, D. N. (2003b). Multiple relationships. In D. N. Bersoff (Ed.), *Ethical conflicts in psychology* (3rd ed., pp. 207–208). Washington, DC: American Psychological Association.

Beutler, L. E., Malik, M., Alimohamed, S., Harwood, T. M., Talebi, H., & Noble, S. (2004). Therapist variables. In M. J. Lambert (Ed.), *Bergin and Garfield's handbook of psychotherapy and behavior change* (pp. 227–306). New York: Wiley.

Biaggio, M., Paget, T. L., & Chenoweth, M. S. (1997). A model for ethical management of faculty-student dual relationships. *Professional Psychology: Research and Practice, 28,* 184–189.

Blevins-Knabe, B. (1992). The ethics of dual relationships in higher education. *Ethics and Behavior, 2,* 151–163.

Boelen, P. A., de Keijser, J., van den Hout, M. A., & van den Bout, J. (2007). Treatment of complicated grief: A comparison between cognitive-behavioral therapy and supportive counseling. *Journal of Consulting and Clinical Psychology, 75,* 277–284.

Boelen, P. A., & Prigerson, H. G. (2007). The influence of symptoms of prolonged grief disorder, depression, and anxiety on quality of life among bereaved adults: A prospective study. *European Archives of Psychiatry and Clinical Neuroscience, 257,* 444–452.

Bonanno, G. A. (1999). Emotional dissociation, self-deception, and adaptation to loss. In C. R. Figley (Ed.), *Traumatology of grieving* (pp. 89–105). Philadelphia: Taylor & Francis.

Bonanno, G. A. (2004). Loss, trauma and human resilience: Have we underestimated the human capacity to thrive after extremely aversive events? *American Psychologist, 59,* 20–28.

Bonanno, G. A., Wortman, C. B., Lehman, D. R., Tweed, R. G., Haring, M., Sonnega, J., et al. (2002). Resilience to loss and chronic grief: A prospective study from preloss to 18-months postloss. *Journal of Personality and Social Psychology, 83,* 1150–1164.

Bonanno, G. A., Wortman, C. B., & Nesse, R. M. (2004). Prospective patterns of resilience and maladjustment during widowhood. *Psychology and Aging, 19,* 260–271.

Bowlby, J. (1969). *Attachment and loss: Vol. 1. Attachment.* New York: Basic.

Bowlby, J. (1980). *Attachment and loss: Vol. 3. Loss, sadness and depression.* New York: Basic.

Bowlby, J. (1988). *A secure base: Parent–child attachment and healthy human development.* New York: Basic.

Braun, K. L., & Nichols, R. (1997). Death and dying in four Asian American cultures: A descriptive study. *Death Studies, 21,* 327–359.

Brodsky, S. L. (1991). *Testifying in court: Guidelines and maxims for the expert witness.* Washington, DC: American Psychological Association.

Brodsky, S. L. (1999). *The expert expert witness: More maxims and guidelines for testifying in court.* Washington, DC: American Psychological Association.

Brody, J. E. (2004, January 27). Often, time beats therapy for treating grief. *New York Times,* p. F7.

Bryant, C. D. (Ed.). (2003). *Handbook of death and dying* (2 vols.). Thousand Oaks, CA: Sage.

Buckman, R. (1992). *How to break bad news: A guide for health care professionals.* Baltimore, MD: Johns Hopkins University Press.

Burian, B. K., & O'Connor Slimp, A. (2000). Social dual-role relationships during internship: A decision-making model. *Professional Psychology: Research and Practice, 31,* 332–338.

Burke, C. A. (1995). Until death do us part: An exploration into confidentiality following the death of a client. *Professional Psychology: Research and Practice, 26,* 278–280.

Byock, I. (1997). *Dying well: Peace and possibilities at the end of life.* New York: Riverhead.

Byock, I. (2004). *The four things that matter most: A book about living.* New York: Simon & Schuster.

Calhoun, L. G., & Tedeschi, R. G. (2001). Posttraumatic growth: The positive lessons of loss. In R. A. Neimeyer (Ed.), *Meaning reconstruction and the experience of loss* (pp. 157–172). Washington, DC: American Psychological Association.

Calhoun, L. G., & Tedeschi, R. G. (Eds.). (2006). *Handbook of posttraumatic growth: Research and practice.* Mahwah, NJ: Lawrence Erlbaum.

Calo, T. J. (2005). The generativity track: A transitional approach to retirement. *Public Personnel Management, 34,* 301–312.

Campbell, C. D., & Gordon, M. C. (2003). Acknowledging the inevitable: Understanding multiple relationships in rural practice. *Professional Psychology: Research and Practice, 34,* 430–434.

Caplan, A. L. (2004). Transplantation at any price? *American Journal of Transplantation, 4,* 1933–1934.

Casarett, D., Kapo, J., & Caplan, A. (2005). Appropriate use of artificial nutrition and hydration—Fundamental principles and recommendations. *New England Journal of Medicine, 353,* 2607–2612.

Cavanagh, K., & Shapiro, D. A. (2004). Computer treatment for common mental health problems. *Journal of Clinical Psychology, 60,* 239–251.

Cavanagh, K., Zack, J. S., Shapiro, D. A., & Wright, J. H. (2003). Computer programs for psychotherapy. In S. Goss & K. Anthony (Eds.), *Technology in counseling and psychotherapy: A practitioner's guide* (pp. 143–164). Hampshire, England: Palgrave Macmillan.

Centers for Disease Control and Prevention. (2008). *U.S. Public Health Service Syphilis Study at Tuskegee: The Tuskegee timeline.* Retrieved September 1, 2008, from http://www.cdc.gov/Tuskegee/timeline.htm

Chan, J., Draper, B., & Banerjee, S. (2007). Deliberate self-harm in older adults: A review of the literature from 1995–2004. *International Journal of Geriatric Psychiatry, 22,* 720–732.

Chenneville, T. (2000). HIV, confidentiality, and duty to protect: A decision-making model. *Professional Psychology: Research and Practice, 31,* 661–670.

Christakis, N. A., & Asch, D. A. (1995). Physician characteristics associated with decisions to withdraw life support. *American Journal of Public Health, 85,* 367–372.

Clarke, D. M. (1999). Autonomy, rationality and the wish to die. *Journal of Medical Ethics, 25,* 457–462.

Clinebell, H. (1981). *Contemporary growth therapies.* Nashville, TN: Abingdon.

Cochrane, J. B., Levy, M. R., Fryer, J. E., & Oglesby, C. A. (1990–1991). Death anxiety, disclosure behaviors, and attitudes of oncologists toward terminal care. *Omega, 22,* 1–12.

Colbach, E. M. (1981). Integrity checks on the witness stand. *Bulletin of the American Academy of Psychiatry and the Law, 9,* 285–288.

Committee on Legal Issues, American Psychological Association. (2006). Strategies for private practitioners coping with subpoenas or compelled testimony for client records or test data. *Professional Psychology: Research and Practice, 37,* 215–222.

Committee on the Revision of the Specialty Guidelines for Forensic Psychology. (2008). *Specialty guidelines for forensic psychology.* Retrieved July 6, 2008, from http://www.ap-ls.org/links/22808sgfp.pdf

Cook, J. E., & Doyle, C. (2002). Working alliance in online therapy as compared to face-to-face therapy: Preliminary results. *CyberPsychology and Behavior, 5,* 95–105.

Corless, I. B. (2001). The HIV-AIDS patient: Holier than thou. In R. B. Gilbert (Ed.), *Healthcare and spirituality: Listening, assessing, caring* (pp. 189–200). Amityville, NY: Baywood.

Cozzens, D. (2004). *Sacred silence: Denial and the crisis in the church.* Collegeville, MN: Liturgical Press.

Curlin, F. A., Nwodim, B. A., Vance, J. L., Chin, M. H., & Lantos, J. D. (2008). To die, to sleep: US physicians' religious and other objections to physician-assisted suicide, terminal sedation, and withdrawal of life support. *American Journal of Hospice and Palliative Medicine, 25,* 112–120.

Currier, J. M., Neimeyer, R. A., & Berman, J. S. (2008). The effectiveness of psychotherapeutic interventions for bereaved persons: A comprehensive quantitative review. *Psychological Bulletin, 134,* 648–661.

Curtis, J. R. (2005). Interventions to improve care during withdrawal of life-sustaining treatments. *Journal of Palliative Medicine, 8*(Suppl. 1), S116–S131.

Curtis, J. R., & Rubenfeld, G. D. (2005). Improving palliative care for patients in the intensive care unit. *Journal of Palliative Medicine, 8,* 840–854.

Daubert v. Merrell Dow Pharmaceuticals, Inc., 509 U.S. 579 (1993).

Davies, D. J. (2003). Cremation. In C. D. Bryant (Ed.), *Handbook of death and dying* (Vol. 2, pp. 767–774). Thousand Oaks, CA: Sage.

Davis, C. G., Wohl, M. J. A., & Verberg, N. (2007). Profiles of posttraumatic growth following an unjust loss. *Death Studies, 31,* 693–712.

Dayton, T. (1994). *The drama within: Psychodrama and experiential therapy.* Deerfield Beach, FL: Health Communications.

Delmonico, F. L., & Graham, W. K. (2006). Direction of the Organ Procurement and Transplantation Network and United Network for Organ Sharing regarding the oversight of live donor transplantation and solicitation for organs. *American Journal of Transplantation, 6,* 37–40.

Diekema, D. S. (2003). Taking children seriously: What's so important about assent? *American Journal of Bioethics, 3,* 25–26.

Diekema, D. S. (2004). Parental refusals of medical treatment: The harm principle as threshold for state intervention. *Theoretical Medicine, 25,* 243–264.

Diekema, D. S. (2006, August). *Medical decision-making for children.* Paper presented at University of Washington conference on health care ethics, Seattle, Washington.

Doka, K. J. (1989). *Disenfranchised grief: Recognizing hidden sorrow.* New York: Wiley.

Donchin, A. (2004). Feminist bioethics. *Stanford encyclopedia of philosophy.* Retrieved August 26, 2007, from http://plato.stanford.edu/entries/feminist-bioethics/

Draper, B., Winfield, S., & Luscombe, G. (1997). The older psychiatrist and retirement. *International Journal of Geriatric Psychiatry, 12,* 233–239.

Driscoll, J. M. (1992). Keeping covenants and confidence sacred: One point of view. *Journal of Counseling and Development, 70,* 704–708.

Dyck, A. J. (2002). *Life's worth: The case against assisted suicide.* Grand Rapids, MI: Eerdmans.

Easterling, L. W., Gamino, L. A., Sewell, K. W., & Stirman, L. S. (2000). Spiritual experience, church attendance and bereavement. *Journal of Pastoral Care, 54,* 263–275.

Ekman, P., & Friesen, W. V. (2003). *Unmasking the face: A guide to recognizing emotions from facial clues.* Cambridge, MA: Malor.

Engel, G. L. (1961). Is grief a disease? *Psychosomatic Medicine, 23,* 18–22.

Erikson, E. H. (1963). *Childhood and society* (2nd ed.). New York: Norton.

Erlangsen, A., Bille-Brahe, U., & Jeune, B. (2003). Differences in suicide between the old and the oldest old. *Journal of Gerontology: Social Sciences, 58B,* S314–S322.

Ersek, M., Kagawa-Singer, M., Barnes, D., Blackhall, L., & Koenig, B. A. (1998). Multicultural considerations in the use of advance directives. *Oncology Nursing Forum, 25,* 1683–1690.

Ethics Committee of the American Psychological Association. (1986). Report of the Ethics Committee: 1985. *American Psychologist, 41,* 694–697.

Everly, G. S., & Mitchell, J. (2003). *Critical incident stress management (CISM): Individual crisis intervention and peer support* (2nd ed.). Ellicott City, MD: International Critical Incident Stress Foundation.

Everly, G. S., Phillips, S. B., Kane, D., & Feldman, D. (2006). Introduction to and overview of group psychological first aid. *Brief Treatment and Crisis Intervention, 6,* 130–136.

Everstine, L., Everstine, D. S., Heymann, G. M., True, R. H., Frey, D. H., Johnson, H. G., et al. (1980). Privacy and confidentiality in psychotherapy. *American Psychologist, 35,* 828–840.

Farber, E. W., & McDaniel, J. S. (1999). Assessment and psychotherapy practice implications of new combination antiviral therapies for HIV disease. *Professional Psychology: Research and Practice, 30,* 173–179.

Farley, M. (1985). *Feminist theology and bioethics.* In S. E. Lammers & A. Verhey (Eds.), *On moral medicine: Theological perspectives in medical ethics* (2nd ed., pp. 90–103). Grand Rapids, MI: Eerdmans.

Federal Rules of Evidence for United States Courts. (1975). St. Paul, MN: 195–198.

Feminist Therapy Institute. (2000). *Feminist therapy code of ethics.* Retrieved February 17, 2008, from http://feminist-therapy-institute.org/ethics.htm

Fenichel, M., Suler, J., Barak, A., Zelvin, E., Jones, G., Munro, K., et al. (2002). Myths and realities of online clinical work. *CyberPsychology and Behavior, 5,* 481–497.

Fieldsteel, N. D. (2005). When the therapist says goodbye. *International Journal of Group Psychotherapy, 55,* 245–279.

Figley, C. (1995). Compassion fatigue as secondary traumatic stress disorder: An overview. In C. R. Figley (Ed.), *Compassion fatigue: Coping with secondary traumatic stress disorder in those who treat the traumatized* (pp. 1–20). New York: Brunner/Mazel.

Fisher, C. B., & Fried, A. L. (2003). Internet-mediated psychological services and the American Psychological Association Ethics Code. *Psychotherapy: Theory, Research, Practice, Training, 40,* 103–111.

Flores, G. (2006). Language barriers to health care in the United States. *New England Journal of Medicine, 355,* 229–231.

Fortner, B. V., & Neimeyer, R. A. (1999). Death anxiety in older adults: A quantitative review. *Death Studies, 23,* 387–411.

Fraley, R. C., & Bonanno, G. A. (2004). Attachment and loss: A test of three competing models on the association between attachment-related avoidance and adaptation to bereavement. *Personality and Social Psychology Bulletin, 30,* 878–890.

Frank, J. D., & Frank, J. B. (1991). *Persuasion and healing: A comparative study of psychotherapy* (3rd ed.). Baltimore, MD: Johns Hopkins University Press.

Frantz, T. T., Farrell, M. M., & Trolley, B. C. (2001). Positive outcomes of losing a loved one. In R. A. Neimeyer (Ed.), *Meaning reconstruction and the experience of loss* (pp. 191–209). Washington, DC: American Psychological Association.

Friedmann, H., & Kohn, R. (2008). Mortality, or probability of death, from a suicidal act in the United States. *Suicide and Life-Threatening Behavior, 38,* 287–301.

Gabbard, G. O. (2000). *Psychodynamic psychiatry in clinical practice* (3rd ed.). Washington, DC: American Psychiatric Press.

Galea, S., Ahern, J., Resnick, H., Kilpatrick, D., Bucuvalas, M., Gold, J., et al. (2002). Psychological sequelae of the September 11 terrorist attacks in New York City. *New England Journal of Medicine, 346,* 982–987.

Gamble, S. J. (2002). Self-care for bereavement counselors. In N. B. Webb (Ed.), *Helping bereaved children: A handbook for practitioners* (pp. 346–362). New York: Guilford.

Gamino, L. A. (2003). Critical incident stress management and other crisis counseling approaches. In M. Lattanzi-Licht & K. J. Doka (Eds.), *Living with grief: Coping with public tragedy* (pp. 123–138). Washington, DC: Hospice Foundation of America.

Gamino, L. A., Easterling, L. W., & Sewell, K. W. (2003). The role of spiritual experience in adapting to bereavement. In G. R. Cox, R. A. Bendiksen, & R. G. Stevenson (Eds.), *Making sense of death: Spiritual, pastoral, and personal aspects of death, dying and bereavement* (pp. 13–27). Amityville, NY: Baywood.

Gamino, L. A., Hogan, N. S., & Sewell, K. W. (2002). Feeling the absence: A content analysis from the Scott & White Grief Study. *Death Studies, 26,* 793–813.

Gamino, L. A., & Sewell, K. W. (2004). Meaning constructs as predictors of bereavement adjustment: A report from the Scott & White Grief Study. *Death Studies, 28,* 397–421.

Gamino, L. A., Sewell, K. W., & Easterling, L. W. (1998). Scott & White Grief Study: An empirical test of predictors of intensified mourning. *Death Studies, 22,* 333–355.

Gamino, L. A., Sewell, K. W., & Easterling, L. W. (2000). Scott & White Grief Study—Phase II: Toward an adaptive model of grief. *Death Studies, 24,* 633–660.

Gamino, L. A., Sewell, K. W., Hogan, N. S., & Mason, S. L. (2008, May). *Who seeks grief counseling? Findings from Scott & White Grief Study.* Paper presented at meeting of Association for Death Education and Counseling, Montreal, Quebec, Canada.

Geyer, M. C. (1994). Dual role relationships and Christian counseling. *Journal of Psychology and Theology, 22,* 187–195.

Gilbert, R. B. (2003). Living, dying, and grieving in the margins. In G. R. Cox, R. A. Bendiksen, & R. G. Stevenson (Eds.), *Making sense of death: Spiritual, pastoral, and personal aspects of death, dying and bereavement* (pp. 191–203). Amityville, NY: Baywood.

Gilligan, C. (1982). *In a different voice: Psychological theory and women's development.* Cambridge, MA: Harvard University Press.

Glosoff, H. L., Herlihy, S. B., Herlihy, B., & Spence, E. B. (1997). Privileged communication in the psychologist–client relationship. *Professional Psychology: Research and Practice, 28,* 573–581.

Glosoff, H. L., Herlihy, B., & Spence, E. B. (2000). Privileged communication in the counselor–client relationship. *Journal of Counseling and Development, 78,* 454–462.

Goldblum, P. B., & Erickson, S. (2000, February). Understanding AIDS bereavement. *FOCUS: A Guide to AIDS Research and Counseling, 15,* 1–5.

Goldsmith, B., Morrison, R. S., Vanderwerker, L. C., & Prigerson, H. G. (2008). Elevated rates of prolonged grief disorder in African Americans. *Death Studies, 32,* 352–365.

Gostin, L. O. (2002). *Public health law and ethics: A reader.* Retrieved January 21, 2008, from http://www.publichealthlaw.net/Reader/docs/Tarasoff.pdf

Gottlieb, M. C. (1993). Avoiding exploitive dual relationships: A decision-making model. *Psychotherapy, 30,* 41–48.

Gottlieb, M. C., Sell, J. M., & Schoenfeld, L. S. (1988). Social/romantic relationships with present and former clients: State licensing board actions. *Professional Psychology: Research and Practice, 19,* 459–462.

Greenberg, S. A., & Shuman, D. W. (1997). Irreconcilable conflicts between therapeutic and forensic roles. *Professional Psychology: Research and Practice, 28,* 50–57.

Gripton, J., & Valentich, M. (2004). Dealing with non-sexual professional–client dual/multiple relationships in rural communities. *Rural Social Work, 9,* 216–225.

Grodin, M. A. (1992). Historical origins of the Nuremberg Code. In G. J. Annas & M. A. Grodin (Eds.), *The Nazi doctors and the Nuremberg Code* (pp. 121–144). New York: Oxford University Press.

Grohol, J. M. (1999). Best practices in e-therapy: Definition and scope of e-therapy. In *Online Mental Health Issues: Current Research and Publications.* Retrieved September 24, 2008, from http://www.ismho.org/builder//?p=page&id=216

Gutheil, T. G., & Gabbard, G. O. (1993). The concept of boundaries in clinical practice: Theoretical and risk management dimensions. *American Journal of Psychiatry, 150,* 188–196.

Gutheil, T. G., & Gabbard, G. O. (1998). Misuses and misunderstanding of boundary theory in clinical and regulatory settings. *American Journal of Psychiatry, 155,* 409–414.

Gutheil, T. G., Hauser, M., White, M. S., Spruiell, G., & Strasburger, L. H. (2003). "The whole truth" versus "the admissible truth": An ethics dilemma for expert witnesses. *Journal of the American Academy of Psychiatry and the Law, 31,* 422–427.

Haas, L. J. (1993). Competence and quality in the performance of forensic psychologists. *Ethics and Behavior, 3,* 251–156.

Haas, L. J., Benedict, J. G., & Kobos, J. C. (1996). Psychotherapy by telephone: Risks and benefits for psychologists and consumers. *Professional Psychology: Research and Practice, 27,* 154–160.

Haidt, J. (2001). The emotional dog and its rational tail: A social intuitionist approach to moral judgment. *Psychological Review, 108,* 814–834.

Handelsman, M. M. (2001). Accurate and effective informed consent. In E. R. Welfel & R. E. Ingersoll (Eds.), *The mental health desk reference: A sourcebook for counselors and therapists* (pp. 453–458). New York: Wiley.

Hardy, K. V. (1989). The theoretical myth of sameness: A critical issue in family treatment and training. In G. W. Saba, B. M. Karrer, & K. V. Hardy (Eds.), *Minorities and family therapy* (pp. 17–34). New York: Haworth.

Harrison Narcotics Tax Act, Publ. L. No. 63–223, Ch. 1, 38 Stat. 785 (1914).

Harvard Medical School. (2008). *A guide to living wills and health care proxies: How to protect your right to make crucial health care decisions.* Boston: Harvard Health.

Hauerwas, S. (1981). *A community of character: Toward a constructive Christian social ethic.* South Bend, IN: University of Notre Dame Press.

Health Insurance Portability and Accountability Act of 1996, 45 C.F.R. §§ 164.508–512. Retrieved April 13, 2006, from http://www.cms.hhs.gov/HIPAAGenInfo/

Hedlund, S. (2005, January/February/March). Death with dignity: The Oregon experience. *Forum, 31*(1), 1–3.

Heilbrun, K. (2001). *Principles of forensic mental health assessment.* New York: Kluwer Academic/Plenum.

Heinlen, K. T., Welfel, E. R., Richmond, E. N., & Rak, C. F. (2003). The scope of webcounseling: A survey of services and compliance with NBCC standards for the ethical practice of webcounseling. *Journal of Counseling and Development, 81,* 61–69.

Herbert, P. B. (2002). The duty to warn: A reconsideration and critique. *Journal of the American Academy of Psychiatry and the Law, 30,* 417–424.

Hickey, K. (2007). Minors' rights in medical decision making. *JONA'S Healthcare Law, Ethics, and Regulation, 9,* 100–104.

Hinrichsen, G. A. (2006). Why multicultural issues matter for practitioners working with older adults. *Professional Psychology: Research and Practice, 37,* 29–35.

Hogan, N. S., Greenfield, D. A., & Schmidt, L. A. (2001). The development and parametric testing of the Hogan Grief Reaction Checklist. *Death Studies, 25,* 1–35.

Hogan, N. S., & Schmidt, L. A. (2002). Testing the grief to personal growth model using structural equation modeling. *Death Studies, 26,* 615–634.

Hogan, N. S., Worden, J. W., & Schmidt, L. A. (2003–2004). An empirical study of the proposed complicated grief disorder criteria. *Omega, 48,* 263–277.

Hogan, N. S., Worden, J. W., & Schmidt, L. A. (2005–2006). Considerations in conceptualizing complicated grief. *Omega, 52,* 81–85.

Holmes, D. L., Rupert, P. A., Ross, S. A., & Shapera, W. E. (1999). Student perceptions of dual relationships between faculty and students. *Ethics and Behavior, 9,* 79–107.

Holst, L. (1991). Withholding nutrition and hydration: Some old and new questions. *Journal of Pastoral Care, 45,* 3–13.

Horowitz, M. (2005–2006). Meditating on complicated grief disorder as a diagnosis. *Omega, 52,* 87–89.

Hubble, M. A., Duncan, B. L., & Miller, S. D. (Eds.). (1999). *The heart and soul of change: What works in therapy.* Washington, DC: American Psychological Association.

Humphry, D. (2007). *Final exit: The practicalities of self-deliverance and assisted suicide for the dying* (3rd ed.). Junction City, OR: Euthansia Research & Guidance Organization.

Ingelfinger, J. R. (2005). Risks and benefits to the living donor. *New England Journal of Medicine, 353,* 447–449.

International Society for Mental Health Online. (2000). *Suggested principles for the online provision of mental health services.* Retrieved September 23, 2008, from http://www.ismho.org/builder/?p=page&id=214

Iserson, K. V. (2001). Commentary: The (partially) educated patient: A new paradigm? *Cambridge Quarterly of Healthcare Ethics, 10,* 154–156.

Jacobs, D. G., Brewer, M., & Klein-Benheim, M. (1999). Suicide assessment: An overview and recommended protocol. In D. G. Jacobs (Ed.), *The Harvard Medical School guide to suicide assessment and intervention* (pp. 3–39). San Francisco: Jossey-Bass.

Jacobs, L. M., Burns, K., & Jacobs, B. B. (2008). Trauma death: Views of the public and trauma professionals on death and dying from injuries. *Archives of Surgery, 143,* 730–735.

Jacobs, S. C. (1999). *Traumatic grief: Diagnosis, treatment and prevention.* Philadelphia: Brunner Mazel.

Jacobs, S. C., Mazure, C., & Prigerson, H. G. (2000). Diagnostic criteria for traumatic grief. *Death Studies, 24,* 185–199.

Jacobs, S. C., & Prigerson, H. G. (2000). Psychotherapy of traumatic grief: A review of evidence for psychotherapeutic treatments. *Death Studies, 24,* 479–495.

Jaffee v. Redmond, 518 U.S. 1 (1996).

Jelinek, S. (2002). The gay-lesbian-bisexual-transgendered patient. In R. B. Gilbert (Ed.), *Healthcare and spirituality: Listening, assessing, caring* (pp. 153–159). Amityville, NY: Baywood.

Jennings, B. (2005). How Americans want to die—grassroots values and cultural diversity. In K. J. Doka, B. Jennings, & C. A. Corr (Eds.), *Living with grief: Ethical dilemmas at the end of life* (pp. 85–99). Washington, DC: Hospice Foundation of America.

John Paul II. (2004, March). *Address of John Paul II to the participants in the International Congress on Life-Sustaining Treatments and Vegetative State: Scientific Advances and Ethical Dilemmas.* Retrieved September 10, 2008, from http://www.vatican.va/holy_father/john_paul_ii/speeches/2004/march/documents/hf_jp-ii_spe_20040320_congress-fiamc_en.html

Johnson, C., & Weeks, O. D. (2001). How to develop a successful aftercare program. In O. D. Weeks & C. Johnson (Eds.), *When all the friends have gone: A guide for aftercare providers* (pp. 5–23). Amityville, NY: Baywood.

Jones, J. (1981). *Bad blood: The Tuskegee syphilis experiment: A tragedy of race and medicine.* New York: Free Press.

Jonsen, A., Siegler, M., & Winslade, W. (2004). *Clinical ethics: A practical approach to ethical decisions in clinical medicine* (6th ed.). New York: McGraw Hill.

Jordan, J. R., & Neimeyer, R. A. (2003). Does grief counseling work? *Death Studies, 27,* 765–786.

Jordan, J. R., & Neimeyer, R. A. (2007). Historical and contemporary perspectives on assessment and intervention. In D. Balk, C. Wogrin, G. Thornton, & D. Meagher (Eds.), *Handbook of thanatology: The essential body of knowledge for the study of death, dying and bereavement* (pp. 213–225). Northbrook, IL: Association for Death Education and Counseling, the Thanatology Association.

Kalichman, S. C. (1999). *Mandated reporting of suspected child abuse: Ethics, law and policy.* Washington, DC: American Psychological Association.

Kalichman, S. C. (2003). *The inside story on AIDS: Experts answer your questions.* Washington, DC: American Psychological Association.

Kamat, V. (2005). The call of the yama and the Hindu funeral. *Family Therapy Magazine, 4,* 28–31.

Kant, I. (1959). *Foundations of the metaphysics of morals* (L. W. Beck, Trans.). Indianapolis, IN: Bobbs-Merrill. (Original work published 1789)

Kaplan, K. (Ed.). (2000). *Right to die versus sacredness of life.* Amityville, NY: Baywood.

Kaplan, R. M. (2004). Shared medical decision-making: A new tool for preventive medicine. *American Journal of Preventative Medicine, 26,* 81–83.

Kato, P. M., & Mann, T. (1999). A synthesis of psychological interventions for the bereaved. *Clinical Psychology Review, 19,* 275–296.

Kelly, M., & Barratt, G. (2007). Retirement: Phantasy and reality—dying in the saddle or facing up to it? *Psychodynamic Practice, 13,* 197–202.

Khulpateea, V. (1998). *Languages of south Asia.* Retrieved September 18, 2008, from http://www.english.emory.edu/Bahri/IndLangs.html

King, J. S., & Moulton, B. W. (2006). Rethinking informed consent: The case for shared medical decision-making. *American Journal of Law and Medicine, 32,* 429–502.

Kirchberg, T. M., & Neimeyer, R. A. (1991). Reactions of beginning counselors to situations involving death and dying. *Death Studies, 15,* 603–610.

Kirkland, K., Kirkland, K. L., & Reaves, R. P. (2004). On the professional use of disciplinary data. *Professional Psychology: Research and Practice, 35,* 179–184.

Kitchener, K. S. (1984). Intuition, critical evaluation and ethical principles: The foundation for ethical decisions in counseling psychology. *Counseling Psychologist, 12,* 43–55.

Kitchener, K. S. (1988). Dual role relationships: What makes them so problematic? *Journal of Counseling and Development, 67,* 217–221.

Klass, D. (2001). The inner representation of the dead child in the psychic and social narratives of bereaved parents. In R. A. Neimeyer (Ed.), *Meaning reconstruction and the experience of loss* (pp. 77–94). Washington, DC: American Psychological Association.

Klass, D., & Marwit, S. J. (1988–1989). Toward a model of parental grief. *Omega, 19,* 31–50.

Klass, D., Silverman, P. R., & Nickman, S. L. (Eds.). (1996). *Continuing bonds: New understandings of grief.* Washington, DC: Taylor & Francis.

Klass, D., & Walter, T. (2001). Processes of grieving: How bonds are continued. In M. S. Stroebe, R. O. Hansson, W. Stroebe, & H. Schut (Eds.), *Handbook of bereavement research: Consequences, coping and care* (pp. 431–448). Washington, DC: American Psychological Association.

Koenig, B. A., & Gates-Williams, J. (1995). Understanding cultural difference in caring for dying patients. *Western Journal of Medicine, 163,* 244–249.

Koenig, H. G., George, L. K., & Peterson, B. L. (1998). Religiosity and remission of depression in medically ill older patients. *American Journal of Psychiatry, 155,* 536–542.

Koocher, G. P. (2003). Ethical and legal issues in professional practice transitions. *Professional Psychology: Research and Practice, 34,* 383–387.

Koocher, G. P. (2005). Basic elements of consent. In G. P. Koocher, J. C. Norcross, & S. S. Hill III (Eds.), *Psychologists' Desk Reference* (2nd ed., pp. 645–646). New York: Oxford University Press.

Koocher, G. P., & Keith-Spiegel, P. (2008). *Ethics in psychology and the mental health professions: Standards and cases* (3rd ed.). New York: Oxford University Press.

Koocher, G. P., & Morray, E. (2000). Regulation of telepsychology: A survey of state attorneys general. *Professional Psychology: Research and Practice, 31,* 503–508.

Kottow, M. H. (1986). Medical confidentiality: An intransigent and absolute obligation. *Journal of Medical Ethics, 12,* 117–122.

Kunkel, A. D., & Dennis, M. R. (2003). Grief consolation in eulogy rhetoric: An integrative framework. *Death Studies, 27,* 1–38.

Kvale, J., Berg, L., Groff, J. Y., & Lange, G. (1999). Factors associated with residents' attitudes toward dying patients. *Family Medicine, 31,* 691–696.

Lambert, M. J. (2004). *Bergin and Garfield's handbook of psychotherapy and behavior change* (5th ed.). New York: Wiley.

Lamers, W. M., Jr. (2007a). Cruzan, Nancy. *Encyclopedia of death and dying.* Retrieved September 11, 2008, from http://www.deathreference.com/Ce-Da/Cruzan-Nancy.html

Lamers, W. M., Jr. (2007b). Quinlan, Karen Ann. *Encyclopedia of death and dying.* Retrieved September 11, 2008, from http://www.deathreference.com/Py-Se/Quinlan-Karen-Ann.html

LaRoche, M. J., & Maxie, A. (2003). Ten considerations in addressing cultural differences in psychotherapy. *Professional Psychology: Research and Practice, 34,* 180–186.

Larson, D. G., & Hoyt, W. T. (2007). What has become of grief counseling? An evaluation of the empirical foundations of the new pessimism. *Professional Psychology: Research and Practice, 38,* 347–355.

Lazarus, A. A. (1994). How certain boundaries and ethics diminish therapeutic effectiveness. *Ethics and Behavior, 4,* 255–261.

Lebacqz, K. (1985). *Bio-ethics: Some challenges from liberation perspectives.* In S. E. Lammers & A. Verhey (Eds.), *On moral medicine: Theological perspectives in medical ethics* (2nd ed., pp. 83–89). Grand Rapids, MI: Eerdmans.

Leibert, T., Archer, J., Jr., Muson, J., & York, G. (2006). An exploratory study of client perceptions of Internet counseling and the therapeutic alliance. *Journal of Mental Health Counseling, 28,* 69–83.

Lens, V. (2007a). Advance directives. *Encyclopedia of death and dying.* Retrieved September 11, 2008, from http://www.deathreference.com/A-Bi/Advance-Directives.html

Lens, V. (2007b). Natural death acts. *Encyclopedia of death and dying.* Retrieved September 11, 2008, from http://www.deathreference.com/Me-Nu/Natural-Death-Acts.html

Lichtenthal, W. G., Cruess, D. G., & Prigerson, H. G. (2004). A case for establishing complicated grief as a distinct mental disorder in *DSM-V. Clinical Psychology Review, 24,* 637–662.

Lindemann, E. (1944). Symptomatology and management of acute grief. *American Journal of Psychiatry, 101,* 141–148.

Lord, J. H. (2006). *No time for goodbyes: Coping with sorrow, anger, and injustice after a tragic death.* Burnsville, NC: Compassion Press.

Maheu, M. M. (2001). Telehealth: Practicing psychotherapy on the Internet: Risk management and great opportunity. *TelehealthNet.* Retrieved September 23, 2008, from http://telehealth.net/articles/njpa.html

Maheu, M. M., & Gordon, B. L. (2000). Counseling and therapy on the Internet. *Professional Psychology: Research and Practice, 31,* 484–489.

Main, M., & Hesse, E. (1990). Parents' unresolved traumatic experiences are related to infant disorganised attachment status: Is frightened and/or frightening parental behavior the linking mechanism? In M. Greenberg, D. Cicchetti, & M. Cummings (Eds.), *Attachment in the preschool years* (pp. 161–185). Chicago: University of Chicago Press.

Manhal-Baugus, M. (2001). E-therapy: Practical, ethical, and legal issues. *CyberPsychology and Behavior, 4,* 551–563.

Manosevitz, M., & Hays, K. F. (2003). Relocating your psychotherapy practice: Packing and unpacking. *Professional Psychology: Research and Practice, 34,* 375–382.

Maris, R. W. (1997). Social and familial risk factors in suicidal behavior. *Psychiatric Clinics of North America, 20,* 519–550.

Marshall, R. D., Amsel, L., Neria, Y., & Jung Suh, E. (2006). Strategies for dissemination of evidence-based treatments: Training clinicians after large-scale disasters. In F. H. Norris, M. J. Friedman, S. Galea, & P. J. Watson (Eds.), *Methods for disaster and mental health research* (pp. 226–239). New York: Guilford.

Martin, T. L., & Doka, K. J. (1999). *Men don't cry…women do: Transcending gender stereotypes of grief.* New York: Routledge.

Martin, T. L., & Wang, W. (2006). A pilot study of the development of a tool to measure instrumental and intuitive styles of grieving. *Omega, 53,* 263–276.

May, R. (1981). *Freedom and destiny.* New York: Norton.

McCullough, D. (2008). *My mother, your mother: Embracing slow medicine, the compassionate approach to caring for your aging loved ones.* New York: Harper Collins.

McGee, T. F. (2003). Observations on the retirement of professional psychologists. *Professional Psychology: Research and Practice, 34,* 388–395.

Medical Reserve Corps. (2008). *About the MRC.* Retrieved August 24, 2008, from http://www.medicalreservecorps.gov/HomePage

Mehrabian, A. (2007). *Non verbal communication.* New Brunswick, NJ: Transaction.

Melnick, J., Nevis, S. M., & Shub, N. (2005). Gestalt therapy methodology. In A. L. Woldt & S. M. Toman (Eds.), *Gestalt therapy: History, theory and practice* (pp. 101–115). Thousand Oaks, CA: Sage.

Mendenhall, T. J. (2006). Trauma-response teams: Inherent challenges and practical strategies in interdisciplinary fieldwork. *Families, Systems and Health, 24,* 357–362.

Meyer, C. (1998). *A good death: Challenges, choices and care options.* Mystic, CT: Twenty-Third Publications.

Middleton, W., Moylan, A., Raphael, B., Burnett, P., & Martinek, N. (1993). An international perspective on bereavement related concepts. *Australian and New Zealand Journal of Psychiatry, 27,* 457–463.

Miletich, L. (2001). Defining the essence of aftercare. In O. D. Weeks & C. Johnson (Eds.), *When all the friends have gone: A guide for aftercare providers* (pp. 25–34). Amityville, NY: Baywood.

Mill, J. S. (1972). *On liberty.* London: Dent. (Original work published 1859)

Millon, T. (1994). *MIPS: Millon Index of Personality Styles manual.* San Antonio, TX: Psychological Corporation/Harcourt Brace.

Milunsky, A. (2003). Lies, damned lies, and medical experts: The abrogation of responsibility by specialty organizations and a call for action. *Journal of Child Neurology, 18,* 413–419.

Miser, W. F. (2005). Educational research: To IRB or not to IRB? *Journal of Family Medicine, 37,* 168–173.

Monahan, J. (1993). Limiting therapist exposure to *Tarasoff* liability: Guidelines for risk containment. *American Psychologist, 48,* 242–250.

Monahan, J., Steadman, H., Silver, E., Appelbaum, P., Robbins, P., Mulvey, E., et al. (2001). *Rethinking risk assessment.* New York: Oxford University Press.

Moscicki, E. K. (1997). Identification of suicide risk factors using epidemiologic studies. *Psychiatric Clinics of North America, 20,* 499–517.

Mossman, D. (1999). "Hired guns," "whores," and "prostitutes": Case law references to clinicians of ill repute. *Journal of the American Academy of Psychiatry and the Law, 27,* 414–425.

Munson, R. (2002). *Raising the dead.* London: Oxford University Press.

Nadeau, J. W. (1998). *Families making sense of death.* Thousand Oaks, CA: Sage.

Nagy, T. F. (2000). *Ethics in plain English: An illustrative casebook for psychologists.* Washington, DC: American Psychological Association.

National Association of Social Workers. (1999). *Code of ethics of the National Association of Social Workers.* Retrieved April 13, 2006, from http://www.socialworkers.org/pubs/code/

National Board for Certified Counselors. (2007). The practice of Internet counseling. In *NBCC ethics information.* Retrieved September 23, 2008, from http://www.nbcc.org/AssetManagerFiles/ethics/internetCounseling.pdf

National Commission for the Protection of Human Subjects of Biomedical and Behavioral Research. (1979). *The Belmont report: Ethical principles and guidelines for the protection of human subjects of research.* Retrieved April 13, 2006, from http://www.hhs.gov/ohrp/humansubjects/guidance/belmont.htm

National Conference of Commissioners on Uniform State Laws. (1980). *Uniform Determination of Death Act.* Chicago, IL: Author.

National Conference of Commissioners on Uniform State Laws. (2006). *Revised Uniform Anatomical Gift Act.* Chicago, IL: Author.

National Institute of Mental Health. (2002). *Mental health and mass violence: Evidence-based early psychological intervention for victims/survivors of mass violence. A workshop to reach consensus on best practices* (NIH Publication No. 02–5138). Washington, DC: U.S. Government Printing Office. Retrieved August 4, 2008, from http://www.nimh.nih.gov/health/publications/massviolence.pdf

National Organ Transplant Act, Publ. L. 98–507 (1984).

National Voluntary Organizations Active in Disaster. (2005). *Early psychological intervention: Points of consensus document.* Retrieved August 4, 2008, from http://www.trynova.org/crt/epi/

Neimeyer, R. A. (1998). *Lessons of loss: A guide to coping.* New York: McGraw-Hill.

Neimeyer, R. A. (2000). Searching for the meaning of meaning: Grief therapy and the process of reconstruction. *Death Studies, 24,* 541–558.

Neimeyer, R. A. (2001). The language of loss: Grief therapy as a process of meaning reconstruction. In R. A. Neimeyer (Ed.), *Meaning reconstruction and the experience of loss* (pp. 261–292). Washington, DC: American Psychological Association.

Neimeyer, R. A., & Gamino, L. A. (2003). The experience of grief and bereavement. In C. D. Bryant (Ed.), *Handbook of death and dying* (Vol. 2, pp. 847–854). Thousand Oaks, CA: Sage.

Neimeyer, R. A., van Dyke, J. G., & Pennebaker, J. W. (2008). Narrative medicine: Writing through bereavement. In H. Chochinov & W. Breitbart (Eds.), *Handbook of psychiatry in palliative medicine* (pp. 454–469). New York: Oxford University Press.

Neimeyer, R. A., Wittkowski, J., & Moser, R. P. (2004). Psychological research on death attitudes: An overview and evaluation. *Death Studies, 28,* 309–340.

Neugarten, B. L., & Datan, N. (1996). The middle years. In D. Neugarten (Ed.), *The meaning of age: Selected papers of Bernice L. Neugarten* (pp. 135–159). Chicago: University of Chicago Press. (Original work published 1974)

Newman, A. (2001). Adolescent consent to routine medical and surgical treatment: A proposal to simplify the law of teenage medical decision-making. *Journal of Legal Medicine, 22,* 501–532.

Nickelson, D. W. (1998). Telehealth and the evolving health care system: Strategic opportunities for professional psychology. *Professional Psychology: Research and Practice, 29,* 527–535.

Nolan, J. R., Nolan-Haley, J. M., Connolly, M. J., Hicks, S. C., & Alibrandi, M. N. (1990). *Black's law dictionary: Definitions of the terms and phrases of American and English jurisprudence, ancient and modern by Henry Campbell Black, M. A.* (6th ed.). St. Paul, MN: West.

Norcross, J. C., & Barnett, J. E. (2008, Spring). Self-care as ethical imperative. *Register Report, 34,* 20–27.

Norcross, J. C., & Guy, J. D. (2007). *Leaving it at the office: A guide to psychotherapist self-care.* New York: Guilford.

Norris, F. H., Friedman, M. J., & Watson, P. J. (2002). 60,000 disaster victims speak: Part II. Summary and implications of disaster mental health research. *Psychiatry, 65,* 240–260.

Nouwen, H. J. M. (1979). *The wounded healer.* New York: Doubleday.

Oates, W. E. (1982). *The Christian pastor* (3rd ed.). Philadelphia: Westminster.

O'Connor Slimp, A., & Burian, B. K. (1994). Multiple role relationships during internship: Consequences and recommendations. *Professional Psychology: Research and Practice, 25,* 39–45.

Omnibus Budget Reconciliation Act, Pub. L. 101–508, 4206, 4751 (1990).

Orlinsky, D. E., Rønnestad, M. H., & Willutzki, U. (2004). Fifty years of psychotherapy process-outcome research: Continuity and change. In M. J. Lambert (Ed.), *Bergin and Garfield's handbook of psychotherapy and behavior change* (pp. 307–389). New York: Wiley.

Osofsky, J. D. (2008). In the aftermath of Hurricane Katrina: A personal story of a psychologist from New Orleans. *Professional Psychology: Research and Practice, 39,* 12–17.

Osterweis, M., Solomon, F., & Green, M. (Eds.). (1984). *Bereavement: Reactions, consequences, and care.* Washington, DC: National Academy Press.

Otto, R., & Heilbrun, K. (2002). The practice of forensic psychology: A look toward the future in light of the past. *American Psychologist, 57,* 5–18.

Parkes, C. M. (1990). Risk factors in bereavement: Implications for the prevention and treatment of pathologic grief. *Psychiatric Annals, 20,* 308–313.

Parkes, C. M. (2001). A historical overview of the scientific study of bereavement. In M. S. Stroebe, R. O. Hansson, W. Stroebe, & H. Schut (Eds.), *Handbook of bereavement research: Consequences, coping and care* (pp. 25–45). Washington, DC: American Psychological Association.

Parkes, C. M., & Weiss, R. S. (1983). *Recovery from bereavement.* New York: Basic.

Patient Self-Determination Act, Publ. L. No. 101–508, secs. 4206 and 4751, 104 Stat. 519 (1990).

Pellegrino, E. D., & Thomasma, D. C. (1993). *The virtue ethics in medical practice.* New York: Oxford University Press.

Pence, G. (2004). *Classic cases in medical ethics: Accounts of cases that have shaped medical ethics, with philosophical, legal and historical backgrounds* (4th ed.). Boston: McGraw Hill.

Pennebaker, J. W. (1997). Writing about emotional experiences as a therapeutic process. *Psychological Science, 8,* 162–166.

Pennebaker, J. W., Zech, E., & Rime, B. (2001). Disclosing and sharing emotion: Psychological, social and health consequences. In M. S. Stroebe, R. O. Hansson, W. Stroebe, & H. Schut (Eds.), *Handbook of bereavement research: Consequences, Coping and Care* (pp. 517–543). Washington, DC: American Psychological Association.

Perlman, H. H. (1957). *Social casework: A problem-solving process.* Chicago: University of Chicago Press.

Pettifor, J. L. (2004). Professional ethics across national boundaries. *European Psychologist, 9,* 264–272.

Piazza, M. (2005, April). *Ritual and mourning: Who has been left out?* Paper presented at the annual meeting of the Association for Death Education and Counseling, Albuquerque, NM.

Pomerantz, A. M., & Handelsman, M. M. (2004). Informed consent revisited: An updated written question format. *Professional Psychology: Research and Practice, 35,* 201–205.

Pope, K. S. (1988). How clients are harmed by sexual contact with mental health professionals: The syndrome and its prevalence. *Journal of Counseling and Development, 67,* 222–226.

Pope, K. S. (1994). *Sexual involvement with therapists: Patient assessment, subsequent therapy, forensics.* Washington, DC: American Psychological Association.

Pope, K. S. (2001). Sex between therapists and clients. In J. Worrell (Ed.), *Encyclopedia of women and gender* (Vol. 2, pp. 955–962). San Diego, CA: Academic Press.

Pope, K. S., & Bouhoutsos, J. C. (1986). *Sexual intimacies between therapists and patients.* Westport, CT: Praeger.

Pope, K. S., Keith-Spiegel, P., & Tabachnick, B. G. (1986). Sexual attraction to patients: The human therapist and the (sometimes) inhuman training system. *American Psychologist, 41,* 147–158.

Pope, K. S., Sonne, J. L., & Greene, B. (2006). *What therapists don't talk about and why: Understanding taboos that hurt us and our clients.* Washington, DC: American Psychological Association.

Pope, K. S., & Vasquez, M. J. T. (2007). *Ethics in psychotherapy and counseling: A practical guide* (3rd ed.). San Francisco: Jossey-Bass.

Pope, K. S., & Vetter, V. A. (1992). Ethical dilemmas encountered by members of the American Psychological Association: A national survey. *American Psychologist, 47,* 397–411.

Powell, T. (1999). Extubating Mrs. K: Psychological aspects of surrogate decision making. *Journal of Law, Medicine and Ethics, 27,* 81–86.

Prigerson, H. G., & Jacobs, S. C. (2001). Traumatic grief as a distinct disorder: A rationale, consensus criteria, and a preliminary empirical test. In M. S. Stroebe, R. O. Hansson, W. Stroebe, & H. Schut (Eds.), *Handbook of bereavement research: Consequences, Coping and Care* (pp. 613–645). Washington, DC: American Psychological Association.

Prigerson, H. G., & Maciejewski, P. K. (2005–2006). A call for sound empirical testing and evaluation of criteria for complicated grief proposed for *DSM-V. Omega, 52,* 9–19.

Prince v. Massachusetts, 321 U.S. 158 (1944).

Public Law 93–348. National Research Act. Retrieved September 2, 2008, from http://history.nih.gov./01docs/historical/documents/PL93-348.pdf

Qaseem, A., Snow, V., Shekelle, P., Casey, D. E., Jr., Cross, T. J., Jr., & Owens, D. K. (2008). Evidence-based interventions to improve the palliative care of pain, dypsnea, and depression at the end of life: A clinical practice guideline from the American College of Physicians. *Annals of Internal Medicine, 148,* 141–146.

Quill, T. E. (1991). Sounding board: Death and dignity: A case of individualized decision making. *New England Journal of Medicine, 324,* 691–694.

Quill, T. E. (1993). Doctor, I want to die. Will you help me? *Journal of the American Medical Association, 270,* 870–873.

Quill, T. E. (2001). *Caring for patients at the end of life: Facing an uncertain future together.* New York: Oxford University Press.

Quill, T. E., & Byock, I. R. (2000). Responding to intractable terminal suffering: The role of terminal sedation and voluntary refusal of food and fluids. *Annals of Internal Medicine, 132,* 408–414.

Quill, T. E., Lee, B. C., & Nunn, S. (2000). Palliative treatments of last resort: Choosing the least harmful alternative. *Annals of Internal Medicine, 132,* 488–493.

Ragusea, A. S., & VandeCreek, L. (2003). Suggestions for the ethical practice of online psychotherapy. *Psychotherapy: Theory, Research, Practice, Training, 40,* 94–102.

Rambachan, A. (2003). The Hindu way of death. In C. D. Bryant (Ed.), *Handbook of death and dying* (Vol. 2, pp. 640–648). Thousand Oaks, CA: Sage.

Rando, T. A. (1993). *Treatment of complicated mourning.* Champaign, IL: Research Press.

Rando, T. A. (2000). *Clinical dimensions of anticipatory mourning: Theory and practice in working with the dying, their loved ones and their caregivers.* Champaign, IL: Research Press.

Raphael, B. (1983). *The anatomy of bereavement.* New York: Basic.

Raphael, B. (1986). *When disaster strikes: How individuals and communities cope with catastrophe.* New York: Basic.

Raphael, B. (2007). The human touch and mass catastrophe: Commentary on "Five Essential Elements of Immediate and Mid-Term Mass Trauma Intervention: Empirical Evidence" by Hobfoll, Watson, et al. *Psychiatry, 70,* 329–336.

Rappeport, J. R. (1993). Ethics, the expert witness, and the search for a higher truth. *Hospital and Community Psychiatry, 44,* 390–391.

Recupero, P. R., & Rainey, S. E. (2005). Informed consent to e-therapy. *American Journal of Psychotherapy, 59,* 319–331.

Redmond, L. M. (1989). *Surviving when someone you love was murdered: A professional's guide to group grief therapy for families and friends of murder victims.* Clearwater, FL: Psychological Consultation and Education Services.

Resnik, D. B. (2001). Patient access to medical information in the computer age: Ethical concerns and issues. *Cambridge Quarterly of Healthcare Ethics, 10,* 147–156.

Richards, T. A. (2001). Spiritual resources following a partner's death from AIDS. In R. A. Neimeyer (Ed.), *Meaning reconstruction and the experience of loss* (pp. 173–190). Washington, DC: American Psychological Association.

Ritchie, E. C. (2003). Mass violence and early intervention: Best practice guidelines. *Primary Psychiatry, 10,* 43–48.

Ritter, R. H., Jr. (1990). The notion of an operational theology: A response to Herbert Anderson. *Journal of Pastoral Care, XLIV,* 283–286.

Ritter, R. H., Jr., Reis, M. D., & Rascoe, T. G. (2007). Interviewing techniques. In R. E. Rakel (Ed.), *Textbook of family medicine* (7th ed., pp. 293–301). New York: Saunders Elsevier.

Ritter, R. H., Jr., Smith, L., Santibanez, L., Ayub, M., & Tayi, R. (2005). A teaching project for training family medicine residents regarding the services of hospital chaplains. *Journal of Pastoral Care and Counseling, 59,* 255–261.

Robbins, J. H. (2006). A psychotherapist retires. *Women and Therapy, 29,* 189–203.

Roberts, D. A. (2003). A taste of heaven here on earth: For the dying and for the accompanier. In G. R. Cox, R. A. Bendiksen, & R. G. Stevenson (Eds.), *Making sense of death: Spiritual, pastoral, and personal aspects of death, dying and bereavement* (pp. 55–69). Amityville, NY: Baywood.

Roberts, R. G. (1997). Reducing malpractice risk. In M. B. Mengel & S. A. Fields (Eds.), *Introduction to clinical skills: A patient-centered textbook* (pp. 355–367). New York: Springer Publishing.

Robertson, J. A. (1999). The dead donor rule. *Hastings Center Report, 29,* 6–14.

Robson, D., & Robson, M. (2000). Ethical issues in Internet counseling. *Counseling Psychology Quarterly, 13,* 249–257.

Rochlen, A. B., Zack, J. S., & Speyer, C. (2004). Online therapy: Review of relevant definitions, debates, and current empirical support. *Journal of Clinical Psychology, 60,* 269–283.

Rocker, G. M., & Curtis, J. R. (2003). Caring for the dying in the intensive care unit. *Journal of the American Medical Association, 290,* 820–822.

Rogers, C. R. (1957). The necessary and sufficient conditions of therapeutic personality change. *Journal of Consulting Psychology, 21,* 95–103.

Roos, S. (2005, January/February/March). Mercy killing, chronic sorrow, and disability. *Forum, 31*(1), 4–5.

Rosser, B. R. S. (2008). Working as a psychologist in the Medical Reserve Corps: Providing mental health relief services in Hurricanes Katrina and Rita. *Professional Psychology: Research and Practice, 39,* 37–44.

Rudd, M. D. (2006). *The assessment and management of suicidality.* Sarasota, FL: Professional Resources Press.

Rudd, M. D., Joiner, T., & Rajab, M. H. (2001). *Treating suicidal behavior: An effective, time-limited approach.* New York: Guilford.

Ruzek, J. I., Brymer, M. J., Jacobs, A. K., Layne, C. M., Vernberg, E. M., & Watson, P. J. (2007). Psychological first aid. *Journal of Mental Health Counseling, 29,* 17–49.

Rynearson, E. K. (1987). Psychological adjustment to unnatural dying. In S. Zisook (Ed.), *Biopsychosocial aspects of bereavement* (pp. 77–93). Washington, DC: American Psychiatric Press.

Rynearson, E. K. (2001). *Retelling violent death.* Philadelphia: Brunner-Routledge.

Rynearson, E. K. (2006). Introduction. In E. K. Rynearson (Ed.), *Violent death: Resilience and intervention beyond the crisis* (pp. xxiii–xxxi). New York: Routledge.

Sacred Congregation for the Doctrine of the Faith. (1980). *Declaration on euthanasia.* Retrieved September 10, 2008, from http://www.vatican.va/roman_curia/congregations/cfaith/documents/rc_con_cfaith_doc_19800505_euthanasia_en.html

Sanders, C. M. (1984). Therapists, too, need to grieve. *Death Education, 8*(Suppl.), 27–35.

Satir, V. (1972). *Peoplemaking.* Palo Alto, CA: Science and Behavior Books.

Schank, J. A., & Skovholt, T. M. (1997). Dual-relationship dilemmas of rural and small-community psychologists. *Professional Psychology: Research and Practice, 28,* 44–49.

Schuck, P. H. (1994). Rethinking informed consent. *Yale Law Journal, 103,* 899–959.

Schultz-Ross, R. A. (1993). Ethics and the expert witness. *Hospital and Community Psychiatry, 44,* 388–389.

Schut, H., Stroebe, M. S., van den Bout, J., & Terheggen, M. (2001). The efficacy of bereavement interventions: Determining who benefits. In M. S. Stroebe, R. O. Hansson, W. Stroebe, & H. Schut (Eds.), *Handbook of bereavement research: Consequences, Coping and Care* (pp. 705–737). Washington, DC: American Psychological Association.

Scott, G. & Huffstutter, P. J. (2008, May 16). L. A. files 'cyber bully' charges against Missouri mother in connection with girl's suicide. *Los Angeles Times.* Retrieved July 3, 2008, from http://www.latimes.com/news/local/la-me-myspace16-2008may16,0,3642392.story

Searight, H. R., & Gafford, J. (2005). Cultural diversity at the end of life: Issues and guidelines for family physicians. *American Family Physician, 71,* 515–522.

Shapiro, F. (1995). *Eye movement desensitization and reprocessing: Basic principles, protocols, and procedures.* New York: Guilford.

Shaver, P. R., & Tancredy, C. M. (2001). Emotion, attachment, and bereavement: A conceptual commentary. In M. S. Stroebe, R. O. Hansson, W. Stroebe, & H. Schut (Eds.), *Handbook of bereavement research: Consequences, coping and care* (pp. 63–88). Washington, DC: American Psychological Association.

Shaw, H. E., & Shaw, S. F. (2006). Critical ethical issues in online counseling: Assessing current practices with an ethical intent checklist. *Journal of Counseling and Development, 84,* 41–53.

Shear, K., Frank, E., Houck, P. R., & Reynolds, C. F. (2005). Treatment of complicated grief: A randomized controlled trial. *Journal of the American Medical Association, 293,* 2601–2608.

Sheehan, M. N. (2008). Artificial nutrition and hydration and the permanently unconscious patient: The Catholic debate [Book review]. *Journal of the American Medical Association, 299,* 1610–1611.

Shuman, D. W. (2004). *Law and mental health professionals-Texas* (3rd ed.). Washington, DC: American Psychological Association.

Shuman, D. W., & Foote, W. (1999). *Jaffee v. Redmond's* impact: Life after the Supreme Court's recognition of a psychotherapist-patient privilege. *Professional Psychology: Research and Practice, 30,* 479–487.

Shuman, D. W., & Greenberg, S. A. (2003). The expert witness, the adversary system, and the voice of reason: Reconciling impartiality and advocacy. *Professional Psychology: Research and Practice, 34,* 219–224.

Shuman, D. W., Greenberg, S. A., Heilbrun, K., & Foote, W. (1998). An immodest proposal: Should treating mental health professionals be barred from testifying about their patients? *Behavioral Sciences and the Law, 16,* 509–523.

Sieger, C. E., Arnold, J. F., & Ahronheim, J. C. (2002). Refusing artificial nutrition and hydration: Does statutory law send the wrong message? *Journal of the American Geriatrics Society, 50,* 544–550.

Silver, R. C., Holman, E. A., McIntosh, D. N., Poulin, M., & Gil-Rivas, V. (2002). Nationwide longitudinal study of psychological responses to September 11. *Journal of the American Medical Association, 288,* 1235–1244.

Simon, R. I. (1995). The natural history of therapist sexual misconduct: Identification and prevention. *Psychiatric Annals, 25,* 90–94.

Simon, R. I., & Gutheil, T. G. (2003). The forensic expert on the road: New hazards along the way. *Psychiatric Annals, 33,* 302–307.

Simon, R. I., & Williams, I. C. (1999). Maintaining treatment boundaries in small communities and rural areas. *Psychiatric Services, 50,* 1440–1446.

Skinner, A., & Zack, J. S. (2004). Counseling and the Internet. *American Behavioral Scientist, 48,* 434–446.

Smart, R. N. (1996). *The religious experience of mankind* (5th ed.). Upper Saddle River, NJ: Prentice Hall.

Smith, M. C. (2004). *O'Connor's Federal Rules * Civil Trials.* Houston, TX: Jones McClure Publishing.

Smyth, J. M., & Pennebaker, J. W. (2008). Exploring the boundary conditions of expressive writing: In search of the right recipe. *British Journal of Health Psychology, 13,* 1–7.

Somberg, D. R., Stone, G. L., & Claiborn, C. D. (1993). Informed consent: Therapists' beliefs and practices. *Professional Psychology: Research and Practice, 24,* 153–159.

Sonne, J. L. (1994). Multiple relationships: Does the new ethics code answer the right questions? *Professional Psychology: Research and Practice, 25,* 336–343.

Sonne, J. L. (2005). *Nonsexual multiple relationships: A practical decision-making model for clinicians.* Retrieved September 16, 2007, from http://kspope.com/site/multiple-relationships.php

Statistics Canada. (2001). *Total population by ethnic origin, for Canada, provinces and territories, 1996 Census.* Retrieved September 18, 2008, from http://www.statcan.ca/english/census96/feb17/eo2can.htm

Steinbrook, R. (2005). Public solicitation of organ donors. *New England Journal of Medicine, 353,* 441–444.

Steinhauer, J. (2008, November 27). Verdict in MySpace suicide case. *New York Times,* p. A25.

Stephen Ministries. (2000). *Media fact sheet; Stephen Ministries St. Louis.* Retrieved August 19, 2007, from http://www.stephenministries.org/PDFs/SSMediaFactSheet.pdf

Stillion, J. M., & McDowell, E. E. (1996). *Suicide across the life span: Premature exits* (2nd ed.). Washington, DC: Taylor & Francis.

Stofle, G. S. (2002). Chat room therapy. In R. C. Hsiung (Ed.), *e-Therapy: Case studies, guiding principles, and the clinical potential of the Internet* (pp. 92–135). New York: Norton.

Strasburger, L. H., Gutheil, M. D., & Brodsky, A. (1997). On wearing two hats: Role conflict in serving as both psychotherapist and expert witness. *American Journal of Psychiatry, 154,* 448–456.

Stroebe, M. S. (2002). Paving the way: From early attachment theory to contemporary bereavement research. *Mortality, 7,* 127–138.

Stroebe, M. S., Hansson, R. O., Stroebe, W., & Schut, H. (2001). Introduction: Concepts and issues in contemporary research on bereavement. In M. S. Stroebe, R. O. Hansson, W. Stroebe, & H. Schut (Eds.), *Handbook of bereavement research: Consequences, coping and care* (pp. 3–22). Washington, DC: American Psychological Association.

Stroebe, M., & Schut, H. (1999). The dual process model of coping with bereavement: Rationale and description. *Death Studies, 23,* 197–224.

Stroebe, M. S., Schut, H., & Stroebe, W. (2005). Attachment in coping with bereavement: A theoretical integration. *Review of Clinical Psychology, 9,* 48–66.

Strong, C. (1995). Respecting the health care decision-making capacity of minors. *Bioethics Forum, 11,* 7–12.

Sue, D. W., & Sue, D. (2003). *Counseling the culturally diverse: Theory and practice* (4th ed.). New York: Wiley.

Suler, J. (2004). The online disinhibition effect. *CyberPsychology and Behavior, 7,* 321–326.

Sullivan, H. S. (1954). *The psychiatric interview.* New York: Norton.

Sulmasy, D. P., Haller, K., & Terry, P. B. (1994). More talk, less paper: Predicting accuracy of substituted judgments. *American Journal of Medicine, 96,* 432–438.

Sulmasy, D. P., Sood, J. R., & Ury, W. A. (2008). Physicians' confidence in discussing do not resuscitate orders with patients and surrogates. *Journal of Medical Ethics, 34,* 96–101.

Tarasoff v. The Regents of the University of California, 551 P.2d 334 (Calif. 1976).

Tedeschi, R. G., & Calhoun, L. G. (1995). *Trauma and transformation.* Thousand Oaks, CA: Sage.

Templer, D. I., Awadalla, A., Al-Fayez, G., Frazee, J., Bassman, L., Connelly, H. J., et al. (2006). Construction of a death anxiety scale—extended. *Omega, 53,* 209–226.

Terry, M. L., Bivens, A. J., & Neimeyer, R. A. (1995). Comfort and empathy of experienced counselors in client situations involving death and loss. *Omega, 32,* 269–285.

Truog, R. D. (2005). The ethics of organ donation by living donors. *New England Journal of Medicine, 353,* 444–446.

Truog, R. D. (2007). Brain death—too flawed to endure, too ingrained to abandon. *Journal of Law, Medicine and Ethics, 35,* 273–281.

Truog, R. D., Campbell, M. L., Curtis, J. R., Haas, C. E., Luce, J. M., Rubenfeld, G. D., et al. (2008). Recommendations for end-of-life care in the intensive care unit: A consensus statement by the American Academy of Critical Care Medicine. *Critical Care Medicine, 36,* 953–963.

Tucillo, J. A., DeFilippis, N. A., Denney, R. L., & Dsurney, J. (2002). Licensure requirements for interjurisdictional forensic evaluations. *Professional Psychology: Research and Practice, 33,* 377–383.

Tuskegee University. (2008). *Research ethics: The Tuskegee Syphilis Study.* Retrieved September 1, 2008, from http://www.tuskegee.edu/global/story.asp?s=1207598

United Network for Organ Sharing. (2004). *How the transplant system works: Matching donors and recipients.* Retrieved September 14, 2008, from http://www.unos.org/Resources/factsheets.asp

U.S. Department of Commerce, Economics and Statistics Administration and U.S. Census Bureau. (2006). *Statistical abstracts of the United States: 2007.* Washington, DC: U.S. Government Printing Office.

U.S. Department of Health and Human Services. (2005). Policy for protection of human research subjects, 45 C.F.R. Part 46.101–409.

U.S. Department of Health and Human Services. (2008). *Fact sheet on the national practitioner data bank.* Retrieved October 22, 2008, from http://www.npdb-hipdb.com/pubs/fs/Fact_Sheet-National_Practitioner_Data_Bank.pdf

U.S. Department of Veterans Affairs. (2008). *Available emblems of belief for placement on government headstones and markers.* Retrieved September 18, 2008, from http://www.cem.va.gov/cem/hm/hmemb.asp

Vaillant, G. E. (1993). *The wisdom of the ego.* Cambridge, MA: Harvard University Press.

Vanderwerker, L. C., & Prigerson, H. G. (2004). Social support and technological connectedness as protective factors in bereavement. *Journal of Loss and Trauma, 9,* 45–57.

Vasquez, M. J. T. (2005). Independent practice settings and the multicultural guidelines. In M. G. Constantine & D. W. Sue (Eds.), *Strategies for building multicultural competence in mental health and educational settings* (pp. 91–108). Hoboken, NJ: Wiley.

Verkerk, M., Lindemann, H., Maeckelberghe, E., Feenstra, E., Hartoungh, R., & De Bree, M. (2004). Enhancing reflection: An interpersonal exercise in ethics education. *Hastings Center Report, 34,* 31–38.

Vigilant, L. G., & Williamson, J. B. (2003). To die, by mistake: Accidental deaths. In C. D. Bryant (Ed.), *Handbook of death and dying* (Vol. 1, pp. 211–222). Thousand Oaks, CA: Sage.

Viorst, J. (1986). *Necessary losses: The loves, illusions, dependencies and impossible expectations that all of us have to give up in order to grow.* New York: Ballantine.

Wagner, B., Knaevelsrud, C., & Maercker, A. (2006). Internet-based cognitive-behavioral therapy for complicated grief: A randomized controlled trial. *Death Studies, 30,* 429–454.

Wagner, L., Davis, S., & Handelsman, M. M. (1998). In search of the abominable consent form: The impact of readability and personalization. *Journal of Clinical Psychology, 54,* 115–120.

Walker, G. C. (2003). Medical euthanasia. In C. D. Bryant (Ed.), *Handbook of death and dying* (Vol. 1, pp. 405–423). Thousand Oaks, CA: Sage.

Walker, M. U. (1998). *Moral understandings: A feminist study in ethics.* New York: Routledge.

Warren, J. J. (2000). When the therapist moves. In J. K. Aronson (Ed.), *Use of the telephone in psychotherapy* (pp. 167–184). Northvale, NJ: J. Aronson.

Weisaeth, L. (2000). Briefing and debriefing: Group psychological interventions in acute stressor situations. In B. Raphael & J. P. Wilson (Eds.), *Psychological debriefing: Theory, practice and evidence* (pp. 43–57). New York: Cambridge University Press.

Weiss, B. D., Senf, J. H., Carter, J. Z., & Rothe, T. C. (1986). Confidentiality expectations of patients in teaching hospital clinics versus private practice offices. *Social Science and Medicine, 23,* 387–391.

Weissman, M. M., Markowitz, J. C., & Klerman, G. L. (2000). *Comprehensive guide to interpersonal psychotherapy.* New York: Basic.

Welfel, E. R. (2006). *Ethics in counseling and psychotherapy: Standards, research, and emerging issues* (3rd ed.). Belmont, CA: Thomson Brooks/Cole.

Welie, J. V. M. (2008, May). *Fed by force of law: Schiavo's shadow over Nebraska and beyond.* Paper presented at the meeting of the Association for Death Education and Counseling, Montreal, Quebec, Canada.

Werth, J. L., Jr. (2005). Concerns about decisions related to withholding/withdrawing life-sustaining treatment and futility for persons with disabilities. *Journal of Disability Policy Studies, 16,* 31–37.

Werth, J. L., Jr., Blevins, D., Toussaint, K. L., & Durham, M. R. (2002). The influence of cultural diversity on end-of-life care and decisions. *American Behavioral Scientist, 46,* 204–219.

Werth, J. L., Jr., Burke, C., & Bardash, R. J. (2002). Confidentiality in end-of-life and after-death situations. *Ethics and Behavior, 12,* 205–222.

Wheeler, S. E. (1996). *Stewards of life: Bioethics and pastoral care.* Nashville, TN: Abingdon.

White, M., & Epston, D. (1990). *Narrative means to therapeutic ends.* New York: Norton.

Wogrin, C. (2007). Professional issues and thanatology. In D. Balk, C. Wogrin, G. Thornton, & D. Meagher (Eds.), *Handbook of thanatology: The essential body of knowledge for the study of death, dying and bereavement* (pp. 371–386). Northbrook, IL: Association for Death Education and Counseling, the Thanatology Association.

Woody, R. H. (1997). Valuing a psychological practice. *Professional Psychology: Research and Practice, 28,* 77–80.

Woody, R. H. (1999). Domestic violations of confidentiality. *Professional Psychology: Research and Practice, 30,* 607–610.

Worden, J. W. (2009). *Grief counseling and grief therapy: A handbook for the mental health practitioner* (4th ed.). New York: Springer Publishing.

Worden, J. W., & Proctor, W. (1976). *PDA: Personal death awareness.* New York: Prentice-Hall.

The World Factbook. (2008). *India.* Retrieved September 18, 2008, from http://www.cia.gov/library/publications/the-world-factbook/geos/in.html#people

World Medical Association. (2000). World Medical Association Declaration of Helsinki: Ethical principles for medical research involving human subjects. *Journal of the American Medical Association, 284,* 3043–3045.

Wortman, C. B., & Silver, R. C. (1989). The myths of coping with loss. *Journal of Counseling and Clinical Psychology, 57,* 349–357.

Wortman, C. B., & Silver, R. C. (2001). The myths of coping with loss revisited. In M. S. Stroebe, R. O. Hansson, W. Stroebe, & H. Schut (Eds.), *Handbook of bereavement research: Consequences, coping and care* (pp. 405–429). Washington, DC: American Psychological Association.

Yalom, I. D. (1980). *Existential psychotherapy.* New York: Basic.

Yalom, I. D., & Leszcz, M. (2005). *The theory and practice of group psychotherapy* (5th ed.). New York: Basic.

Yalom, I. D., & Lieberman, M. A. (1971). A study of encounter group casualties. *Archives of General Psychiatry, 25,* 16–30.

Ybarra, R. (2007, September 9). Organ donation brings life from sorrow: Mother gives up child's kidney, saving Texas teenager. *Waco Tribune-Herald,* p. 3C.

Young, B. H. (2006). The immediate response to disaster: Guidelines for adult psychological first aid. In E. C. Ritchie, P. J. Watson, & M. J. Friedman (Eds.), *Interventions following mass violence and disasters: Strategies for mental health practice* (pp. 134–154). New York: Guilford.

Young, M. A. (2001). *Victim assistance: Frontiers and fundamentals.* Washington, DC: National Organization for Victim Assistance.

Zinnbauer, B. J., Pargament, K. I., Cole, B., Rye, M. S., Butter, E. M., Belavich, T. G., et al. (1997). Religion and spirituality: Unfuzzying the fuzzy. *Journal for the Scientific Study of Religion, 36,* 549–564.

Ziskin, J., Faust, D., & Anderer, S. (2004). *Coping with psychiatric and psychological testimony* (6th ed.). New York: Oxford University Press.

Zisook, S., & Lyons, L. (1988–1989). Bereavement and unresolved grief in psychiatric outpatients. *Omega, 20,* 43–58.

Zuckerman, E. L. (2003). *The paper office: Forms, guidelines, and resources to make your practice work ethically, legally, and profitably* (3rd ed.). New York: Guilford.

Zur, O., & Barnett, J. E. (2008, September/October). Laptops threaten security. *National Psychologist, 17,* 22.

Index